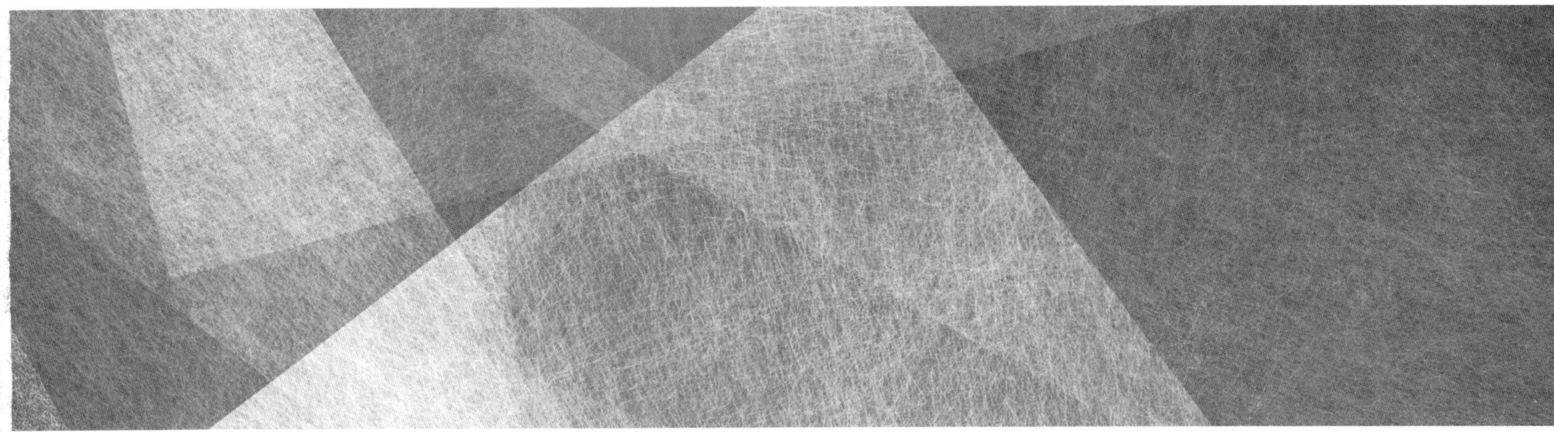

WOMEN'S HEALTH NURSE PRACTITIONER AND MIDWIFERY

CERTIFICATION REVIEW

JoAnn Zerwekh, EdD, RN

President/CEO
Nursing Education Consultants, Inc.
Chandler, Arizona

Adjunct Faculty
Upper Iowa University
Mesa, Arizona

Faculty
University of Phoenix Online
Phoenix, Arizona

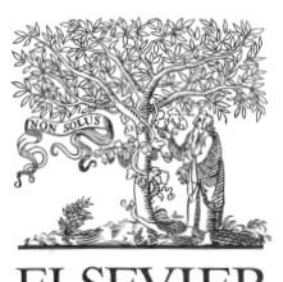

ELSEVIER

Elsevier
3251 Riverport Lane
St. Louis, Missouri 63043

WOMEN'S HEALTH NURSE PRACTITIONER AND MIDWIFERY CERTIFICATION REVIEW
ISBN: 978-0-323-67529-1

Notice

Practitioners and researchers must always rely on their own experience and knowledge in evaluating and using any information, methods, compounds or experiments described herein. Because of rapid advances in the medical sciences, in particular, independent verification of diagnoses and drug dosages should be made. To the fullest extent of the law, no responsibility is assumed by Elsevier, authors, editors or contributors for any injury and/or damage to persons or property as a matter of products liability, negligence or otherwise, or from any use or operation of any methods, products, instructions, or ideas contained in the material herein.

ISBN: 978-0-323-67529-1

Senior Content Strategist: Sandra Clark
Content Development Manager: Lisa Newton
Senior Content Development Specialist: Laura Selkirk
Publishing Services Manager: Catherine Jackson
Senior Project Manager: Kate Mannix
Design Direction: Brian Salisbury

Printed in the United States of America

Last digit is the print number: 9 8 7 6 5 4 3 2 1

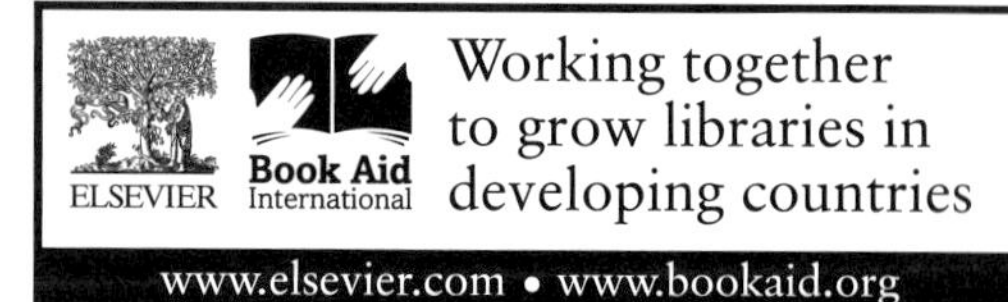

About the Author

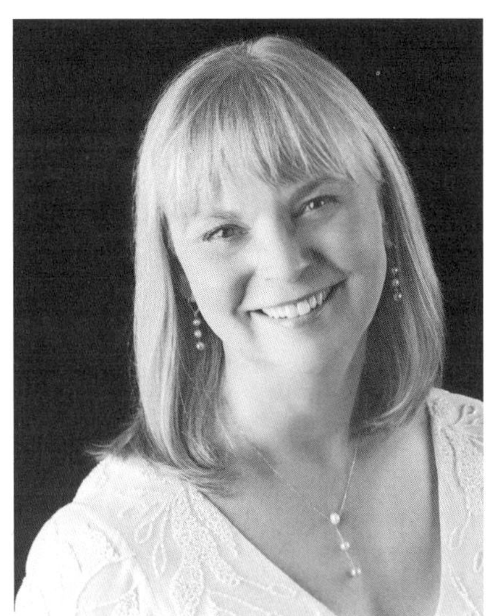

JoAnn Zerwekh has worked as a family nurse practitioner at Carondelet Health Care primary health care clinics in southern Arizona. She taught FNP students at the University of Phoenix and worked for a brief period as the advance practice consultant for the Arizona Board of Nursing. She is the author of numerous publications, including *Family Nurse Practitioner Certification Review, Adult-Gerontology Primary Care Nurse Practitioner Certification Review, Nursing Today: Transition & Trends, Illustrated Study Guide for the NCLEX-RN® Exam,* and *Illustrated Study Guide for the NCLEX-PN® Exam* review books, and the popular *Memory NoteCards of Nursing* and *Memory Notebooks of Nursing*. She is the President/CEO of Nursing Education Consultants, Inc.

Contributors

DEBORAH BAMBINI, PhD, WHNP-BC, CNE, CHSE, ANEF
Professor
Kirkhof College of Nursing
Grand Valley State University
Grand Rapids, Michigan

EMMA VIRGINIA CLARK, MHS, MSN
Certified Nurse Midwife
Family Health and Birth Center
Community of Hope;
Director, Maternal, Newborn, and Child Health
Chemonics International;
Adjunct Faculty
School of Nursing, NM/WHNP Program
Georgetown University
Washington, DC

MICHELLE COLLINS, PhD, CNM, RN-CEFM, FACNM, FAAN, FNAP
Associate Dean of Academic Affairs
Professor, Women, Children and Family Nursing
Rush University College of Nursing
Chicago, Illinois

KELLY ELLINGTON, DNP, WHNP-BC, RNC-OB
Assistant Professor
University of North Carolina Wilmington
Garner, North Carolina

HEIDI COLLINS FANTASIA, PhD, RN, WHNP-BC
Associate Professor and Department Chair
Solomont School of Nursing
Zuckerberg College of Health Sciences
University of Massachusetts
Lowell, Massachusetts

LISA L. FERGUSON, DNP, APRN, WHNP-BC, CNE
Clinical Assistant Professor
College of Nursing
University of Florida
Gainesville, Florida

TAMARA K. JO, RN, MSN, WHNP, NP-C
Nurse Practitioner in Sarcoma
Dana Farber Cancer Institute
Boston, Massachusetts

RENEE O. SPAIN, DNP, MAED, CNM
Clinical Assistant Professor
Clinical Site Coordinator, Nurse Midwifery Education Program
East Carolina University
Greenville, North Carolina

Reviewers

CAROL BAFALOUKOS, DNP, WHNP-BC, FNP-C
Program Chair, Online MSN/FNP Program
University of Phoenix
Phoenix, Arizona

CATHLEEN CROWLEY-KOSCHNITZKI, DNP, CNM, WHNP-BC, FNP-C, PMHNP-BC, CNE
Associate Professor
Chamberlain College of Nursing NP Tracks
PMHNP iTrust Wellness Group
Greenville, South Carolina

DEBRA ILCHAK, DNP, RN, FNP-BC, CNE
Clinical Associate Professor
Edson College of Nursing and Health Innovation
Arizona State University
Phoenix, Arizona

KRISTEN S. MONTGOMERY, PhD, CNM
Nurse Midwife
LocumTenens.com
Moore, South Carolina

SARAH A. OBERMEYER, PhD, CNM, WHNP-BC
Assistant Professor
Azusa Pacific University
Azusa, California

SHELLEY SADLER, RN, MSN, APRN, WHNP-BC
Instructor of Nursing
Morehead State University
Morehead, Kentucky

Preface

With the proliferation of new DNP programs, there is an increasing need for additional reference information and study materials for the certification examinations. Nurse practitioners and midwives are playing a vital role in the health care delivery system in the United States. With the assistance of certified women's health nurse practitioners, midwives, and my editorial expertise in test item writing, the *Women's Health Nurse Practitioner and Midwifery Certification Review* has been developed to assist the advanced practice nurse to prepare for the WHNP and Midwifery certification exams. Extensive efforts have been made to include current information that is representative of the content, based on the blueprints for the certification exams. This book of questions is not intended to be an exhaustive review of the content but an adjunct to the review process.

Test-taking strategies are included in Chapter 1. As a candidate prepares for the certification exam, it is vitally important to be familiar with and to practice good testing strategies. Testing strategies can prevent the candidate from making mistakes and selecting the wrong answer. As the review process begins, a review of the test-taking strategies chapter and the practice of good testing strategies is critical. With many years' experience in the field of testing, I consistently have identified the importance that practice testing plays in the review process. Practice questions give the candidate an opportunity to review questions written from different perspectives. To enhance the review process, answers with complete rationales are provided at the end of each chapter. Not only does the candidate increase his/her knowledge of the subject area, but also, with more practice, testing skills become fine-tuned. Good testing skills make the candidate more comfortable and help decrease the stress associated with certification exams.

The next two chapters are a review of Physical Assessment and Diagnostic Tests. A chapter on Gynecology and Family Planning reviews important concepts related to anatomy and physiology of reproduction, family planning, gynecology disorders, male issues affecting women's health, and pharmacology. A section on Obstetrics contains four chapters on topics related to antepartum care, intrapartum care (midwifery only), postpartum care, and neonatal care (midwifery only). The section on Primary Care provides questions that test information related to health promotion and maintenance and general health supervision. The primary care clinical chapters are developed using a systems approach (i.e., cardiovascular, respiratory, endocrine, etc.). In each of these chapters, the test questions focus on common primary care issues that the women's health nurse practitioner and midwife encounter in their practices. This format assists the candidate to easily locate specific questions. The section on Professional Issues is content specific for the women's health nurse practitioner.

My thanks to the many women's health nurse practitioners and midwives across the country who provided questions and insight into their respective clinical role. I wish to thank Laura Selkirk, my Content Development Specialist, and Sandy Clark, Senior Content Strategist at Elsevier, for their support and suggestions in the preparation of the manuscript. Thank you also goes to the women's health nurse practitioners and midwives who took time from their busy schedules to review the questions for content correctness and clarity.

Acknowledgments

I want to express my appreciation to Sandy Clark at Elsevier and her "can-do" attitude that made the realization of this first edition of the *Women's Health Nurse Practitioner and Midwifery Certification Review* book possible.

I am especially grateful to the many people at Elsevier who assisted with this major revision effort, including the folks who have assisted with the online practice exams. In particular, I want to thank Laura Selkirk in Content; Kate Mannix, Senior Project Manager; Erica Kelley in Marketing; and Brian Salisbury in Design.

I want to thank the contributors and reviewers for their assistance in the revision process. Your current practice and clinical expertise is surely noted in your contribution to this first edition.

I want to thank my adult children, Ashley Garneau and Tyler Zerwekh, and their spouse and significant other (Brian Garneau and Julie Goehring) for their love and support. You make your mother proud by all that you do as successful healthcare professionals. I would also like to thank my stepchildren, Carrie Parks and Matt Masog, for their great friendship, and to express my sorrow at the loss of their father, John Masog, my late husband, who was loved and is missed by all of us.

A special note to my amazing grandchildren (Maddie and Harper Zerwekh; Ben Garneau; Brooklyn and Alexis Parks; Owen, Emmett, and Cole Masog) who have such bright futures; you always put a smile on Grandma's face and make her proud.

JoAnn Zerwekh

Contents

1

Test-Taking Strategies

Certification Exam Information

NCC Exam

For the WHNP/midwife certification exam, the credentialing body is the National Certification Corporation (NCC). The NCC exam is timed, with 3 hours allocated for completion. There are up to 175 questions; 150 test items are counted for scoring, and the remainder of the questions are embedded in the exam as pretest items, which do not count toward the candidate's score (Table 1.1). Each multiple-choice question contains three options from which the candidate must choose the best response. More information can be obtained at the NCC website: http://www.nccwebsite.org.

AMCB Exam

The American Midwifery Certification Board (AMCB) is the credentialing body for the midwifery exam. The AMCB exam consists of a total of 175 questions with a 4-hour time limit (Table 1.2). Each question contains four options from which the candidate must choose the best response. There are some pretest items that are not included in scoring the exam. Those items being pretested are scattered throughout the exam and are not identified. More information can be obtained at the AMCB website: https://www.amcbmidwife.org/amcb-certification.

Note: The practice test items in this book are a combination of both three- and four-option responses to accommodate both credentialing bodies' multiple-choice format.

Testing Strategies

Knowing how to take an exam is a skill that is developed through practice and experience. Being able to take an exam effectively is almost as important as the basic knowledge required to answer the question. Everyone has taken an exam only to find in the review of the exam that questions were missed because of inadequate testing skills.

Nurse practitioner and midwifery programs provide the graduate student with a comprehensive base of knowledge; how you utilize this knowledge will determine your success on a certification exam. The certification exam is an objective test that covers knowledge, understanding, and application of professional nursing theory and practice.

Read the information in this chapter carefully and make sure you understand the strategies discussed. This chapter is designed to help you identify problem areas in testing skills and learn how to use strategy and judgment in selecting correct answers. It is important for you to practice testing skills if you are going to be able to utilize these skills on the certification exam.

1. Do not read extra meaning into the question. The question is asking for specific information; if it appears to be simple "common sense," then assume it is simple. Do not look for a hidden meaning in what appears to be an easy question.

EXAMPLE

The WHNP/midwife understands that the most common form of facial paralysis in the adult patient is:

1. Facial nerve fasciitis.
2. Trigeminal neuralgia.
3. Bell palsy.
4. Herpes zoster.

The correct answer is Option #3. Be careful not to "read into" the question and add pain to the facial paralysis symptom. Instead, concentrate on the question's key words, "the most common form of facial paralysis," which is Bell palsy, a disorder that affects the facial nerve and is characterized by muscle flaccidity of the affected side of the face. Trigeminal neuralgia is a disorder of cranial nerve V that is characterized by an abrupt onset of pain in the lower and upper jaw, cheek, and lips. Herpes zoster affects the dermatomes and does not cause a paralysis, but rather pain, herpetic grouped skin vesicles, and possibly postherpetic neuralgia.

Table 1.1
NCC Percentage of Questions in Content Areas

Gynecology	38%
Obstetrics	28%
Physical assessment and diagnostic testing	12%
Primary care	12%
Pharmacology	9%
Professional issues	1%

NCC, National Certification Corporation.

Data from NCC. (2019). *2019 Candidate guide: women's health care nurse practitioner*. https://www.nccwebsite.org/content/documents/cms/whnp-candidate_guide.pdf.

Table 1.2
AMCB Percentage of Questions in Content Areas

Antepartum	22%
Intrapartum	21%
Postpartum	17%
Newborn	11%
Well woman/gynecology	17%
Women's health/primary care	12%

AMCB, American Midwifery Certification Board.

Data from AMCB. (2019). *AMCB certification exam candidate handbook: nurse-midwifery and midwifery.* https://www.amcbmidwife.org/amcb-certification/candidate-handbook.

2. Read the stem correctly. Make sure you understand exactly what information the question is asking. It is important to understand the question before reviewing the options for the correct answer.

EXAMPLE

Ten days after delivery, a patient is diagnosed with mastitis. Which of the following would the WHNP/midwife expect to find on physical exam?

1. Tender, hard, hot, and reddened area on breast.
2. Dimpled skin on breasts and firm nodules around areola.
3. Decreased milk production, inverted nipple, and firm, inflamed breast tissue.
4. Soft, tender, palpable masses with cracked, and bleeding nipples.

The question asks you to determine findings on a physical exam. The answer is Option 1. A tender, hard, hot, and reddened area on breast over the affected area is typically found with mastitis. The patient with mastitis will also typically be febrile. Dimpled skin (peau d'orange or orange-peel appearance) is a potential sign of breast cancer. Decreased milk production, inverted nipple, and firm breast tissue may be complications of engorgement. Cracked nipples may result from improper positioning or oversuckling. Soft, tender breast masses may be engorged milk ducts.

3. Before considering the options, think about the characteristics of the condition and the critical concepts to consider. Begin by assessing each option regarding the concepts of the condition.

EXAMPLE

A mother who is 3 days postpartum has been complaining of soreness and fullness in her breasts and that she wants to stop breastfeeding her infant until her breasts feel better. The WHNP/midwife:

1. Shows the patient how to apply a breast binder to decrease the discomfort and the production of milk.
2. Tells the patient that breast fullness may be a sign of infection and to stop breastfeeding.
3. Suggests to the patient that she decrease her fluid intake for the next 24 hours to suppress lactation temporarily.
4. Explains to the patient that the breast discomfort is normal, and that the infant's sucking will promote the flow of milk.

Formulate in your mind critical information for the care of this patient. Think to yourself, "Is it normal to have fullness and soreness in the breasts during the first 3 days of lactation?" If you are unsure, go back and reassess the question. In this instance Option #4 is correct. Initially, breast soreness may occur for about 2 to 3 minutes during each feeding until the let-down reflex is established.

4. Identify what type of response the question is asking. A positive stem requires identification of three false items and one correct answer.

EXAMPLE

How soon after exposure should patients who believe they have been exposed to HIV have an HIV antibody test?

1. The next day and 2 months later.
2. 6 months after exposure and again at 12 months.
3. 6 to 12 weeks after exposure and again at 6 months.
4. 4 weeks and 12 weeks later.

The correct answer is Option #3. This question requires you to identify three incorrect responses and one correct response. The HIV antibody develops between 6 and 12 weeks after exposure. Because of the variability of antibody development, it is recommended that the test be repeated in 6 months to confirm the findings.

5. Identify questions that require identification of something the WHNP/midwife should not or would not do (i.e., an unsafe action, contraindication, or inappropriate action).

EXAMPLE

A 48-year-old patient presents to the clinic complaining of hot flashes, no menses for 14 months, insomnia, crying spells, irritability, decreased libido, and fatigue. At the end of her history and physical, she begins to cry and tells the WHNP/midwife that she "thinks she's going crazy." She then begs the WHNP/midwife to tell her what is wrong. Which action is inappropriate for the WHNP/midwife to do at this point?

1. Obtain laboratory tests, including follicle stimulating hormone and luteinizing hormone.
2. Discuss hormone replacement therapy, including risks and benefits and short- and long-term treatment strategies.
3. Provide antidepressant therapy and a referral for counseling sessions for depression.

4. Provide written information regarding menopause and options for treatment of symptoms.

The correct answer is Option #3. These symptoms are classic for menopausal syndrome, although some depressive symptoms are listed. Antidepressant therapy and counseling for depression at this stage of treatment is not appropriate. Testing, teaching, and treatment in this case should be aimed at the menopause. The depressive symptoms will undoubtedly improve with greater understanding and treatment of the menopausal symptoms.

6. Questions may also be analytical. These questions may ask the nurse practitioner to identify findings and statements that are consistent or inconsistent with the patient's presenting problem, and/or differentiate between them.

EXAMPLE

A multigravida who is at 30 weeks gestation calls the WHNP/midwife complaining of vaginal bleeding, abdominal pain, and uterine contractions. On physical exam, no watery discharge is noted, and the uterus feels hard. The WHNP/midwife suspects:

1. Placental abruption.
2. Placenta previa.
3. Molar pregnancy.
4. Ectopic pregnancy.

Before you examine the options in this question, it is important to think about the types of prenatal vaginal bleeding and when do they occur during the pregnancy. The correct answer is Option #1. Symptoms of placental abruption are bright-red vaginal bleeding, board-like uterus on palpation, uterine contractions, and uterine tenderness and pain. Vaginal bleeding is not always present, that is, concealed abruption. Placenta previa is painless bleeding and occurs in the second and third trimester. Ectopic pregnancy occurs during the first trimester. Molar pregnancy or gestational trophoblastic disease would not progress to 30 weeks gestation.

7. Identify key words that affect your understanding of the question. Make sure you understand exactly what information the question is asking. Be aware of questions in the stem, such as *except*, *contraindicated*, *avoid*, *least*, *not applicable*, and *does not occur*. These words change the direction of the question. It may help to rephrase the question in your own words to better understand what information is being requested.

EXAMPLE

A patient complains of intolerable itching in the pubic hair. On exam, the WHNP/midwife notes erythematous papules and tiny white specks in the pubic hair. The differential diagnosis includes all *except*:

1. Pediculosis pubis.
2. Scabies.
3. Impetigo.
4. Atopic dermatitis.

Rephrase the question and look for the three conditions associated with itching, "What are the three differential diagnoses for pruritus or itching in the pubic hair?" Intense itching is characteristic of pediculosis pubis, scabies, and atopic dermatitis. Impetigo starts out as a tender erythematous papule and progresses through a vesicular to a honey-crusted stage with no itching. The correct answer is Option #3 because impetigo is not in the differential diagnosis with conditions that are characterized by itching.

8. As you read the options, eliminate the options you know are not correct. This will help narrow the field of choice. When you select an answer or eliminate a distracter, you should have a specific reason for doing so. Do not try to predict a correct answer; it is distressing if the answer you want is not a selection.

EXAMPLE

A young adult patient, G2 P1 A0 L1, 10 weeks' gestation with intrauterine pregnancy (IUP), is seen for her first obstetric intake history and physical. She knows when she conceived and denies any vaginal bleeding or abdominal pain. The patient has a soft, nontender fundus that measures 14 cm; adnexal exam negative for mass or tenderness; no fetal heart rate (FHR) audible with doptone. What is the most likely diagnosis seen on ultrasound?

1. Fibroid uterus. *(No, a fibroid could cause the uterus to enlarge, but it is generally accompanied by firmness to palpation of the uterus.)*
2. Multiple gestations. *(Yes, multiple gestations will cause the uterus to enlarge faster than normal. FHR may be inaudible with the doptone at 10 weeks' gestation.)*
3. Ectopic pregnancy. *(No, ectopic pregnancy could be the cause of an inaudible FHR, but is usually accompanied by adnexal tenderness, a mass, or vaginal bleeding.)*
4. 14-week viable IUP. *(No, a 14-week viable IUP should have an audible FHR with the doptone.)*

After systematically evaluating the options, Option #2 is the correct answer.

9. Identify similarities in the distracters. Frequently, three distracters will contain similar information, and one will be different. The different one may be the correct answer.

EXAMPLE

An older adult patient is encouraged to increase protein intake. The addition of which of these foods to 100 mL of milk will provide the greatest amount of protein?

1. 50 mL of light cream and 2 tbsp of corn syrup.
2. 30 g of powdered skim milk and 1 egg.
3. 1 small scoop (90 g) of ice cream and 1 tbsp of chocolate syrup.
4. 2 egg yolks and 1 tbsp of sugar.

Options #1, #3, and #4 all contain a simple sugar. The correct answer, Option #2, has the greatest amount of protein. Notice that three of the options are similar, and the one that is different is the correct answer. This strategy is not a substitute for basic knowledge but may help you figure out the answer.

10. Select the most comprehensive answer. All options may be correct, but one will include the other three options or will need to be considered first.

EXAMPLE

The WHNP/midwife is planning to teach a client with newly diagnosed gestational diabetes about the condition. Before the WHNP/midwife provides instruction, what is most important to evaluate? The patient's:

1. Required dietary modifications.
2. Understanding of carbohydrate counting.
3. Ability to administer insulin.
4. Present understanding of gestational diabetes.

Options #1, #2, and #3 are certainly important considerations in diabetic education for the newly diagnosed pregnant patient. However, they cannot be initiated until the WHNP/midwife evaluates the patient's knowledge of gestational diabetes, which is the reason that Option #4 is the correct answer. When two options appear to say the same thing, only in different words, then look for another answer; that is, eliminate the options that you know are incorrect. Options #1 and #2 both refer to the client's understanding of nutrition.

11. Select the best answer that is most specific to what the question asks. All options may be correct, but one is more specific or essential to the question being asked.

EXAMPLE

A 16-week pregnant patient comes into the clinic and complains of an abnormally thick vaginal discharge. She notes increased discomfort when she urinates. On exam she has a copious amount of thick discharge that is on the external labia and also in the vaginal vault. A potassium hydroxide (KOH) wet prep test is negative. This is most consistent with candidiasis infection. What is the best option for treatment?

1. Diflucan 500 mg x 1 dose.
2. Miconazole 100 mg vaginally for 4 days.
3. Clotrimazole 100 mg vaginal tablet x 7 days.
4. Clindamycin 300 mg twice a day x 7 days.

The correct answer is Option #3. Clotrimazole 100 mg vaginal tablet x 7 days would be an appropriate treatment for candidiasis. Diflucan should not be used in pregnancy, it is a class C category drug, but there are some case reports of birth defects in women who were exposed to doses above 400 mg for long periods during the first trimester. Miconazole is a good choice for treatment, but it should be used for at least 7 days; a 4-day course is too short. Clindamycin is the correct medication and dose for bacterial vaginosis but not for a Candida infection. Recognize key words that identify the question that is asking for a priority of care—first, initial, essential, best, and most.

12. Watch questions in which the options contain several items to consider. After you are sure you understand what information the question is requesting, evaluate each part of the option. Is it appropriate to what the question is asking? If an option contains one incorrect item, the entire option is incorrect. All items listed in the selection must be correct if the option is to be the answer to the question.

EXAMPLE

The biophysical profile includes which of the following parameters?

1. Fetal breathing movements, fetal muscle tone, and amniotic fluid volume.
2. Ultrasonography, alpha-fetoprotein screening, and fetal heart reactivity.
3. Amniocentesis, amniotic fluid volume, and nonstress test.
4. Contraction stress test, nonstress test, and gross fetal movement.

The correct answer is Option #1. In a methodical evaluation of the findings in the options, you can eliminate Options #2, #3, and #4. The biophysical profile includes observation of fetal respiratory movement, fetal tone, gross fetal movement, measurement of amniotic fluid volume, and fetal heart reactivity. Each parameter is given a score of 0 or 2; the scores from all parameters are then added together, the normal is 8 to 10. Ultrasonography, alpha-fetoprotein screening, nonstress testing, and stress test are not part of this profile.

13. Be alert to relevant information contained in previous questions. Sometimes as you are answering questions, you will find information similar to the question being tested. Previous questions may assist you in identifying relevant information in the current question. This strategy is particularly helpful when the student is answering paper–and–pencil tests.

EXAMPLE

The Advisory Committee of Immunization Practices (ACIP) recommends that healthy older adults receive the Tdap vaccination:

1. Every 5 years.
2. At age 75 years.
3. At age 65 years.
4. Every 10 years.

The correct answer to this question is Option #3. ACIP approved the use of Tdap (tetanus toxoid, reduced diphtheria toxoid, and acellular pertussis) for all adults aged 65 years and older. Boostrix should be used for adults aged 65 years and older; however, ACIP concluded that either vaccine (Boostrix or Adacel) administered to a person 65 years or older is immunogenic and would provide protection. In another question involving immunizations, you read the following question (see next example):

EXAMPLE

In taking the history of an alert older adult, the WHNP/midwife determines the patient is an avid gardener and spends much time outside. Also, she is soon to be a grandmother for the first time. The patient had a pneumococcal vaccination last year but cannot remember whether a tetanus vaccination was ever administered. A health maintenance recommendation for this patient would be to obtain:

1. Pneumococcal vaccine.
2. Tdap/Td vaccine.
3. Hepatitis B vaccine.
4. No recommendation.

The correct answer is Option #2. A clue to the correct answer may be found in the previous question. Older adults who enjoy gardening and outdoor activities should have a Tdap/Td booster once, as recommended by the ACIP, and especially they should be immunized to protect newborn grandchildren. As part of standard wound management care to prevent tetanus, a tetanus toxoid–containing vaccine might be recommended for wound management in adults aged 19 years and older if 5 years or more have elapsed since last receiving the vaccine. If a tetanus booster is indicated, Tdap is preferred over Td for wound management in adults aged 19 years and older who have not received Tdap previously. Td should be administered every 10 years.

When you are taking the test on a computer, it is more difficult to remember previous questions because you may not be able to go back and change answers or review previous questions; therefore this strategy is often most helpful for those students taking paper–and–pencil tests.

14. Evaluate priority questions carefully. Frequently, all answers are appropriate to the situation. You need to decide which actions you should do first.

EXAMPLE

The midwife is evaluating an infant 8 hours after delivery. The infant was full term, weighed 10 lbs. at birth, and is being breastfed. The mother has a history of gestational diabetes during the pregnancy. What findings indicate the need for further evaluation?

1. Blood glucose of 50 mg/dL with glucose screening strips.
2. Respirations of 70 breaths/min, tremors, and jitteriness.
3. Bilirubin level 3 mg/dL.
4. No passage of meconium stool.

The correct answer is Option #2. Early signs of hypoglycemia are jitteriness, poor muscle tone, tremors, and symptoms of respiratory difficulty and are a priority for further evaluation. The blood sugar of 50 mg/dL is within normal limits at this time (40–60 mg/dL the first 24 hours). If blood sugar levels are less than 45 mg/dL on the screening strip, a follow-up serum glucose should be done. The meconium stool should be passed within the first 24 hours, and the bilirubin level is normal.

Techniques to Increase Critical Thinking Skills

Memory aids and Mindmapping™ are tools that assist in drawing associations from other ideas with the use of visual images. **Mnemonics** are words, phrases, or other techniques that help you remember information. **Imagery** is a tool that helps you identify a problem and visualize a mental picture. Learning content that uses these techniques will assist you to recall information more effectively.

Mindmapping™ is a method of organizing important information that is in sharp contrast to the traditional outline format. A thought or concept is written in the center of the page, and images and color are added to information as ideas begin to flow from the center focus (Fig. 1.1).

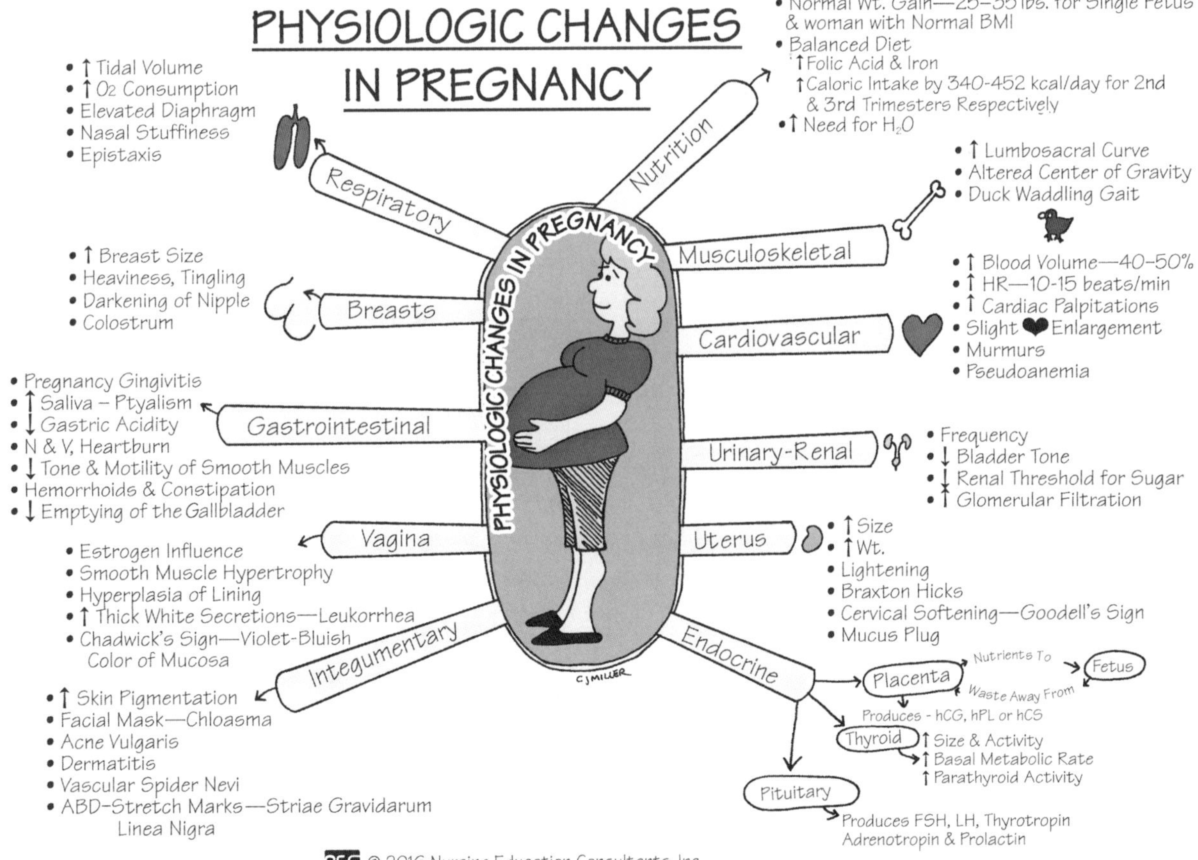

Fig. 1.1 Example of Mindmapping™: physiologic changes in pregnancy. *BMI*, Body mass index; *FSH*, follicle-stimulating hormone; *hCG*, human chorionic gonadotropin; *LH*, luteinizing hormone. (From Zerwekh, J., Garneau, A., & Miller, C. J. (2017). *Digital collection of the memory notebook of nursing* (4th ed.). Chandler, AZ: Nursing Education Consultants, Inc.)

Acronyms help you recall specific information through word associations or letter arrangements. Examples of these are the "Oral Contraceptives–What to report…ACHES" (Fig. 1.2).

Acrostics are catchy phrases in which the first letter of each word stands for something to recall. For example, in remembering information about a nonstress test, think of "nonreactive nonstress is not good" (Fig. 1.3).

Memory aids/images are pictures or caricatures that help you recall information more effectively (Fig. 1.4), such as the picture of a cap for caput succedaneum.

Rhymes are phrases or words spoken in a rhythmic or musical manner that increase recall, such as the rhyme for hypoglycemia versus hyperglycemia (Fig. 1.5). Another rhyme, "fingers, nose, penis, toes," identifies the areas in which lidocaine with epinephrine is contraindicated as a local anesthetic. Books and electronic resources are available on these helpful aids (see References at the end of the book).

Testing Skills For Paper–and–Pencil Tests

Because your certification exams are available on computer, the following skills are applicable for *paper–and–pencil tests*, which you may encounter as a student in your program.

1. Go through the exam and mark all answers that you know are correct. This ensures you have adequate time to answer the questions you know. Then go back and evaluate those questions for which you did not readily recognize the answer.
2. Do not indiscriminately change answers. If you go back and change an answer, you should have a specific reason for doing so. You may remember information and realize you answered the question incorrectly. Frequently, test-takers "talk themselves out of" the correct answer and change it to an incorrect one.
3. After you have completed the exam, go back, and check your booklet and make sure all questions are answered. Be sure to answer all questions, even if you must guess at some.

Successful Test Taking

1. Listen carefully to the instructions given at the beginning of the exam. Make sure you understand all information given and exactly how to mark your answers and/or how to use the keyboard and mouse. Adjust the computer screen for optimum viewing.
2. Watch your timing. Do not spend too much time on one question. It is particularly important that you practice

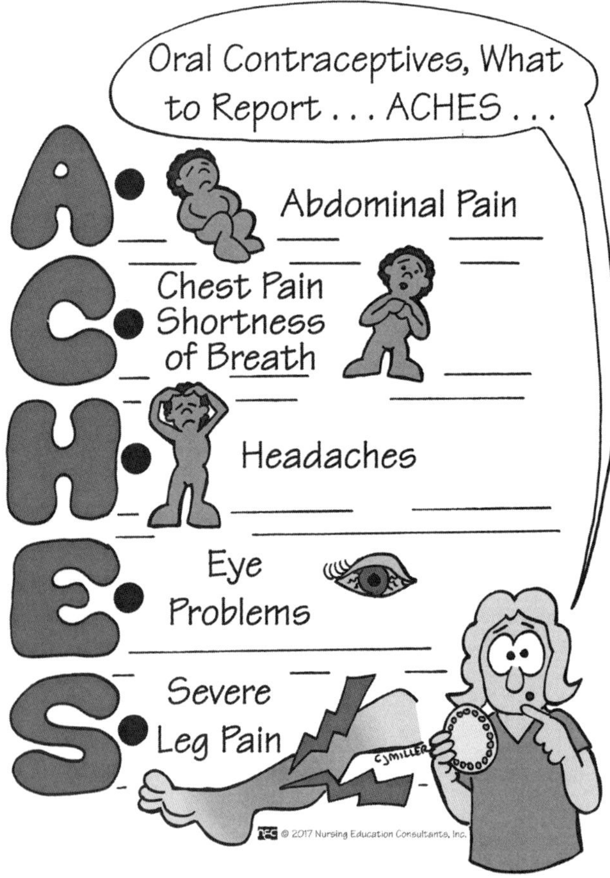

Fig. 1.2 Oral contraceptives (ACHES): what to report. (From Zerwekh, J., Garneau, A., & Miller, C. J. (2017). *Digital collection of the memory notebook of nursing* (4th ed.). Chandler, AZ: Nursing Education Consultants, Inc.)

NON-STRESS TEST
3 Negatives in a Row to Interpret Results of Non-Stress Test
N Non-Reactive
N Non-Stress is
N Not Good
I must meet criteria to pass a non-stress test and be called "reactive." No need to study for this test, I only need to be healthy.
© 2016 Nursing Education Consultants, Inc.

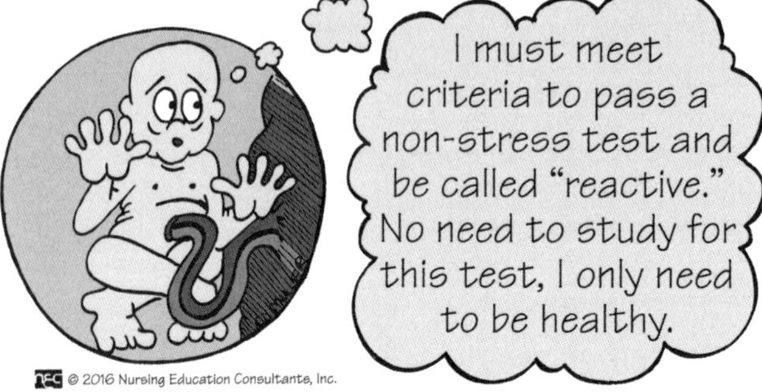

Fig. 1.3 Nonstress test. (From Zerwekh, J., Garneau, A., & Miller, C. J. (2017). *Digital collection of the memory notebook of nursing* (4th ed.). Chandler, AZ: Nursing Education Consultants, Inc.)

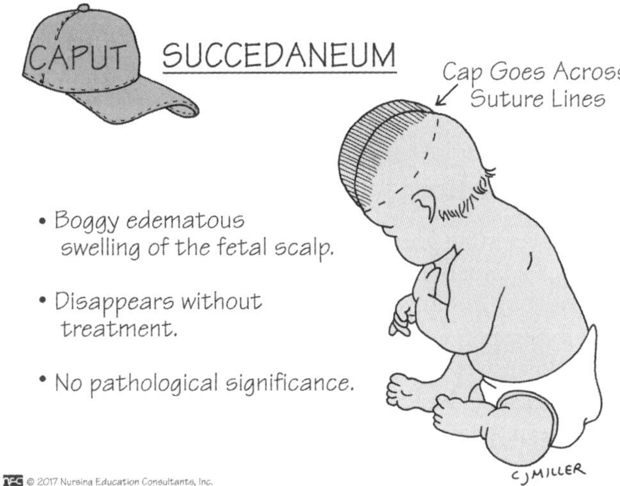

Fig. 1.4 Caput succedaneum. (From Zerwekh, J., Garneau, A., & Miller, C. J. (2017). *Digital collection of the memory notebook of nursing* (4th ed.). Chandler, AZ: Nursing Education Consultants, Inc.)

BLOOD SUGAR MNEMONIC

HOT & DRY = SUGAR HIGH

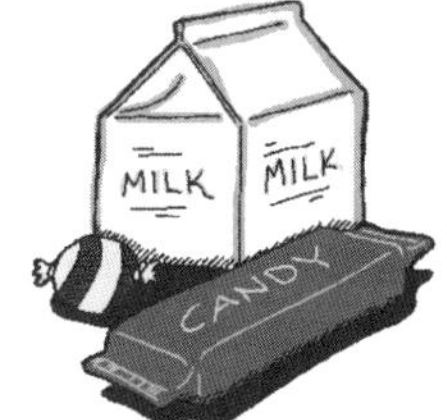

COLD & CLAMMY = NEED SOME CANDY

Fig. 1.5 Blood sugar rhyme. (From Zerwekh, J., Garneau, A., & Miller, C. J. (2017). *Digital collection of the memory notebook of nursing* (4th ed.). Chandler, AZ: Nursing Education Consultants, Inc.)

your timing on the sample exams. You may not be able to review your questions and answers on completion of the computerized test; therefore watch your timing on the computerized tests and make use of a computer clock if it is available.
3. Be aware of your "first hunch" because it is frequently the correct answer. Sometimes information is processed by the brain without your awareness. If something about an answer "feels right" or if you have a "gut feeling" about an answer, pay attention to it.
4. Eliminate options that assume the patient "would not understand" or "is ignorant of" the situation or those that "protect them from worry." For example, "The patient should not be told she has cancer because it would upset her too much."
5. Be aware of options that contain the words *always* and *never*.
6. There is no pattern of correct answers. Both computerized and paper-and-pencil exams are compiled by a computer and the position of the correct answers is selected at random.
7. Watch the length of the options to consider. The number of words required to adequately state the correct answer is sometimes longer than the other options.

Decrease Anxiety

Your activities on the day of the exam strongly influence your level of anxiety. By carefully planning ahead, you will be able to eliminate some anxiety-provoking situations. If you are a diabetic or have special needs, contact the certification agency ahead of time to plan to have accommodations that you may require.

1. Visit the exam site before the day of the exam. Evaluate travel time, parking, and time to reach the designated area. Be sure to get an early start to allow for extra time.
2. If you have to travel some distance to the exam site, try to spend the night in the immediate vicinity.
3. Do something pleasant the evening before the exam. This is not the time to "crash study."
4. Anxiety is contagious. If those around you are extremely anxious, avoid contact with them before the exam.
5. Make your meal before the test a light, healthy one.
6. Avoid eating highly spiced or different foods. This is not the time for a gastrointestinal upset.
7. Wear comfortable clothes. This is not a good time to wear tight clothing or new shoes.
8. Wear clothing of moderate weight. It is difficult to control the temperature to keep everyone comfortable. Take a sweater or wear layered clothes. You may not be allowed to remove any garments once you are seated for the exam.
9. Wear soft-soled shoes; this decreases the noise in the testing area.
10. Make sure you have the papers and proper identification that are required to gain admission to the exam site. If you wear reading glasses, do not forget to bring them with you.
11. Do not take study materials to the exam site. You will not be able to take such materials with you into the exam area.
12. Do not panic when you encounter content with which you are unfamiliar in a question. Use good test-taking strategies, select an answer, and continue. Remember, you are not going to know all of the correct answers.
13. Reaffirm to yourself that you know the material. It is not time for any self-defeating behavior or negative self-talk. You will pass! Build your confidence by visualizing yourself in 6 months working in the area you desire. Create that mental picture of where you want to be and who you want to be—a certified WHNP/midwife. Use your past successes to bring positive energy and "vibes" to your certification. **You can do it!**

Study Habits

Enhancing Study Skills

- Decide on a realistic study schedule; write it down and stick with it.
- Divide the review material into segments—pediatrics, well woman, cardiac, and so forth.
- Prioritize the segments; review first the areas in which you seem deficient or weak.
- Identify areas that will require additional review.
- Establish a realistic schedule; study in short segments or "bursts." Avoid marathon sessions.
- Plan on achieving your study goal several days before the exam.
- Do not study when you are tired or when there are frequent distractions or interruptions.
- Review general concepts of practice from a variety of resources.

Group Study

- Keep the group limited to three to five people.
- Group members should be mature and serious about studying.
- The group should agree on the planned study schedule.
- If the group makes you anxious, or if you do not think the group meets your study needs, do not continue to participate.

Testing Practice

- Include testing practice in your schedule.
- Select approximately 50 questions for a practice testing session of 1 hour. This will allow you to evaluate the pace of the exam (i.e., approximately 1 question per minute).
- Try to answer the questions as if you were taking the real exam. Do not look up the correct answer immediately after answering the question. Complete all questions you have selected, then go back and grade the questions.
- Utilize the testing strategies described in this chapter.
- Evaluate the practice exam for problem areas: testing skills and knowledge base.
- Evaluate the questions you answer incorrectly. Review the rationale for the right answer and understand why you missed it.
- Utilize the questions at a later point to review the information again.

2

Physical Assessment

Health History

1. Which statement is accurate about conducting a physical exam on an older adolescent?
   1. Provide a previsit screening tool or questionnaire to allow the adolescent to identify and write down concerns prior to the start of the visit.
   2. Have the adolescent's parent remain in the room during the health history and review of systems.
   3. Explain to the adolescent that everything that is discussed will remain confidential.
   4. Use a gentle confrontational approach when the adolescent is silent or unable to express specific words about physical changes occurring.

2. The WHNP/midwife is constructing a pedigree chart during a clinical visit. What is the purpose of obtaining a pedigree diagram?
   1. Record of growth and development milestones.
   2. Sexual orientation (lesbian, gay, bisexual, transgender) and sexual development.
   3. Genetic and familial health problems.
   4. Cultural variation and ethnic background.

3. The WHNP/midwife is asking questions during a review of systems and understands that constitutional symptoms include:
   1. Increased heart rate, bounding pulse, dizziness.
   2. Pruritic rash, malaise, diminished visual acuity.
   3. Weight, height, body mass index.
   4. Pain, fever, malaise.

4. An adult patient with cerebral palsy and minimal cognitive dysfunction is seen at the clinic. The WHNP/midwife understands that health history information should:
   1. Be obtained only from the past medical record.
   2. Be obtained from the patient's family member and/or caregiver.
   3. Involve the patient to the limit of their ability.
   4. Involve the community group home where the patient resides.

5. When communicating with adolescents, the WHNP/midwife needs to be sensitive to the adolescent's:
   1. Reluctance to talk.
   2. Desire to be in control.
   3. Need for detailed instructions.
   4. Urge to communicate.

6. The WHNP/midwife is conducting an admission assessment interview with an adult Native-American client. Which therapeutic approach would be most effective?
   1. Use a soft voice with open-ended statements and reflective technique; avoid direct constant eye contact.
   2. Convey an open, friendly attitude; ask direct questions; touch the client occasionally for reassurance.
   3. Touch the client frequently for reassurance as a nonverbal supportive behavior, along with smiling or making a sardonic face to express a negative comment.
   4. Talk in a loud voice; maintain unbroken eye contact when asking direct questions and use minimal gestures.

7. The WHNP/midwife is preparing to conduct an interview with a non-English speaking client. An interpreter is scheduled. Which of the following actions are appropriate?
   1. Watch the client's verbal and nonverbal communication.
   2. Speak and look directly to the interpreter.
   3. Use accurate medical terminology so client understands situation.
   4. Have the interpreter paraphrase the client's communication to facilitate the pace of the interview.

8. Which of the following describes how cultural diversity may affect a client's health?
   1. Diabetes and cancer have higher occurrence rates among white people than among African-Americans.
   2. Asian-Americans have a low incidence of stomach and liver cancers.
   3. African-Americans have an increased incidence of hypertension, which is easily controlled by the beta-adrenergic blocker propranolol.
   4. White people may self-treat their depression with over-the-counter alternative remedies, such as St. John's wort.

Physical Exam

General

9. Which statement is accurate about common changes occurring because of aging that are considerations during a physical assessment?
   1. Tenting of the skin is a good indicator of hydration status.
   2. The whispered voice test is a helpful aid in screening for loss of hearing.
   3. Third and fourth heart sounds are uncommon.
   4. Increased sensitivity to touch and exaggerated vibratory sense in the lower extremities is noted.

10. **QSEN** A WHNP/midwife is assessing a 47-year-old patient who has come to the office for an annual well-woman exam. One of the first physical signs of aging is:
    1. Having more frequent aches and pains.
    2. Diminished eyesight, especially close vision.
    3. Increasing loss of muscle tone.
    4. Diminished hearing or taste.

11. When assessing for dehydration in an older adult, which finding resulting from aging may provide unreliable physical assessment evidence?
    1. Poor skin turgor.
    2. Slight elevated temperature.
    3. Very dry mucous membranes.
    4. Swollen, furrowed tongue.

Reproductive

12. The major influence on the timing of puberty is:
    1. Exposure to light.
    2. Genetics.
    3. General health.
    4. Nutrition.

13. A 14-year-old girl is seen in the clinic by the WHNP/midwife because she has not achieved menarche. Physical exam reveals axillary and pubic hair and breast buds that developed 10 months ago with increased size of areola. Based on these findings, the most appropriate intervention would be:
    1. Bone age studies.
    2. Labs for luteinizing hormone and follicle-stimulating hormone levels.
    3. Chromosome analysis to rule out Turner syndrome.
    4. Reassurance that she is developing normally.

14. A 16-year-old girl is seen by the WHNP/midwife for a sports physical. The exam reveals increased quantity of pubic hair covering the labia and mons and the areola area forms a secondary mound on breast contour. Using the Tanner scale, the WHNP/midwife would record these findings as:
    1. Tanner stage I.
    2. Tanner stage II.
    3. Tanner stage III.
    4. Tanner stage IV.

15. An 11-year-old girl who has just begun to show signs of breast development asks the WHNP/midwife when she will start having periods like her friends. The WHNP/midwife's response is based on the knowledge that:
    1. The average age of menarche is 12.8 years.
    2. Most girls will have a growth spurt following the onset of menarche.
    3. Menarche usually occurs approximately 3 to 6 months after the onset of breast development.
    4. Menarche usually occurs approximately 18 to 24 months after the onset of breast development.

16. A teenage girl with curly pubic hair on the mons pubis and breast enlargement without secondary contour would be classified on the Tanner scale (stages) as:
    1. Tanner stage I.
    2. Tanner stage II.
    3. Tanner stage III.
    4. Tanner stage IV.

17. The development of the male sexual characteristics in utero is dependent on:
    1. Estrogen.
    2. Progesterone.
    3. Prolactin.
    4. Testosterone.

18. The production of sperm usually begins during the:
    1. Eighth week of gestation.
    2. Beginning of puberty.
    3. End of puberty.
    4. Eighth month of gestation.

19. What is true about the developmental process of sperm or spermatozoa?
    1. Each mature sperm contains 23 chromosomes.
    2. Sperm become motile immediately at maturation.
    3. Spermatogenesis takes place in the prostate.
    4. Higher than normal body temperature contributes to normal sperm production.

20. What substance is produced by the testes?
    1. Alkaline phosphate.
    2. Gonadotropin.
    3. Testosterone.
    4. Acid phosphate.

21. The WHNP/midwife understands the following about birth defects and growth and developmental problems in infants of mothers who have prenatal alcohol exposure:
    1. If alcohol is ingested late in the pregnancy, there is a higher incidence of postmaturity syndrome.
    2. The practice of drinking alcohol while eating a meal significantly reduces the risk of fully expressed fetal alcohol syndrome.
    3. If alcohol is ingested in large amounts early in the pregnancy, there is an increased incidence of fully expressed clinical features of fetal alcohol syndrome.
    4. Growth retardation is associated with early trimester alcohol consumption and postmaturity syndrome.

22. In response to a young adult man's question concerning the production of sperm, the WHNP/midwife knows that sperm is produced in the:
    1. Epididymis.
    2. Vas deferens.
    3. Prostate.
    4. Seminiferous tubules.

23. An adolescent girl with breast budding and sparse, straight, lightly pigmented pubic hair along medial border of labia is at which Tanner stage of sexual maturity?
    1. Stage I.
    2. Stage II.
    3. Stage III.
    4. Stage IV.

24. Precocious puberty is defined as:
    1. Onset of puberty before age 8 in girls and 9 in boys.
    2. Onset of puberty before age 5 in girls and 7 in boys.
    3. Onset of puberty before age 10 in girls and 12 in boys.
    4. Onset of puberty for either sex before older siblings enter into puberty.

25. What finding is considered a normal surface characteristic of the cervix?
    1. Small, yellow, raised round area on cervix.
    2. Red patches with occasional white spots.
    3. Friable, bleeding tissue at opening of cervical os.
    4. Irregular granular surface with red patches.

26. When describing the findings from a normal breast exam, what should the WHNP/midwife document on the patient record?
    1. Left nipple everted, several coarse black hairs arising from areola, enlarged axillary lymph nodes palpated bilaterally, tender nodes in supraclavicular area.
    2. No dimpling or retraction; 1-cm hard, fixed, stellate mass noted next to nipple with scant nipple discharge; no pain or tenderness on palpation.
    3. Right breast slightly larger and denser than left with no nipple discharge, right areola dark pink in color and inverted, left areola dark brown in color and everted, breasts tender to palpation with no axillary nodes noted.
    4. Pendulous breasts with no dimpling, retraction, nipple discharge, or areas of discoloration; numerous small nevi near areola with Montgomery tubercles noted, no supraclavicular or axillary lymph nodes palpated.

Urinary

27. A basic urogenital evaluation in the older adult with complaints of new onset incontinence should include:
    1. History, physical exam, postvoid residual, and urinalysis (UA).
    2. Postvoid residual, blood urea nitrogen, serum creatinine, and UA.
    3. History, physical exam, serum glucose, blood urea nitrogen, serum creatinine, and UA.
    4. Urodynamic/endoscopic/imaging tests, UA, and serum creatinine.

28. When taking a history on voiding patterns in adults, the WHNP/midwife should consider:
    1. Adults normally void q2 to 3 hours in a 24-hour period (8–12 times a day).
    2. Urge sensation to void occurs when the bladder fills to 200 to 300 mL.
    3. Normally, 15 to 20 minutes pass between first urge to void and reaching functional capacity.
    4. Adults typically reach functional (comfortable) capacity at 200 to 300 mL and normally experience some leakage if voiding is delayed.

29. The WHNP/midwife expects which findings on exam of an older adult patient with dehydration?
    1. Tongue furrows and skin tenting over the clavicle.
    2. Specific gravity of urine 1.004.
    3. Pulse rate 58 beats/min (strong, regular) and blood pressure 100/62 mm Hg.
    4. Geographic tongue and reduced saliva pool.

Endocrine

30. With nearly 70% of the adult population being overweight, including obesity, it is important to distinguish a bulge of subcutaneous fat at the base of the neck from a goiter. Which of the following statements is true regarding how to differentiate them?
    1. Swallowing cannot be relied on, as both tissues move up and down when drinking fluid.
    2. Fat layers remain in a fixed position, but a thyroid gland moves up and down while drinking.
    3. Goiters are typically visibly defined from the lateral position of observation.
    4. Fatty tissue appears to be less prominent when observed from the side compared with an enlarged thyroid.

31. What is the correct procedure for palpation of a patient's thyroid gland?
   1. Stand behind the patient, hyperextend the head, and palpate both sides simultaneously.
   2. Have the patient lower the chin and tilt the head slightly toward the side being evaluated.
   3. Hyperextend the head and have the patient lean away from the side being evaluated.
   4. Have the patient lean away from the side being examined and take a swallow of water.

32. When a patient sips water and swallows, the thyroid gland:
   1. Moves downward and slightly posterior and feels smooth on palpation.
   2. Elongates and enlarges during the swallow and immediately returns to a resting position.
   3. Moves slightly out during the sipping and backward during the swallowing.
   4. Moves upward during the swallow and feels symmetric and smooth to palpation.

33. Which characteristics of skin, hair, and nails are correctly listed for the thyroid condition?
   1. Thin nails and coarse and dry but warm skin are associated with hyperthyroidism.
   2. Thicker nails, coarse skin, and hair that breaks off easily are linked with hypothyroidism.
   3. Fine hair, coarse skin, and onycholysis of the nails are found with hyperthyroidism.
   4. Puffy facies, brittle nails, and hyperpigmented skin are associated with hypothyroidism.

34. Select the facial feature description linked with the correct endocrine pathology:
   1. Coarse facial features, heavier brow line, and prominent jaw: acromegaly.
   2. "Moon face," extra hair growth on the upper lip and chin with acne on the back and chest: acromegaly.
   3. Wide-eyed look with nervous tic and bulging eyes: hypothyroidism.
   4. Lid lag, moist skin, periorbital puffiness: hypothyroidism.

35. Which finding would alert the WHNP/midwife that a patient might be experiencing a problem with the endocrine system?
   1. Coagulation abnormalities and fatigue.
   2. Growth abnormalities and glucose intolerance.
   3. Hypoxia and jaundice.
   4. Steatorrhea and abdominal distention.

36. An adult patient is being evaluated for hypoglycemia because of a blood sugar level of 58 mg/dL. The WHNP/midwife would begin the differential diagnosis by:
   1. Deciding if the hypoglycemia is fasting or postprandial.
   2. Ascertaining if it is related to alcohol use.
   3. Deciding if the patient has other medical problems.
   4. Reassuring the patient that it is a benign problem.

37. An older adult female patient complains of lethargy, cold intolerance, weight gain, and yellowing of the palms. The most important laboratory study ordered by the WHNP/midwife in diagnosing this condition is:
   1. Complete blood count.
   2. Liver enzymes.
   3. Thyroid panel.
   4. Cardiac enzymes.

Cardiac

38. The WHNP/midwife is performing a physical exam on a healthy adult woman. On auscultation, the stethoscope would be placed in which areas to best hear the characteristic heart sounds S_1 and S_2?
   1. S_1 is best heard at the apex and S_2 at the base of the heart.
   2. Both are heard equally well at the right midclavicular line.
   3. On the left side, S_1 is at the area of the pulmonic valve and S_2 at the aortic valve.
   4. Both sounds are best heard at Erb point.

39. On the basis of a general assessment of an adult patient, the WHNP/midwife determines the presence of the apical impulse at the point of maximal impulse (PMI) on the patient's chest wall. Where on the chest wall is the PMI normally found?
   1. Second intercostal space at the midclavicular line on the left side.
   2. Right lower sternal border, fifth intercostal space.
   3. Left side at the fifth intercostal space on the midclavicular line.
   4. Left fifth intercostal space, lateral to the midclavicular line.

40. The WHNP/midwife is auscultating the carotid arteries for bruits. What is the correct procedure?
   1. Use the diaphragm of the stethoscope.
   2. Use the bell of the stethoscope.
   3. Place the stethoscope 1 inch off the area above the sternocleidomastoid muscle.
   4. Position the patient at a 30° angle and press firmly, using the bell of the stethoscope.

Respiratory

41. The WHNP/midwife knows that normal breath sounds that have a low pitch, soft intensity, and that are heard best on inspiration over the posterior lung fields are called:
   1. Bronchial.
   2. Vesicular.
   3. Bronchovesicular.
   4. Rhonchi.

42. When auscultating for vocal resonance in a patient with possible consolidation of lung tissue, the WHNP/midwife tells the patient to say "99," and the voice remains loud and distinct over the area of suspected consolidation. This is called:
    1. Tactile fremitus.
    2. Bronchophony.
    3. Whispered pectoriloquy.
    4. Egophony.

43. The WHNP/midwife understands that in percussion of the lungs, hyperresonance is:
    1. A normal finding in the adult patient.
    2. Common when the lungs are hyperinflated, such as with chronic emphysema.
    3. Characterized by soft intensity, high pitch, short duration, and extremely dull quality.
    4. Characterized by loud intensity, high pitch, medium duration, and dull quality.

44. What is the correct procedure when percussing the anterior and posterior chest?
    1. Percuss the entire right side of the anterior chest and move to the left side.
    2. Begin at the upper left side of the posterior chest and compare with the respective anterior side, moving from front to back.
    3. Percuss systematically and symmetrically the intercostal spaces of the posterior chest, moving from the left to the right side, and then percuss the anterior chest.
    4. Percuss the posterior chest, and then measure for diaphragmatic excursion on the anterior chest.

45. When assessing for tactile fremitus, the WHNP/midwife knows that increased fremitus:
    1. Occurs when there is an obstruction in the transmission of vibrations.
    2. Occurs with consolidation or compression of lung tissue.
    3. Is the symmetric transmission of vibration through the chest wall.
    4. Is found in emphysema.

46. On assessment of the patient's respiratory status, crepitation is felt over the third rib at the midaxillary line on the left side. What is the interpretation of this finding?
    1. There is consolidation of fluid in the left lower lobe of the lung.
    2. Severe inflammation is present on the visceral pleural surfaces of the left lung.
    3. An increase in pressure has occurred in the pleural cavity of the right lung.
    4. Air is present in the subcutaneous tissue.

47. When the lateral diameter of the chest is the same size as the anterior-posterior (AP) diameter, the WHNP/midwife correctly identifies this finding as a:
    1. A normal finding in a younger adult.
    2. Pectus carinatum.
    3. Pectus excavatum.
    4. Suggestive of obstructive lung disease.

48. A WHNP/midwife performing a lung assessment using percussion is aware that:
    1. Percussion is best performed lateral to medial and inferior to superior beginning in the anterior chest.
    2. Percussion should start medial to lateral moving superior to inferior beginning in the posterior chest.
    3. Patient positioning is not important to the effectiveness of the assessment.
    4. Patients should not raise their arms while the nurse practitioner is percussing laterally as this causes movement of the ribcage.

HEENT (Head, Eyes, Ears, Nose, and Throat)

49. The WHNP/midwife is examining lymph nodes in the neck. Which nodes are palpated in the anterior triangle of the neck?
    1. Posterior cervical chain.
    2. Anterior superficial chain.
    3. Periauricular lymph nodes.
    4. Supraclavicular lymph nodes.

50. When using an ophthalmoscope, the WHNP/midwife:
    1. Holds the ophthalmoscope in the right hand (uses right eye) while examining the patient's left eye.
    2. Starts the exam with the ophthalmic lens set at zero.
    3. Begins in a position 1 inch from the eye to check the red light reflex.
    4. Examines the anterior chamber in a well-lighted room and asks the patient to focus on an object.

51. The WHNP/midwife observes lid lag in a patient with:
    1. Myasthenia gravis.
    2. Hyperthyroidism.
    3. Hordeolum.
    4. Chalazion.

52. The WHNP/midwife is examining an older adult patient. There is a glossy white circle around the pupils of the eyes with yellowing of the sclera, and the pupils have a decreased reaction to the direct light reflex. The patient has a history of presbyopia. What is the correct interpretation of these findings?
    1. Beginning development of cataracts with a significant decrease in visual acuity.
    2. Expected changes in the eyes as a result of the aging process.
    3. Decrease in depth perception and early eye changes associated with glaucoma.
    4. Visual changes secondary to long-term treatment with digoxin and corticosteroids.

53. The WHNP/midwife is preparing to examine the eyes of an adult patient. To examine the retinal vessels and assess for hemorrhages, the WHNP/midwife uses which aperture on the ophthalmoscope?
    1. Small aperture.
    2. Red-free filter.
    3. Slit.
    4. Grid.

54. When testing the eyes for the presence of a normal consensual response, the WHNP/midwife:
    1. Shines the light into the patient's pupil and observes the rate of pupillary constriction.
    2. Directs the light into one pupil and observes for the constriction or response of the other pupil.
    3. Holds a card in front of one eye and has the patient focus on a fixed object, removes the card, and observes movement of the newly uncovered eye.
    4. Asks the patient to focus on an object, and then directs a light source to the bridge of the nose while observing for symmetric reflection in both eyes.

55. On ophthalmic exam, there appears to be a narrowing or blocking of the vein at the point where an arteriole crosses over it. The significance of this finding is:
    1. The need to evaluate the patient for chronic hypertension.
    2. The possibility of increased ocular pressure associated with glaucoma.
    3. Its association with papilledema, causing decreased venous drainage.
    4. It may represent a small embolus in the retinal vessels.

56. When examining the eyes, the WHNP/midwife determines that the pupils constrict when a patient shifts their gaze from a far object to a near one. This is interpreted as:
    1. Accommodation.
    2. Intact extraocular motor nerves.
    3. Appropriate consensual response.
    4. Visual acuity within normal limits.

57. When examining the ears of an adult patient, the WHNP/midwife determines that the tympanic membrane (TM) is pearl gray, shiny, and translucent. This is interpreted as:
    1. Scarring from previous infections.
    2. Decreased circulation to the membrane.
    3. Presence of serous fluid behind the membrane.
    4. Normal characteristics of the adult ear.

58. When assessing the TM, specific landmarks are determined and described according to the face of a clock. Where are the normal landmarks for the right TM located?
    1. Direct light reflex located at the 5 to 6 o'clock position and malleus at the 1 to 2 o'clock position, with the umbo in the center.
    2. Manubrium slanted to the left, with malleus at the 10 o'clock position.
    3. Direct light reflex in center of membrane, with malleus at the 9 o'clock position.
    4. Umbo is to the left of the center, with anterior malleolar folds at the 10 o'clock position.

59. During a routine physical exam, a WHNP/midwife notes three horizontal creases across the lower bridge of the nose in an adolescent patient. What should be the next appropriate response?
    1. Refer the patient to the dermatologist for further evaluation.
    2. Assume that the finding is normal and continue with the exam.
    3. Prescribe fexofenadine (Allegra) for the patient.
    4. Ask the patient about symptoms of sneezing, rhinorrhea, congestion, tearing, and itching of the nose/eyes/ears.

60. The WHNP/midwife understands that the nasal mucosa:
    1. Is dark pink, smooth, and moist.
    2. Is pale and translucent in appearance.
    3. Is pale and boggy.
    4. Is red and swollen.

Integumentary

61. What are common findings noted when assessing the skin of a pregnant patient?
    1. Petechiae.
    2. Thick, brittle nails.
    3. Senile lentigines.
    4. Chloasma.

62. During a teaching session, the WHNP/midwife instructs the patient regarding normal skin lesions in the older population. These would include:
    1. Seborrheic dermatitis.
    2. Senile keratosis.
    3. Senile lentigo.
    4. Squamous cell.

63. The WHNP/midwife describes an annular skin lesion as usually arranged in:
    1. Groups of vesicles erupting unilaterally.
    2. A line.
    3. A pattern of merging together, not discrete.
    4. A circle, or ring shaped.

64. When assessing an adult's hydration status, the best place to evaluate skin turgor on an adult is:
    1. Just below the clavicle.
    2. Below the scapula on the back.
    3. On the inside of the forearm.
    4. On the back of the hand.

65. On exam of a patient's skin, the WHNP/midwife finds a lesion that is approximately 0.75 cm in diameter, brown, circumscribed, flat, and nonpalpable. What is the correct term for this lesion?
   1. Macule.
   2. Papule.
   3. Nodule.
   4. Wheal.

66. The history and physical of a patient indicate past occurrences of lichenification. The WHNP/midwife identifies the characteristics of this lesion as:
   1. Dried, crusty exudate, slightly elevated.
   2. Rough, thickened epidermis, accentuated skin markings.
   3. Keratinized cells shaped in an irregular pattern with exfoliation.
   4. Loss of epidermis with hollowed-out area and dermis exposed.

67. Clubbing of the nails commonly occurs in patients with chronic respiratory conditions. The WHNP/midwife assesses for this condition by:
   1. Evaluating the nail for transverse depressions and ridges.
   2. Placing the patient's hands together with palms inward and index fingers aligned.
   3. Placing nail beds of each index finger together to determine angle of nail plate.
   4. Determining if there is diffuse discoloration of the nail bed from decreased oxygenation.

68. A circumscribed, elevated lesion greater than 1 cm in diameter and containing clear serous fluid is best described as a:
   1. Papule.
   2. Vesicle.
   3. Bulla.
   4. Pustule.

69. In performing a skin assessment, the WHNP/midwife understands that the following characteristic of a mole would necessitate immediate intervention:
   1. A 5-mm, symmetric, uniformly brown mole on the thigh that has not changed in appearance for more than 5 years.
   2. Multiple small (1–3 mm) flat moles across the upper back that are dark brown in color, round, and have smooth edges.
   3. A 3-cm, waxy papule with a "stuck-on" appearance, noted on the face.
   4. A new, 5- to 6-mm brown mole with an irregular red border that is occasionally pruritic.

Musculoskeletal

70. During the history, which of the following questions would best assist the WHNP/midwife in diagnosing osteoarthritis (OA) versus rheumatoid arthritis (RA)?
   1. "Is your joint pain symmetric and localized?"
   2. "Does your morning stiffness usually last several hours?"
   3. "Have you experienced fatigue, weakness, and weight loss?"
   4. "Is your joint pain asymmetric and worse with movement and relieved by rest?"

71. Bouchard nodes are associated with which of the following conditions?
   1. Rheumatoid arthritis.
   2. Osteoporosis.
   3. Osteoarthritis.
   4. Reiter syndrome.

72. An older adult woman complains of stiffness and pain in both her hands and left knee shortly after waking that worsens in the afternoon. She feels some relief with rest. On exam, the WHNP/midwife notices the presence of Heberden nodes. Which of the following is most likely?
   1. Osteoporosis.
   2. Rheumatoid arthritis.
   3. OA.
   4. Reiter syndrome.

Neurology

73. Which statement is accurate regarding pain assessment in the very old adult?
   1. Pain perception varies from what is usually expected in the adult patient.
   2. Pain symptoms are more dramatic and specific as the patient ages.
   3. Older adults often exaggerate pain symptoms.
   4. Dull pain is often felt as sharp, stabbing pain.

74. QSEN During the physical exam of an older patient, the WHNP/midwife indicates an understanding of deviations in the neurologic system from the normal aging process with which abnormal clinical finding?
   1. Decrease in short-term memory.
   2. Decrease in deep tendon and superficial reflexes.
   3. Decreased sense of touch.
   4. Positive Romberg sign.

Gastrointestinal and Liver

75. The WHNP/midwife is preparing to examine the abdomen of a patient. What is the correct sequence in which to conduct the exam?
    1. Inspection, palpation, percussion, auscultation.
    2. Palpation, percussion, auscultation, inspection.
    3. Percussion, palpation, auscultation, inspection.
    4. Inspection, auscultation, percussion, palpation.

76. When obtaining a history from a 21-year-old female adult patient with abdominal pain, which of the following should initially be assessed?
    1. Food effects on the pain.
    2. Location and onset of the pain.
    3. Change of pain with bowel movements.
    4. First day of last menstrual period.

77. To test for a positive obturator sign in a patient with abdominal pain, the WHNP/midwife:
    1. Passively flexes the right thigh at the hip, and medially rotates the leg from the 90° hip/knee flexion position.
    2. Asks the patient to take a deep breath while palpating in the abdominal right upper quadrant.
    3. Places his or her right hand above the patient's knee and has the patient raise the leg.
    4. Palpates the right abdomen one-third the distance from the anterior superior iliac spine to the umbilicus.

Hematology

78. On physical exam, a palpable, firm, nontender supraclavicular lymph node is noted on the left side of the body. The finding is consistent with a diagnosis of:
    1. Bacterial infection draining from the internal jugular chain.
    2. Thoracic or abdominal malignancy.
    3. Inflammation of the tonsils and adenoids.
    4. Non-Hodgkin lymphoma.

79. The term "shotty" is often used to describe lymph nodes that are:
    1. Tender, mobile, and greater than 5 mm.
    2. Small and pellet-like.
    3. Discrete and cystic.
    4. Irregular, soft, and fixed to surrounding tissue.

Mental Health

80. QSEN The WHNP/midwife understands the following concerning direct questioning about intimate partner violence (IPV) in the home:
    1. Direct questioning should be avoided for fear of offending the patient.
    2. It should be a routine component of history taking with all patients presenting as an initial visit to primary care clinicians.
    3. Direct questioning should be used only when there are obvious findings noted on physical exam.
    4. It should be used only once per year when the patient is seen for a routine physical exam.

81. When receiving records from another agency, the WHNP/midwife notes on the summary sheet that the patient has a dual diagnosis. This means the patient has:
    1. Both manic and depressive symptoms of bipolar affective disorder.
    2. Two closely related psychiatric disorders (e.g., panic disorder and bulimia nervosa).
    3. Coexistence of both a psychiatric disorder (e.g., depression) and a substance abuse disorder (e.g., alcohol dependence).
    4. Coexistence of a personality disorder (e.g., borderline personality) and a psychiatric disorder (e.g., panic disorder).

82. QSEN In taking a history from a patient with depression, which is the most important question for the WHNP/midwife to ask?
    1. Have you ever experienced hallucinations, delusions, or illusions?
    2. Have you ever been hospitalized in a psychiatric facility?
    3. Do you regularly take antidepressants or other medications?
    4. Have you thought about or attempted suicide?

2 Answers and Rationales

Health History

1. (1) Providing a previsit screening tool or questionnaire to allow the older adolescent to identify and write down concerns prior to the start of the visit is a helpful open-ended approach to assist the WHNP/midwife to phrase questions in an appropriate way to promote a sense of partnership that encourages communication. Adolescents may be reluctant to talk and have a clear need for confidentiality. All adolescent patients should be given the opportunity to discuss their concerns privately. Every effort should be made to maintain confidentiality; however, it is important to explain that there are limits on what can be kept confidential during the clinical visit. It should be explained that information that suggests that the adolescent's safety or the safety of another is at risk may be reasons for the WHNP/midwife to "break" confidentiality. Adolescents do not respond well to confrontation or any type of "forced" conversation to express how they are feeling.

2. (3) A pedigree chart is a diagram of family information using a standardized set of symbols (squares representing males and circles females). A dark symbol is used to indicate someone affected with a genetic condition, and unfilled symbols for those who are unaffected; carriers of a condition are often indicated by a gray symbol. The pedigree chart should have at least three generations noted. The pedigree chart is an important component of a family history and can provide information regarding diseases that are transmitted or occur in family generations. It can be used as a diagnostic tool to help guide decisions about genetic testing for the patient and at-risk family members.

3. (4) A constitutional symptom is defined as a symptom that affects the general well-being or general status of a patient. Examples include weight loss, shaking, chills, fever, pain, and vomiting. Constitutional symptoms tend to be nonspecific to a particular disease and because of this, they are not useful in diagnosis of conditions as are nonconstitutional symptoms. The other options all have specific measures and indicators, such as increased heart rate, rash, diminished acuity, and body mass index.

4. (3) The patient with a history of cerebral palsy with minimal cognitive dysfunction should be fully involved in the health history interview to the best of their ability. Support from the patient's family and/or caregiver may be encouraged; however, the focus should be on the patient by speaking directly to them. Additional information from past medical records and the community group home can be obtained either prior to (preferable) or following the health history interview.

5. (1) Adolescents may be reluctant to talk with a health care provider and if they are willing to communicate, they often have a need for confidentiality. All adolescent patients should be given the opportunity to discuss their concerns privately. Explain to the adolescent and parent that during the clinical visit, you will be asking the parent to leave the room to provide an opportunity for the adolescent to communicate confidentially. It is important with motivational interviewing to show concern for the adolescent's perspective, as often it has not been acknowledged, which leads to a desire to be in control. Avoid assumptions, judgments, and lectures. When possible, ask open-ended questions beginning with less sensitive issues and then proceeding to more sensitive ones.

6. (1) Indigenous cultures, such as the Native-American culture, place special significance on the place of humans in the natural world. That culture emphasizes the importance of a holistic body-mind-spirit and living in harmony with nature. Using a soft voice with open-ended statements that reflect a cooperative, sharing style rather than competitive or intrusive approaches would be the preferred therapeutic approach (i.e., a passive style would be best received). Also, some Native-American cultures use silence to a far greater degree, which should not be mistaken for belligerence or sullenness, but likened more to a common response in dealing with strangers or noted as a sign of wisdom. The other options would be more effective to use with clients of a Western culture orientation.

7. (1) Watch and listen to client's nonverbal communication when client is talking. During the interview, look and speak with client, not interpreter. Pace a conversation so there is time for the client's response to be interpreted. Do not ask the interpreter to paraphrase or insert their meaning into the client's words. Ask the client for feedback and clarification at regular intervals. Use brief, concise sentences and simple language—avoid technical terms and slang language.

8. (4) Many cultural factors affect a client's approach to health and health care. Alternative remedies, such as St. John's wort, are used for self-treatment of depression. For most cancers, certain racial and ethnic groups have lower survival rates than white people. Hypertension has a higher rate of occurrence in African-Americans, and they are at greater risk of developing heart disease, end-stage renal disease, and stroke than the general population. Asian-Americans have a higher incidence

of stomach and liver cancers. Ethnic groups respond differently to medications. White people are more sensitive to the effects of beta-adrenergic blockers, such as propranolol, whereas African-Americans are less responsive to this drug group.

Physical Exam

9. (2) High-frequency hearing loss (presbycusis) is a common age-related change with hearing. The whispered voice test is a simple test that can be useful in hearing assessment during a clinic visit, if older patients do not identify that they have difficulty hearing. It is the only test that does not require any equipment. Older adult patients with sensorineural hearing loss will have difficulty with the whispered voice test because their hearing loss is usually in the high-frequency range. A whisper is a high-frequency sound and is used to detect high-tone loss. Because of thinning of the skin, tenting is not a good indicator of hydration status. Fourth heart sounds are common. There is a decreased or absent vibratory sense of the lower extremities, testing unnecessary.

10. (2) Refractive errors are the most frequent eye problems in the United States. Blurred vision results from an inappropriate length of the eye and/or shape of the eye or cornea, and almost all errors—myopia (nearsightedness), hyperopia (farsightedness), astigmatism (distorted vision at all distances), and presbyopia (a form of farsightedness that usually occurs between 40 and 45 years of age)—can be corrected by eyeglasses, contact lenses, or, in some cases, surgery.

11. (1) Because of changes in skin collagen and loss of skin elasticity with aging, poor skin turgor, which is often used as a sign of dehydration in younger individuals, is unreliable in older adults. The patient's body temperature may be elevated due to dehydration, or the elevation may be a result of an inflammatory or infectious process. Mucous membranes are often not noticeably dry until severe dehydration is present. The tongue may be swollen and furrowed in the older adult who is dehydrated.

12. (2) Genetics is the primary determinant of the timing of puberty. Factors such as geographic location, exposure to light, nutritional status, and health status play a role, but genetics is the major influence.

13. (4) Menarche usually occurs approximately 18 to 24 months after the onset of breast development. Bone age and laboratory studies are not necessary because development is within normal limits. Findings do not indicate a chromosomal abnormality, so chromosome analysis is unnecessary.

14. (4)

Tanner Stage	Pubic Hair
I	None
II	Countable, straight, increased pigmentation and length
III	Darker, begins to curl, increased quantity on mons pubis
IV	Increased quantity, coarser texture, labia and mons well covered
V	Adult distribution, with feminine triangle and spread to medial thighs
	Breast Development
I	None
II	Breast bud present, increased areolar size
III	Further enlargement of breast, no secondary contour
IV	Areolar area forms secondary mound on breast contour
V	Mature, areolar area is part of breast contour, nipples project

15. (4) Menarche usually occurs approximately 18 to 24 months after the onset of breast development. Although the average age of menarche is 12.8 years, this should not be the basis for the WHNP/midwife's response. Most girls have a growth spurt at Tanner stage IV.

16. (3)

Tanner Stage	Pubic Hair
I	None
II	Countable, straight, increased pigmentation and length
III	Darker, begins to curl, increased quantity
IV	Increased quantity, coarser texture, covers most of pubic area
V	Adult distribution, spread to medial thighs and lower abdomen
	Genital Development
I	Prepubertal
II	Testicular enlargement, slight rugation of scrotum
III	Further testicular enlargement, penile lengthening begins
IV	Testicular enlargement continues, increased rugation of scrotum, increased penile length
V	Adult genitalia

17. (4) The most important sex hormone during embryonic development is the primary male sex hormone, testosterone. Testosterone is produced by the gonads of the genetic male embryo, causing the male gonads to develop into two testes, which produce sperm. The other hormones are female hormones. Estrogen, the major female hormone, is produced by the ovaries (ovarian follicle and corpus luteum) and cortices of the adrenal glands and placenta during pregnancy. Progesterone, the second major female hormone, is produced by the corpus luteum. Prolactin is an anterior pituitary hormone and one of the somatotropic hormones that are secreted by lactotropic cells. Prolactin is also responsible for milk production in the female.

18. (3) Between the ages of 9 and 12 years, the gonads produce more of the sex hormones, which trigger sexual maturation or puberty. Puberty in males begins at approximately age 11 and lasts for 2 to 3 years, ending with the first ejaculation that contains mature sperm.

19. (1) Each mature sperm develops from mitotic division of diploid (46-chromosome) germ cells (spermatogonium) found on the basement membrane of each seminiferous tubule and becomes primary spermatocytes with 23 chromosomes each. Each of these two cells further divides into two more cells (spermatids), each of which has 23 chromosomes. Motility depends on the biochemicals in semen and in the female reproductive tract. Sperm production needs a temperature that is less than normal body temperature by at least 1°F to 2°F. Elevated temperature (hyperthermia) can cause irregular sperm formation.

20. (3) The testes have two functions: production of gonadotropin (androgens and testosterone) and production of gametes (sperm). The sperm are produced in the seminiferous tubules of the testes. The androgens and testosterone are produced mainly by Leydig cells of the testes (androgens and testosterone are also produced by the adrenal glands). Gonadotropin hormone is produced and secreted by the anterior pituitary gland.

21. (3) Large amounts of alcohol early in the pregnancy have the most devastating effects on the maturing fetus. There is no safe, established dose for alcohol in pregnancy. Food consumption along with alcohol intake does not reduce the risk of defects. Ingesting alcohol in the later months of pregnancy is associated with an increased incidence of premature and small-for-gestational-age neonates.

22. (4) Sperm is produced in the seminiferous tubules of the testes.

23. (2) Tanner has five stages of sexual maturity for both boys and girls. Stage I for both is preadolescent, and stage V for both is mature or adult development. Stages II, III, and IV chronicle development of breasts, pubic hair distribution, penis, and testes. This young girl is demonstrating characteristics of Tanner stage II.

Tanner Stage	Pubic Hair
I	None
II	Countable, straight, increased pigmentation and length
III	Darker, begins to curl, increased quantity on mons pubis
IV	Increased quantity, coarser texture, labia and mons well covered
V	Adult distribution, with feminine triangle and spread to medial thighs
	Breast Development
I	None
II	Breast bud present, increased areolar size
III	Further enlargement of breast, no secondary contour
IV	Areolar area forms secondary mound on breast contour
V	Mature, areolar area is part of breast contour, nipples project

24. (1) Precocious puberty is defined as beginning at age 8 for girls and at age 9 for boys.

25. (1) A nabothian cyst (Naboth follicle) is a small, white or yellow, raised, round area on the cervix and is considered to be a normal variant. The surface of the cervix should be smooth and may have a symmetric, reddened circle around the os (squamocolumnar epithelium, or ectropion). The other options are all unexpected, abnormal findings.

26. (4) Long-standing nevi and Montgomery tubercles are normal findings; pendulous breast is only a description of size, which is important to note. Enlarged lymph nodes and tender supraclavicular nodes are potential cause for concern. A fixed stellate mass with nipple discharge is not normal, and although asymmetry might be normal, the different colors of the areolae and unilateral nipple inversion could represent a problem.

27. (1) A basic evaluation of urinary incontinence should include a history and physical; there are systemic reasons for incontinence, which include neurologic, gastrointestinal, as well as genitourinary/reproductive organ

impairments. Measurement of postvoid residual either by pelvic ultrasound (bladder scan) or catheterization is done to determine retention and potential overflow incontinence. UA may indicate urinary tract infection as the cause of incontinence. The other tests may be performed based on the findings from the initial evaluation, including 3-incontinence questionnaire and voiding diaries.

28. (2) Adults normally void four to six times in a 24-hour period (q4–6 hours). Most adults usually do not awaken to void at night unless they have a medical problem (e.g., benign prostatic hypertrophy, urge incontinence, or diuretic therapy). The feeling of the bladder filling occurs at approximately 90 to 150 mL, with the first urge sensation at 200 to 300 mL. Normally, 1 to 2 hours pass between the first urge to void and reaching functional capacity. Adults typically reach functional (comfortable) capacity at 300 to 600 mL and should *never* experience leakage if voiding is delayed.

29. (1) Signs of dehydration in the older adult are skin tenting over the clavicle, concentrated urine (specific gravity >1.025), oliguria, sunken eyes, lack of axillary moisture, orthostatic blood pressure changes, tachycardia, dry mucous membranes of mouth and nose, and absent or small saliva pool. In the obese older adult patient who has lost weight, tenting of the forehead is not always a reliable clinical sign because of excessive loss of subcutaneous fat. As the older patient becomes dehydrated, aqueous humor of the eye also decreases. Gentle palpation of the eyeball will reveal a boggy versus a firm eyeball, a useful assessment tool in these patients. It is important to examine the mouth because it reveals reliable assessment data in the older adult suspected of dehydration. A geographic tongue (patchy papillary loss that causes a map-like appearance) should not be confused with tongue furrows and tongue coating.

30. (2) Goiters are typically not visible from the lateral aspect in most patients without regard to weight. When examining, inspection from the side to identify any enlargement between the cricoid cartilage and the suprasternal notch is helpful. Any prominence noted in this area should be measured with a ruler and recorded. If the prominence is larger than 2 mm (0.08 inch), there is a high likelihood of goiter. A small goiter is one to two times the normal size of the thyroid, and a large goiter is more than twice normal size.

31. (2) When examining the thyroid, it is important that the patient relax the sternocleidomastoid muscles, which is done by having the patient tilt toward the side being evaluated.

32. (4) The thyroid gland is fixed to the cricoid cartilage and superior portion of the trachea, and thus ascends during swallowing. This assists the WHNP/midwife to distinguish thyroid structures from other neck masses. The gland's size, degree of enlargement, consistency, surface characteristics, and the presence of nodules or bruits are noted during the exam.

33. (2) Puffiness of the face and the skin around the eyes (periorbital), as well as dry, thickened skin, with coarse, breakable hair are linked with chronic low thyroid states. Classic signs of hyperthyroidism are onycholysis (brittle nails, Plummer nails), warm, velvety skin, fine hair with hair loss, and pretibial edema. Onycholysis is the loosening or separation of a fingernail or toenail from its nail bed and is associated with fungal infections, trauma, and hyperthyroidism.

34. (1) Coarse facial features, heavier brow line, and prominent jaw are associated with acromegaly. Other findings include frontal skull bossing (prominent, protruding forehead), mandibular overgrowth, maxillary widening, teeth separation, malocclusion, overbite, and skin thickening on the face (tongue, lips, and nose). Moon face, as well as extra hair growth on the upper lip and chin with acne on the back and chest, are typical Cushing characteristics. A wide-eyed look with nervous tic, bulging eyes (exophthalmos), lid lag, and warm, moist skin are associated with hyperthyroidism. Periorbital puffiness is associated with hypothyroidism.

35. (2) Growth abnormalities are associated with anterior pituitary dysfunction and glucose intolerance with diabetes related to pancreatic dysfunction. Coagulation abnormalities and fatigue would be associated with hematologic dysfunction. Hypoxia would be associated with oxygenation problems and jaundice with liver or biliary problems. Steatorrhea is associated with malabsorption syndrome, cystic fibrosis, and other issues of the exocrine pancreas.

36. (1) True hypoglycemia can be organized around whether it is fasting or postprandial. Postprandial hypoglycemia may be caused by early adult-onset diabetes or postgastrectomy syndrome. Fasting hypoglycemia is most often caused by excessive doses of insulin, sulfonylureas alone, or with biguanides and thiazolidinediones.

37. (3) The symptoms of lethargy, cold intolerance, weight gain, and yellowing of the palms suggest hypothyroidism, and thyroid studies (e.g., thyroid stimulating hormone) would be most useful. A complete physical would be performed, and liver etiology is still a differential. Xanthoderma (yellowing of palms) typically occurs only due to a coexisting carotenemia. Thyroid etiology is the "most likely" choice because cold intolerance is given.

38. (1) S_1 is heard loudest at the apex (characteristic "lub" sound) and S_2 at the base (characteristic "dub" sound). Each sound should be assessed carefully regarding the intensity of the sound in each area. The S_2 second heart sound has two components: A_2 is produced by aortic valve closure, and P_2 is produced by pulmonic valve closure.

39. (3) The PMI represents the thrust and contraction of the left ventricle. The left ventricle lies behind the right ventricle and extends to the left, forming the left border of the heart.

40. (2) The correct procedure is to listen for carotid bruits with the bell of the stethoscope, which brings out low-frequency sounds and filters out high-frequency sounds. The bell should be placed very lightly on the neck with just enough pressure to seal the edge.

41. (2) Vesicular breath sounds are normal, low-pitched, low-intensity sounds heard in the peripheral lung fields. Inspiration is 2.5 times longer than the expiratory phase. Bronchial breath sounds, normally heard over the trachea and larynx, are high-pitched loud sounds with a shortened inspiratory and lengthened expiratory phase. Bronchovesicular breath sounds that are heard mainly where fewer alveoli are located, which is over the second intercostal space anteriorly and between the scapulae posteriorly, have a moderate pitch and intensity with equal duration of expiratory and inspiratory sounds. Rhonchi is an adventitious breath sound and is usually not heard during normal respiration.

42. (2) Greater clarity and increased loudness of spoken sounds are defined as bronchophony. If bronchophony is extreme (e.g., in the presence of consolidation of the lungs), even a whisper can be heard clearly and intelligibly through the stethoscope (whispered pectoriloquy). During auscultation, if the patient is speaking, their voice is normally heard as soft, muffled, and indistinct. When you ask the patient to say "99," during auscultation, you will hear an abnormally clear distinct sound of "99," if there is lung consolidation. Whispered pectoriloquy is exaggerated bronchophony and is heard through a stethoscope when the patient whispers a series of words (e.g., "one-two-three"). In egophony, the spoken voice has a nasal or bleating quality when heard through a stethoscope, and the spoken "e-e-e" sounds like "a-a-a." Tactile fremitus is a palpable vibration of the thoracic wall that is produced when the patient speaks.

43. (2) Hyperresonance is a percussion assessment finding suggestive of air trapping, which can be found in obstructive lung conditions, such as emphysema. It is characterized by very loud intensity, very low pitch, long duration, and a booming quality. It is not a normal finding.

44. (3) Both the anterior and posterior chest should be percussed systematically and symmetrically at 4- to 5-cm intervals over the intercostal spaces, moving from left to right. Begin posteriorly with patient sitting with head bent forward and arms folded. As percussion moves laterally and anteriorly have the patient lift their arms up. Care is needed to ensure percussion is done in the intercostal spaces moving superior to inferior and medial to lateral. Diaphragmatic excursion is usually only measured on the posterior chest.

45. (2) Consolidation or compression of lung tissue will cause an increase in fremitus, which is noted with lobar pneumonia. Decreased fremitus occurs with obstruction of vibration, such as in emphysema, pneumothorax, or obstructed bronchus. Symmetric transmission of vibration is a normal finding.

46. (4) Crepitation or crepitus (also called subcutaneous emphysema) usually results from air bubbles under the skin caused by a leakage of air into the subcutaneous tissue. Infection by a gas-producing organism is a less common cause. Crepitation always requires attention. Severe inflammation of the pleural surface would not have a palpable abnormality. Fluid consolidation would cause an increased asymmetric fremitus on palpation.

47. (4) The adult chest is usually symmetrical and the AP diameter is often half the lateral diameter. Pigeon chest (pectus carinatum) is a forward protrusion of the sternum with the ribs sloping back. Funnel chest (pectus excavatum) is a depression of the sternum. Barrel chest occurs when the AP diameter equals the transverse diameter and is usually a sign of advancing obstructive lung disease.

48. (2) Percussion should start posteriorly and move from medial to lateral and superior to inferior. As the practitioner moves laterally, the patient is asked to raise their arms to make lateral access easier. The percussion assessment should start with the patient sitting with their head lowered and their arms folded in front.

49. (2) The conceptualization of triangles is useful in determining the location of palpable lymph nodes in the neck. The sternocleidomastoid muscle is the division between the anterior (containing the anterior superficial cervical chain) and the posterior (containing the posterior cervical chain) triangles. The trapezius muscle marks the posterior border of the posterior triangle. The supraclavicular nodes are palpated in the angle formed by the clavicle and the sternocleidomastoid muscle.

50. (2) The correct use of the ophthalmoscope involves using the right hand and right eye to examine the patient's right eye. The room should be semidarkened for best visualization. The examiner initially inspects the lens and vitreous body from a distance of approximately 12 inches (at

zero setting) and moves closer to the eye, usually rotating the lenses to the positive numbers (+15 to +20), which assists in focusing on near objects.

51. (2) Lid lag occurs in patients with hyperthyroidism and is evaluated by having the patient follow the examiner's finger as it is slowly moved up and down. The patient has lid lag if sclera can be seen above the iris as the patient looks downward. Ptosis is a drooping lid margin that falls at the pupil or below and may indicate an oculomotor lesion or myasthenia gravis. A chalazion is a chronic, sterile, lipogranulomatous inflammatory lesion of the meibomian gland, whereas a hordeolum is an acute inflammation of one of the glands in the eyelid.

52. (2) Yellowing of the sclera and arcus senilis (also known as corneal arcus) is a benign, yellow-whitish ring around the limbus and is seen in the older adult due to age-related physiologic changes. Cataracts occur as a result of opacity of the lens of the eye that causes partial or total blindness. The visual acuity and depth perception of the patient cannot be determined from the information provided.

53. (2) The red-free filter is used to visualize the vessels and hemorrhages in better detail by improving contrast. This setting will make the retina look black and white. The small aperture is used when the pupil is very constricted; the slit is used to examine contour abnormalities of the cornea, lens, and retina; and the grid is used for estimating the size of lesions found in the fundal area.

54. (2) A light beam shining onto one retina causes pupillary constriction in both that eye, termed the *direct reaction* to light, and in the opposite eye, referred to as the *consensual reaction.*

55. (1) Chronic hypertension stiffens and thickens arteries, resulting in arteriovenous nicking. Intraocular pressure cannot be determined from an ophthalmic exam. Papilledema is associated with swelling around the optic disc with blurred margins. Small emboli are represented by an abrupt impediment or severe narrowing of an arteriole not associated with where the retinal veins and arteries cross.

56. (1) Accommodation is the ability of the lens to change shape. Changes in pupil size when focusing from near to distant objects (and vice versa) tests for accommodation. *Extraocular movements* refer to the ability to move the eye in six cardinal directions. Consensual response is constriction of the eye in response to light being shined in the opposite eye. The Snellen eye chart is used to determine visual acuity.

57. (4) The normal TM is thin, translucent, shiny, and slightly concave with a pearl gray or pale pink appearance. This describes the normal characteristics of the TM. There is no evidence indicating scarring, presence of fluid, or decreased circulation to the membrane.

58. (1) Direct light reflex located at the 5 to 6 o'clock position and malleus at the 1 to 2 o'clock position, with the umbo in the center, describes the correct position for the landmarks on the right ear. The manubrium slants to the right with the malleus at the 1 to 2 o'clock position for the right ear. The direct light reflex in the center of the membrane with the malleus at the 9 o'clock position describes the correct position for the left ear. The umbo is in the center with the anterior folds at the 1 to 2 o'clock position for the right ear.

59. (4) The WHNP/midwife recognizes the nasal crease to be a result of uncontrolled allergic rhinitis, which may be seasonal or perennial as the patient repeatedly wipes the nose with palm. Dermatologic evaluation is not necessary. The finding is not normal. Before treatment is prescribed, a thorough history on allergic rhinitis should be obtained.

60. (1) The nasal mucosa is normally dark pink, smooth, and moist. A pale, boggy mucosa suggests chronic allergy. A red and swollen mucosa suggests acute allergic rhinitis. The normal secretion is mucoid. Purulent, crusty, or bloody secretions are abnormal.

61. (4) Chloasma is hyperpigmentation occurring on the face of a pregnant woman. Both structural and functional changes occur in the skin. Older adults often have senile lentigines (liver spots), which are brown macules found on the backs of the hands, forearms, and face caused by localized mild epidermal hyperplasia in association with increased numbers of melanocytes and increased melanin production. Petechiae are reddish purple spots (usually 1–2 mm) of bleeding under the skin that may occur from numerous causes but are not associated with early pregnancy. The nails become thin and brittle, with marked ridging with aging.

62. (3) The senile lentigo is a gray-brown, irregular, macular lesion on sun-exposed areas of the face, arms, and hands that are normal skin lesions. The other lesions are common abnormal skin lesions in the older adult.

63. (4) The term "annular" stems from the Latin word "annulus," meaning ringed. Lesions are circular or ovoid patches with a red periphery and central clearing (e.g., tinea corporis). Multiple groups of vesicles erupting unilaterally following the course of cutaneous nerves are described as herpetiform or zosteriform (herpes zoster). Linear lesions are arranged in a line (allergic contact

dermatitis to poison ivy). Confluent lesions merge and are not discrete (scarlet fever rash).

64. (1) On an adult, the best place is just below the clavicle or on the abdomen. The best place to evaluate skin turgor for hydration status in children is the fleshy part of arms or legs because a child with a distended abdomen may have a tight abdomen, which appears to have adequate turgor, even though the child may actually be dehydrated.

65. (1) A macule is less than 1 cm in diameter, nonpalpable, flat, and brown, red, purple, or tan (freckles, flat moles, rash of rubella). A papule is elevated and palpable (warts, pigmented nevi). A nodule is 1 to 2 cm in diameter, solid, elevated, and deeper (lipoma). A wheal is elevated and irregular and has a variable diameter (insect bites, urticaria).

66. (2) Lichenification occurs with chronic irritation, often of an exposed extremity (chronic dermatitis). Crusts are dried exudate (impetigo); scales are heaps of keratinized cells from exfoliation (psoriasis); and loss of epidermis is excoriation, as seen in an abrasion (repetitive scratching or picking).

67. (3) The angle between the nail plate and the proximal nail fold when viewed from the side is greater than 180° and should form a diamond in clubbed nails. Normal nails form a 160° angle and should form a diamond shape between them when the nail beds of the index fingers are placed together. Transverse ridges and grooves may occur from trauma. Placing the palms together provides no assessment data. Diffuse discoloration may result from a fungal infection or an injury.

68. (3) Bulla is the correct term. A papule is solid. A vesicle is less than 1 cm in diameter, and a pustule contains a purulent exudate.

69. (4) The appearance of a new mole with high-risk features, including irregular border, color changes, and changes in sensation (e.g., pruritus), would necessitate immediate biopsy and/or referral to a dermatologist. Uniform moles, those that are symmetric and have smooth borders, and those not showing signs of change can be followed with annual skin assessments. Seborrheic keratosis is a benign skin growth, usually on sun-exposed areas, and appearing as waxy or "stuck-on" that requires no treatment.

70. (4) Signs and symptoms of OA include asymmetric joint pain exacerbated by movement and relieved by rest. Stiffness is of short duration (<15 minutes) after inactivity or in the morning. Pain may be described as aching and poorly localized. The other questions are indicative of RA.

71. (3) Bouchard nodes are bony enlargements of the middle joints of the fingers, also the proximal interphalangeal joints on the hands noted in clients with osteoarthritis. RA affects the small joints, metacarpophalangeal, leading to Boutonnière and swan-neck deformities, carpal bones of wrist, second to fifth metatarsophalangeal, and thumb interphalangeal joints. Reiter syndrome, also known as reactive arthritis, is the classic triad of conjunctivitis, urethritis, and arthritis occurring after an infection, particularly those in the urogenital or gastrointestinal tract. Osteoporosis is characterized by low bone mass, deterioration of bone tissue, and disruption of bone architecture that leads to compromised bone strength and an increased risk of fracture.

72. (3) Signs of OA are characterized by slowly developing joint pain, including stiffness of joints, typically worse in the afternoon and early evening. Usually, pain is worse with activity and improves with rest. A visible physical finding of OA are Heberden nodes (bony overgrowths), which are found on the distal interphalangeal joint and are hard, nontender nodules usually 2 to 3 cm in diameter but sometimes encompassing the entire joint.

73. (1) Pain is both highly prevalent and undertreated in the older adult population. Pain may be unreliably reported because, with age, its perception varies from the expected. Pain symptoms may be less dramatic, vague, or nonspecific. The severe pain is usually associated with pancreatitis, for example, may be perceived as a dull ache, and the perception of pain during a cardiac event (myocardial infarction) may be minimal. Some patients may not report chronic pain symptoms because they attribute them to getting older or feel that nothing can be done to relieve the pain, especially because they have lived with the chronic pain for such a long time that it becomes part of their daily living.

74. (4) Romberg sign indicates the inability to maintain balance, which indicates a need for further evaluation. A decrease in short-term memory, deep tendon and superficial reflexes, and sense of touch are normal age-related changes. If it affects the patient's functional ability, a decrease in short-term memory would be considered a deviation. Also, the testing strategy of looking for similarities in the options applies here, as the three incorrect responses all relate to a decrease in a body function with age.

75. (4) Inspection and auscultation should be conducted first to prevent eliciting pain and undue guarding. The WHNP/midwife should auscultate and listen to the abdomen before percussing and palpating it because palpation may alter the frequency of bowel sounds. If the exam is painful initially, the patient will be uncomfortable, which will not allow the examiner to continue.

76. (4) Although all the information is important in determining the cause of abdominal pain, for a young female patient of childbearing age, ascertaining whether the patient is pregnant is a priority. A possibility of pregnancy would alter the testing that might need to be ordered, so a pregnancy test should be ordered. Additionally, abdominal pain may be from pelvic inflammatory disease or related gynecologic disorders. The WHNP/midwife should obtain a gynecologic, pregnancy, and recent sexual history, including dates of last two normal menstrual periods, condom use and other birth control use, and timing of last sexual intercourse. Food effects are important to ascertain because it may lead to a diagnosis of dietary intolerances. Location and associated symptoms are valuable to narrow down the differential diagnoses of the pain. Abrupt onset of pain has differential diagnoses that are different from pain that is recurrent/chronic, having occurred at least for 3 weeks. Acute pain can be visceral, parietal, or referred. Visceral pain originates in the hollow abdominal organs due to contraction, distention, or stretching of the organ, and is usually felt along the midline of the abdomen. Parietal pain results from inflammation of the peritoneum, is usually severe, and noted at the site of the originating disorder. Referred pain is usually noted distal to the site and is caused by innervation along the spinal level of the site. Referred pain may feel superficial or deep sensation. Change in bowel habits may indicate an intestinal origin if there is relief, even if only temporary. Pain not affected by a bowel movement or passing gas is not likely intestinal/colonic pain and may be related to other sources, such as kidney/bladder or the musculoskeletal system.

77. (1) Passive flexion and medial rotation of the right leg causes right hypogastric pain, a positive obturator sign, which suggests an inflamed appendix. A positive Murphy sign, severe pain, and a brief inspiratory arrest, results when a patient takes a deep breath while the examiner applies pressure over the right upper quadrant suggestive of cholecystitis. The Psoas sign is positive with pain on pushing against the hand or with the patient on the left side extending and elevating of the right. When contraction or extension of the psoas muscle causes pain, it is a sign of inflammation of the psoas muscle and a sign of appendicitis. McBurney point tenderness is in the right lower quadrant 2 inches from the anterior superior spinous process of ilium and is associated with acute appendicitis.

78. (2) A Virchow node in the left supraclavicular region is of concern because of the high correlation with abdominal or thoracic malignancy. Infections and inflammatory conditions produce tender, inflamed lymph nodes.

79. (2) "Shotty," or small and pellet-like, lymph nodes that are movable, cool, nontender, discrete, and less than 1 cm in diameter are usually considered normal and often represent enlargement of the lymph nodes following a viral infection. They feel like BBs or buckshot under the skin that move under the examiner's fingers when palpated. If shotty nodes are found in the epitrochlear or supraclavicular regions, they require additional evaluation. A fixed, or nonmovable, lymph node is cause for concern.

80. (2) The personal nature of IPV often influences a victim's decision to report the crime, thus victimizations by intimate partners are highly underreported for both men and women. Given the lack of harm and potential benefits of screening, routine screening is recommended on initial visits to primary care clinicians, to obstetrician-gynecologists, to the emergency department, and on hospital admission. All pregnant women and patients presenting with concerning symptoms or signs, including women with injuries, women with chronic unexplained abdominal pain, women with sexually transmitted diseases, older adults with evidence of neglect, and older adults with injuries, should be asked about IPV. For those patients who screen positive, the WHNP/midwife should offer resources, reassure confidentiality, and provide close follow-up.

81. (3) Dual diagnosis involves both a psychiatric diagnosis and a substance abuse diagnosis.

82. (4) Although it is important to know whether the patient has ever experienced hallucinations, delusions, or illusions and had ever been hospitalized in a psychiatric facility, the single most important factor to ascertain is whether or not the patient has contemplated suicide. In addition, determination of a specific plan and the means to do it are also involved in the questioning about suicidal ideation. Asking a patient whether or not he or she is suicidal does not increase the risk of the patient committing suicide. It is also important for the WHNP/midwife to determine whether the patient regularly takes antidepressants or other medications. Patients may have stopped taking their antidepressants, causing an acute exacerbation of their depression, or started another medication that may be causing an increase in their depression.

3

Diagnostic Tests

Reproductive

1. When obtaining a cervical specimen for a conventional slide Papanicolaou (Pap) smear, what procedure should the WHNP/midwife implement?
   1. Lubricates the speculum with a non–water-soluble lubricant to assist in the insertion of the instrument.
   2. Uses a cotton-tipped applicator when obtaining the cervical cells from a prenatal patient.
   3. Uses warm water to lubricate the speculum to assist in the insertion of the instrument.
   4. Completes the bimanual portion of the exam first to determine the relative position of the cervix to assist in the comfortable insertion of the speculum.

2. To promote physical patient comfort before performing a pelvic exam, which action should the WHNP/midwife implement?
   1. Ask the patient to bear down slightly as the speculum is inserted.
   2. Have the patient empty her bladder.
   3. Explain each step of the procedure in a calm manner.
   4. Carefully reassure the patient that the exam will only take a few minutes.

3. The primary role of a breast ultrasound is to:
   1. Screen for breast cancer.
   2. Definitively diagnose breast cancer.
   3. Determine if a breast lesion is cystic or solid.
   4. Locate small lesions before surgery.

4. When is the optimal time to perform a hysterosalpingogram (HSG)?
   1. During menses.
   2. Immediately after ovulation.
   3. After menses, but before ovulation.
   4. 3 to 4 days before menses.

5. A WHNP/midwife is reviewing information regarding the use of mammography in clinical practice. Which statement regarding mammography is inaccurate?
   1. It detects all breast cancers.
   2. It should be accompanied by a breast exam.
   3. A negative mammography result should not delay biopsy of a clinically suspicious mass.
   4. It is a cost-effective method to screen for breast cancer.

6. The use of potassium hydroxide (KOH) when doing a wet mount assists in the diagnosis of:
   1. Bacterial vaginosis and *Candida* vaginitis.
   2. Trichomoniasis and chlamydia cervicitis.
   3. Syphilis and gonorrhea.
   4. Herpes simplex and condyloma.

7. The WHNP/midwife is reviewing the laboratory results of 21-year-old patient seen recently for a Pap smear: Classification: high-grade squamous intraepithelial lesion; endocervical cells seen; adequate smear. The WHNP/midwife phones the patient and tells her which of the following?
   1. "Your Pap smear was normal. Follow-up in 1 year, or sooner if problems arise."
   2. "Your Pap smear shows invasive cancer. I would like you to see a gynecologic oncologist for treatment."
   3. "Your Pap smear shows abnormal tissue that needs to be evaluated. Please schedule an appointment for a colposcopy."
   4. "Your Pap smear shows a minor abnormality. Sometimes this can signify a disease process just beginning. Please schedule another Pap smear in 4 months for follow-up."

8. A 27-year-old patient reports the desire to become pregnant. She and her husband have had regular, unprotected intercourse for more than 1 year. The WHNP/midwife completes a thorough history and gynecologic exam, which appear normal. What diagnostic test might be ordered early in the workup?
   1. HSG.
   2. Tests for antisperm antibodies.
   3. Semen analysis.
   4. Endometrial biopsy.

9. In an infertility workup, what is the best way to evaluate ovulation?
   1. HSG.
   2. Postcoital test.
   3. Endometrial biopsy.
   4. Basal body temperature (BBT) chart.

10. Which test is the "gold standard" for the diagnosis of chlamydial infection?
    1. Use of KOH wet mount "whiff" test.
    2. Presence of inflammatory cells in Pap smear.
    3. Direct fluorescent antibody test.
    4. Culture with special media and collection technique.

11. Which is the most accurate statement regarding a reactive serologic test for syphilis?
    1. All reactive serologic tests require confirmation with a treponemal test.
    2. Reactive serologic tests are highly suspicious for active syphilis.
    3. A false-positive serologic test, although rare, can be unnecessarily traumatizing to a patient.
    4. A reactive serologic test most likely implies the need for re-treatment.

12. In the evaluation of a young adult with amenorrhea and normal secondary sex characteristics, the purpose of the progesterone challenge is to determine the presence of:
    1. Endogenous estrogen.
    2. Thyroxine (T_4).
    3. Prolactin.
    4. Adequate body fat.

13. A 65-year-old woman reports to the clinic stating she has been experiencing intermittent vaginal bleeding over the last 2 months. Her last menstrual period was more than 10 years ago. Her last Pap smear at the clinic 9 months ago was within normal limits (WNL). She is not taking any hormonal products. She is sexually active with occasional complaints of dyspareunia. What is the most appropriate response of the WHNP/midwife at this time?
    1. Order complete blood count (CBC) and thyroid-stimulating hormone (TSH) and repeat Pap smear.
    2. Schedule laparoscopy.
    3. Schedule endometrial biopsy.
    4. Schedule pelvic/transvaginal ultrasonography.

Pregnancy

14. At an initial prenatal visit occurring in the first trimester, which blood test is not recommended?
    1. Antibody screen.
    2. Rubella.
    3. Maternal serum alpha-fetoprotein.
    4. Hepatitis B (HBV) surface antigen.

15. The most common indication for genetic counseling is:
    1. Maternal age.
    2. Drug exposure during the first trimester.
    3. Increased maternal alpha-fetoprotein.
    4. History of previous stillbirth.

16. The WHNP/midwife schedules a 38-year-old primigravida patient for an amniocentesis at 16 weeks' gestation. The WHNP/midwife would explain that the purpose of this procedure is to:
    1. Assess for the possibility of twins.
    2. Determine the bilirubin level.
    3. Perform genetic studies.
    4. Assess lecithin/sphingomyelin (L/S) ratio.

17. Management of a patient after an amniocentesis includes assessing for:
    1. Increased fetal activity.
    2. Elevated temperature.
    3. Spontaneous rupture of the membranes.
    4. Abnormal lung sounds.

18. The WHNP/midwife is discussing the monitoring of the growth of twins during the pregnancy with a patient in the first trimester. Which test would the practitioner explain to the patient?
    1. Nonstress test (NST).
    2. Sonogram.
    3. L/S ratio.
    4. Amniocentesis.

19. The WHNP/midwife managing a pregnant patient with sickle cell trait would include which information in the plan?
    1. CBC each trimester.
    2. Weekly NST.
    3. Urine cultures each trimester.
    4. Frequent ultrasounds for growth.

20. Screening based on American College of Obstetricians and Gynecologists (ACOG) guidelines for gestational diabetes mellitus (GDM) during pregnancy includes:
    1. 1-hour postprandial 100 g glucose screen for all women at 24 to 28 weeks' gestation.
    2. 3-hour, 150 g glucose tolerance test (GTT) at initial visit for all women with GDM history.
    3. 1-hour postprandial 50 g glucose screen at initial visit for women at risk.
    4. Glycosylated hemoglobin A1C for all women at 24 to 28 weeks' gestation.

21. A 23-year-old (G3 P0) woman has a 50 g glucose load with a 1-hour postprandial glucose screen result of 210 mg/dL. What is the next appropriate step for the WHNP/midwife to take?
    1. Order 3-hour 100 g GTT.
    2. Order fasting blood sugar.
    3. Order A1C.
    4. Refer immediately for diabetic treatment.

22. A teenager returns to the clinic for contraceptive follow-up after being on a low-dose oral contraceptive for 3 months. She complains of amenorrhea for 2 months, urinary frequency, and leukorrhea. Vaginal exam reveals the uterus to be approximately 6 cm and presence of the Chadwick sign. The first diagnostic test indicated should be:
    1. Pregnancy test.
    2. CBC.
    3. Microscopic urinalysis.
    4. Culture for gonorrhea and chlamydia.

23. The recommended screening test for GDM is:
    1. 3-hour GTT.
    2. 1-hour postprandial 50 g glucose screen.
    3. 2-hour postprandial blood sugar measurement.
    4. Random blood sugar measurement.

24. A 28-year-old woman is seen by the WHNP/midwife for an office visit. Her last menstrual period was 8 weeks ago; she is complaining of left lower quadrant abdominal pain, spotting, and fatigue. Her pelvic exam reveals cervical os closed, minimal blood in vaginal vault, uterus minimally enlarged, mild cervical motion tenderness, left adnexal fullness and tenderness, and right adnexa WNL. Vital signs are stable. The serum pregnancy test is positive. What is the most cost-effective and useful test for the WHNP/midwife to order?
    1. Abdominopelvic computed tomography (CT) scan.
    2. Barium enema.
    3. Pelvic ultrasound.
    4. Flat plate of abdomen.

25. The biophysical profile includes which of the following parameters?
    1. Fetal breathing movements, fetal tone, fetal movement, NST, and amniotic fluid volume.
    2. Ultrasonography, alpha-fetoprotein screening, contraction stress test, and fetal heart reactivity.
    3. Amniocentesis, amniotic fluid volume, and NST.
    4. Contraction stress test, NST, and gross fetal movement.

26. A physiologic reason for a nonreactive NST is:
    1. Fetal hypoxia.
    2. Maternal drug use.
    3. Fetal inactivity or sleep.
    4. Congenital heart defect.

27. A 35-year-old woman came into the office 1 week ago and stated that she had been trying to get pregnant. She had a serum beta human chorionic gonadotropin (HCG) test that was positive. Since then she felt okay, but she is concerned that she had some slight vaginal bleeding. A repeat beta HCG serum test is ordered, and it has not increased since the last test 1 week ago. What has most likely happened with her pregnancy?
    1. Normal pregnancy.
    2. A multiple gestational pregnancy.
    3. Ectopic or nonviable intrauterine pregnancy.
    4. Confirms patient was never pregnant.

28. Women should be screened for gestational diabetes at what point(s) in the pregnancy?
    1. At the first prenatal visit.
    2. Between 24 and 28 weeks gestation and at the first prenatal visit if deemed at risk.
    3. Between 28 and 32 weeks gestation.

29. A woman presents at 33 weeks gestation with a complaint of decreased fetal movement over the previous 24 hours. An NST is completed. Which of the following patterns denotes a reactive NST reading?
    1. 1 acceleration 10 beats above the baseline lasting 10 seconds over 30 minutes.
    2. 2 accelerations 10 beats above the baseline lasting 10 seconds over 20 minutes.
    3. 1 acceleration 15 beats above the baseline lasting 15 seconds over 30 minutes.
    4. 2 accelerations 15 beats above the baseline lasting 15 seconds over 20 minutes.

30. Which of the following would *not* be an indication for weekly biophysical profile testing?
    1. Maternal concern.
    2. Type 1 diabetes.
    3. Mild intrauterine growth restriction.
    4. Hyperemesis gravidarum.

Urinary

31. Which of the following patients should be evaluated for urodynamic studies?
    1. Patient with history of stress incontinence and urge incontinence.
    2. Patient with recent surgery for bladder suspension.
    3. Patient with initial incontinence episode after total knee replacement.

32. The WHNP/midwife is evaluating blood chemistries on a patient who is experiencing an increase in blood pressure. She has no previous history of hypertension or other chronic disease. Which serum laboratory value would be most concerning?
    1. Serum creatinine 4.2 mg/dL.
    2. Blood urea nitrogen 30 mg/dL.
    3. Serum potassium 4.5 mEq/L.
    4. Serum osmolarity 290 mOsm/kg.
33. The WHNP/midwife understands the following regarding urine culture and sensitivity testing.
    1. A conventional threshold is growth of greater than 100,000 colony-forming units (CFU)/mL from a midstream-catch urine sample.
    2. In symptomatic patients, a smaller number of bacteria (between 5 and 10 CFU/mL of midstream urine) are recognized as an infection.
    3. Immediately place the urine culture and sensitivity specimen on ice after patient clean-catch collection.
    4. A negative urine culture result is typically greater than 100,000 CFU/mL.

34. The WHNP/midwife is evaluating a urinalysis report of a young women presenting for her annual physical exam. Which findings are considered abnormal?
    1. Specific gravity 1.015.
    2. Large numbers of epithelial cells and casts.
    3. WBCs (≤5).
    4. Few red blood cells (RBCs) (≤2).

Cardiac

35. When ordering a lipid profile on a patient, the WHNP/midwife should teach the patient to eat a typical diet over the next week and:
    1. Eat a normal breakfast the morning of the lipid profile blood draw.
    2. Fast for 8 to 12 hours as directed before the lipid profile is drawn.
    3. There are no restrictions on alcohol consumption for this blood test.
    4. Take any current medications with a few sips of water before the blood test.

36. A 45-year-old woman's lipid profile results are sent to the WHNP/midwife with the following levels: total cholesterol, 287 mmol/L; high-density lipoprotein, 30 mg/dL; and low-density lipoprotein, 165 mg/dL. On the basis of interpretation of these findings, the WHNP/midwife should first do which of the following?
    1. Initiate treatment with low-dose statins.
    2. Discuss adherence to a heart-healthy diet and regular aerobic physical activity.
    3. Assess the 10-year arteriosclerotic cardiovascular disease risk.
    4. Refer to cardiologist.

Respiratory

37. A throat culture is indicated for the following suspected cause of pharyngitis:
    1. Rhinovirus and coronavirus infection.
    2. Group A β-hemolytic streptococci.
    3. Mononucleosis.
    4. *Candida albicans.*

38. A young adult patient is seeing the WHNP/midwife to obtain routine vaccine testing for a nursing program. This patient has had the bacillus Calmette-Guerin vaccine administered in another country. The WHNP/midwife knows that:
    1. A tuberculin skin test is not sufficient to test for latent tuberculosis (TB) infection.
    2. Ordering an interferon-gamma release assay is preferred because of the vaccine.
    3. The student does not need to be tested because they received the vaccine.
    4. A TB titer is the most accurate way of reviewing the effectiveness of immunity.

39. When interpreting purified protein derivative skin tests in a patient with a history of IV drug abuse, the WHNP/midwife identifies positive results in individuals with:
    1. Redness or erythema at the site.
    2. Induration reaction ≥5 mm.
    3. Induration reaction ≥10 mm.
    4. Induration reaction ≥15 mm.

40. A 65-year-old obese patient presents to the clinic with difficulty breathing. On exam, there is a low suspicion of a pulmonary embolus. Which of the following should the WHNP/midwife use to rule out the likelihood of a pulmonary embolus?
    1. Decreased platelets.
    2. Normal fibrin D-dimer.
    3. Normal chest x-ray.
    4. Normal aPTT.

41. The WHNP/midwife identifies clubbing on a patient during an exam. Based on this finding, which three diagnostic tests/assessment techniques would be ordered?
    1. Imaging studies of the hands.
    2. Orthostatic blood pressures.
    3. Pulse oximetry reading.
    4. Electrocardiogram.
    5. Chest x-ray.

HEENT (Head, Eye, Ear, Nose, and Throat)

42. During a physical exam, the WHNP/midwife notes xanthelasma. What laboratory test will the nurse order?
    1. Erythrocyte sedimentation rate (ESR).
    2. CBC.
    3. Thyroid profile.
    4. Lipid profile.

43. The Rinne test is performed to compare bone conduction (when the tuning fork is placed on the mastoid bone) with air conduction (when the tuning fork is held near the ear). A normal Rinne test is described as:
    1. Equal conduction through the mastoid bone and ear canal.
    2. Air conduction is greater than bone conduction.
    3. Bone conduction is twice as long as air conduction.
    4. Sound is clearer with bone conduction than with air conduction.

Endocrine

44. What blood test can be drawn to help identify whether the patient has type 1 or type 2 diabetes?
    1. Hemoglobin A1C.
    2. Glycosylated fructose.
    3. C-peptide level.
    4. Apo A versus Apo B.

45. The laboratory value that points most directly to parathyroid abnormality is:
    1. Low TSH.
    2. Elevated calcium.
    3. Elevated magnesium.
    4. Depressed phosphate.

46. The treatment goal for glycemic control in a person with type 2 diabetes is to achieve and maintain a hemoglobin A1C level of:
    1. Less than 10%.
    2. 6% to 9%.
    3. Less than 7%.
    4. Greater than 8%.

47. An adult woman presents to the WHNP/midwife's office complaining of fatigue, weakness, and weight gain over the past 4 months. Physical exam reveals elevated blood pressure, facial and supraclavicular fullness, hirsutism noted on the face, proximal muscle weakness, and facial and truncal distribution of acne. Appropriate laboratory tests the WHNP/midwife should order include:
    1. Antinuclear antibody (ANA) and rheumatoid factor.
    2. Three-hour GTT and lipid profile.
    3. RBC count and a calcium level.
    4. Dexamethasone suppression test, urinary-free cortisol level, and TSH and T_4.

48. The WHNP/midwife would anticipate which laboratory values in the patient with Graves disease?
    1. TSH levels to be increased.
    2. TSH levels to be decreased.
    3. TSH levels to be WNL.
    4. T_4 levels to be decreased.

49. An adult patient presents to the WHNP/midwife for evaluation of polyuria, polydipsia, and weight loss. Which laboratory result would require immediate intervention by the WHNP/midwife?
    1. A1C of 14%.
    2. Serum glucose of 150 mg/dL.
    3. A1C of 6.0%.
    4. Serum glucose of 65 mg/dL.

50. To make the diagnosis of diabetes, the patient must have two fasting plasma glucose levels documented on two occasions greater than or equal to:
    1. 200 mg/dL.
    2. 140 mg/dL.
    3. 126 mg/dL.
    4. 110 mg/dL.

51. A middle-aged woman presents with agitation, confusion, fever, tachycardia, and diaphoresis. Her daughter states that nausea, vomiting, and abdominal pain preceded these symptoms. The patient has no history of cardiac disease, diabetes, or substance abuse. She was started on an "antidrug" 2 weeks prior, and is scheduled for some form of throat surgery next week (per her daughter). Based on this history, the WHNP/midwife immediately orders:
    1. TSH, T_4.
    2. Urinalysis.
    3. Spinal tap.
    4. CT of the head.

52. A patient with Graves disease is to have radioactive iodine (I^{131}) therapy. Which information is important for the WHNP/midwife to include when teaching about this treatment?
    1. Patients are highly radioactive for approximately 7 days after treatment and need to be isolated.
    2. Patients should not become pregnant during or after receiving this therapy because of the teratogenic effects to the fetus that occur due to chromosomal abnormalities.
    3. Patients may become hypothyroid after this treatment, and therefore need to have regular TSH and T_4 levels drawn, with the potential for thyroid hormone replacement.
    4. This therapy is contraindicated in patients with cardiac disease.

Musculoskeletal

53. Which diagnostic test provides a general indicator that inflammation is occurring within the musculoskeletal system?
    1. Serum amyloid A (SAA) proteins.
    2. Antinuclear antibodies.
    3. ESR.
    4. Hemoglobin A1C.

54. The screening bone mineral density (DEXA) report ordered for a 60-year-old postmenopausal woman shows a result of −1.5 SD (standard deviation) at the hip. She gives a past history of myocardial infarction 1 year ago and wrist fracture at age 32. What option would *not* be considered for this patient?
    1. Counsel on smoking cessation and alcohol consumption.
    2. Initiate therapy with continuous conjugated estrogen 0.625 mg and medroxyprogesterone acetate 2.5 mg.
    3. Initiate therapy with raloxifene (Evista).
    4. Encourage weight-bearing exercises and increased calcium intake.

55. An older adult patient complains of fatigue, weakness, lightheadedness, and anorexia. She also complains of hot, swollen proximal interphalangeal and metacarpophalangeal joints. These symptoms occurred 5 months ago and recurred a few days ago. Which laboratory findings would be most conclusive of these assessments?
    1. High mean corpuscular volume (MCV), low serum ferritin.
    2. Normal MCV, high serum ferritin.
    3. Elevation in uric acid level.
    4. Elevation in WBC count.

56. Which of the following T-scores is indicative of osteoporosis?
    1. T-score of 0 to −1.0.
    2. T-score of −1.0 to −2.0.
    3. T-score of −2.5 or less.
    4. T score of +1.0 or less.

57. A WHNP/midwife has just reviewed DEXA report for a 65-year-old postmenopausal woman and noted normal findings. Which interval timeframe should be utilized for repeated DEXA screening so as to have more predictive value with regard to fracture risk?
    1. Greater than 2 years.
    2. DEXA should be performed on an annual basis.
    3. In 2 years from the date of the initial screening test.
    4. There is no need for repeated testing.

Gastrointestinal and Liver

58. In preparing a patient for a colorectal screening, the WHNP/midwife should instruct the patient to:
    1. Eat at least two servings of meat daily before collecting samples.
    2. Avoid aspirin, iron, and antiinflammatory medications.
    3. Avoid taking extra vitamin and mineral supplements before the test.
    4. Eat extra servings of high-fiber foods and water to ensure good samples.

59. A 25-year-old woman comes in complaining that her girlfriend (partner) has been diagnosed with acute hepatitis B (HBV) and she is afraid she may have it also. When testing the patient, the WHNP/midwife would determine a diagnosis of acute HBV infection from the following blood test results:
    1. Negative HBV surface antigen and positive HBV core antibody.
    2. Negative HBV surface antigen and positive HBV surface antibody.
    3. Positive HBV surface antigen and positive HBV core antibody.
    4. Negative HBV core antibody and negative HBV surface antibody.

60. The WHNP/midwife is seeing a healthy 80-year-old woman who has never had colon cancer screening. What is the most appropriate approach for her?
    1. Because she is over 75 years of age, she does not need any screening.
    2. Recommend screening with CT colonography.
    3. Recommend testing with fecal occult blood and if positive then perform a colonoscopy.
    4. Recommend screening with a colonoscopy.

61. Which laboratory testing would **not** be useful when evaluating elevated liver function tests (transaminases)?
    1. Iron studies: ferritin and iron saturation.
    2. Chronic hepatitis panel for HB and HC.
    3. ANA and smooth muscle antibodies.
    4. Vitamin D level.

62. The WHNP/midwife is explaining a patient's laboratory work following an acute hepatitis A virus (HAV) infection. What is the significance of a positive anti-HAV immunoglobulin G (IgG)?
    1. Indicates immunity to HAV.
    2. Indicates an acute HAV infection.
    3. Indicates patient needs HAV vaccine.
    4. Indicates patient has not had the HAV vaccine.

Hematology

63. A female patient with iron deficiency would most likely present with which of the following lab values?
    1. Hematocrit (Hct) 30%, serum iron 18, MCV 70, decreased transferrin, increased ferritin.
    2. Hct 22%, serum iron 18, MCV 60, increased transferrin, increased ferritin.
    3. Hct 22%, serum iron 18, MCV 70, increased transferrin, decreased ferritin.
    4. Hct 22%, serum iron 18, MCV 90, decreased transferrin, increased ferritin.

64. Which test is most important for diagnosing iron deficiency anemia?
    1. Direct Coombs.
    2. Serum folate level.
    3. Serum ferritin.
    4. RBC count.

65. A macrocytic, normochromic anemia is diagnosed in an older adult woman. What should be the next test(s) ordered?
    1. Serum iron and total iron-binding capacity (TIBC) levels.
    2. Bone marrow biopsy.
    3. Colonoscopy.
    4. Vitamin B_{12} and RBC/folate levels.

66. The WHNP/midwife would suspect disseminated intravascular coagulation (DIC) if the patient's laboratory results, including prothrombin time (PT), indicated:
    1. Increased PT, decreased platelet count, and decreased fibrinogen.
    2. Decreased PT, increased hematocrit, and increased fibrinogen.
    3. Increased platelet count, decreased hematocrit, and increased PT.
    4. Increased platelet count, increased hematocrit, and decreased PT.

67. After confirming the diagnosis of iron deficiency anemia in an older adult female patient based on CBC, peripheral smear, serum iron, TIBC, and serum ferritin, what would be the next essential test for the WHNP/midwife to order?
    1. Fecal occult blood test (FOBT) × 3.
    2. PT/partial PT.
    3. Liver function tests.
    4. Endoscopy.

68. The definitive test for the diagnosis of sickle cell anemia is:
    1. CBC with a peripheral smear.
    2. Bone marrow biopsy and aspiration.
    3. Hemoglobin electrophoresis.
    4. Hemoglobin and hematocrit.

69. A patient has a microcytic and hypochromic anemia and was placed on iron supplementation with no change in the anemia. Recent laboratory tests note a normal ferritin and iron levels with continued microcytic and hypochromic anemia findings. What laboratory test will be used in the differential diagnosis to distinguish this anemia?
    1. Sickledex.
    2. CBC.
    3. Reticulocyte count.
    4. Hemoglobin electrophoresis.

70. Which of the following would be a prudent decision by the WHNP/midwife?
    1. If the reticulocyte count is 100,000 mcg/L, then refer to a hematologist.
    2. If the MCV is above 100 fL, then order vitamin B_{12} and folate tests.
    3. If the MCV is below 50 fL, then order a platelet count.
    4. If the hemoglobin is less than 8 g/dL, then refer to a hematologist.

71. In ordering laboratory tests to screen for a bleeding disorder, the WHNP/midwife would order all *except*:
    1. CBC and differential.
    2. PT and aPTT.
    3. Fibrinogen level.
    4. Hemoglobin electrophoresis.

3 Answers and Rationales

Reproductive

1. (3) Lubricants, other than water, should not be used if a cervical specimen is being obtained for conventional Pap smear analysis; some can alter the appearance of the cells and affect cytologic accuracy. For a liquid-based Pap test, in addition to the use of water, the posterior blade of the speculum may also be lubricated with a small amount of water-based lubricant before insertion. The endocervical cell retrieval is diminished with use of a cotton-tipped applicator and is not recommended in any female patient regardless of pregnancy status. The bimanual exam is performed after the internal vaginal exam.

2. (2) To aid in the exam, an empty bladder provides comfort for the patient and assists the WHNP/midwife in making a more accurate assessment during the bimanual portion of the exam. Asking the patient to bear down slightly while the speculum is inserted and explaining each step of the procedure helps reduce the patient's anxiety, which ultimately may help achieve comfort.

3. (3) A breast ultrasound is used to determine whether a lesion is solid or cystic. Ultrasound misses 50% of lesions less than 2 cm. The test is not sensitive enough to be used for routine screening and cannot replace mammography. The definitive diagnosis of breast cancer is the breast biopsy.

4. (3) The HSG is used to document the presence of a normal uterine cavity and the patency of the fallopian tubes. A contrast dye is injected into the uterus and radiographs are taken to assess anatomy. The best time to do this test is 2 to 5 days after menses, but before ovulation.

5. (1) Mammography is the best screening tool used to assess for malignancy, but it does have limitations in that there are false-positive and false-negative readings, according to the American Cancer Society. Therefore physical findings should not delay diagnostic testing in the presence of a clinically suspicious mass, even if a negative test result was obtained. It should be used in conjunction with a breast exam. It is a cost-effective screening test.

6. (1) KOH lyses epithelial and white blood cells (WBCs), making it easier to visualize *Candida albicans* (yeast). *Candida* cells are resistant and remain intact. KOH also assists with diagnosing bacterial vaginosis by alkalinizing vaginal discharge, causing a distinct fishy odor. This is a positive amine or whiff test.

7. (3) The Pap smear is a screening test for cervical cancer and precancerous states. The diagnostic test needed to confirm the diagnosis of a high-grade lesion is the colposcopy with guided biopsies. The results of this test are clearly abnormal and must be addressed. Waiting 1 year could be deleterious to the patient's health. This is not a Pap smear report that one would choose to redo in 4 months; the patient needs a diagnostic test, not another screening test. Because this is not a diagnosis of cervical cancer on this Pap smear, referral to a gynecologic oncologist is premature at this time.

8. (3) All the tests listed may be included in the workup for infertility. Because male factors account for 35% to 40% of infertility, a semen analysis should be done early in the workup. HSG and endometrial biopsy require scheduling at specific times of the menstrual cycle. Tests for antisperm antibodies would be done if the postcoital test revealed abnormalities.

9. (4) The BBT chart is an easy and inexpensive tool to evaluate for ovulation. Patients should be instructed on the first visit how to use a BBT thermometer and record the findings on a BBT chart. The remaining choices are usually included in an infertility workup, but do not evaluate the presence of ovulation.

10. (4) Culture is a definitive method of diagnosis. It is a collected cervical specimen, and the results take approximately 2 to 6 days to obtain. Blood titers and a urine screen can also be used to diagnose a chlamydial infection. The direct fluorescent antibody is fast and has good sensitivity and specificity.

11. (1) Serologic tests are used as screening tests, but positive results require follow-up with a treponemal test to detect specific antibodies.

12. (1) A positive withdrawal bleed after a progesterone challenge indicates adequate levels of endogenous estrogen. A serum prolactin level should be obtained as part of the amenorrhea workup in addition to a serum pregnancy test. A diagnosis of anovulation can be made on the basis of the successful withdrawal bleed and normal prolactin levels. Low body fat and abnormal T_4 levels can also lead to amenorrhea, but do not affect the progesterone challenge test.

13. (3) If bleeding resumes after 1 year of amenorrhea in a postmenopausal woman or persists longer than 6 months after hormone replacement therapy (HRT) initiation,

further evaluation is necessary. The most common cause of this abnormal finding is endometrial atrophy, but more serious pathology must be definitively ruled out. An endometrial biopsy should be scheduled to further evaluate the cause of bleeding.

Pregnancy

14. (3) Routine prenatal laboratory studies include CBC, blood type and Rh, antibody screen, HBV surface antigen, syphilis screen, and rubella immune status. The maternal serum alpha-fetoprotein is done between 15 and 20 weeks. Before this time, the fetus produces little alpha-fetoprotein, and results would be inaccurate.

15. (1) The largest group of women who potentially benefit from genetic counseling are those age 35 and older. The primary cause of congenital abnormalities in women older than age 35 years is chromosomal abnormalities. The other answers are all reasons for genetic counseling, but to a much lesser degree.

16. (3) The woman's age places her at risk for an infant with Down syndrome. Amniocentesis for L/S ratio is performed in the third trimester for fetal lung maturity and amniocentesis for bilirubin level (delta optical density) is performed for a pregnancy complicated by isoimmunization.

17. (3) Damage to the membranes is a possibility and a high-priority situation. Fever would not be an immediate problem. Fetal heart rate is monitored, not activity.

18. (2) The ultrasound test (sonogram) is used to assess growth of the fetus and position of the placenta and fetus. The NST is used to observe the response of the fetal heart rate to activity. The L/S ratio determines whether there is sufficient surfactant. An amniocentesis is performed to obtain amniotic fluid for analysis later in the pregnancy, if indicated.

19. (3) Sickle cell trait occurs in 8% of African-Americans. These women are asymptomatic, not anemic, and usually have no problems, except under conditions of hypoxia. There is no difference in perinatal outcome, and these women do not require frequent ultrasounds or NSTs. They are at increased risk for asymptomatic bacteriuria and require a urine culture each trimester.

20. (3) This is standard screening for women at risk of GDM. The ACOG recommends a two-step screening method that has been used for many years. The first step is a screen consisting of a 50 g oral glucose load, followed by a plasma glucose measurement 1 hour later. An initial positive screening result is followed by step 2, a 3-hour (100 g) oral GTT on another day. The ACOG recommends use of the two-step screening procedure because there is no evidence that the one-step method leads to clinically significant improvement in maternal or newborn outcomes. This glucose screen should also be done for all other pregnant women between 24 and 28 weeks of gestation.

21. (4) An elevated result, greater than 200 mg/dL, on the glucose challenge is considered diagnostic, alleviating the need for an oral GTT or fasting blood sugar.

22. (1) This clinical picture is highly indicative of pregnancy, especially the presence of the Chadwick sign.

23. (2) The recommended screening test for gestational diabetes is a blood sugar measurement 1 hour after 50 g of glucose at 24 to 28 weeks' gestation. If the result of this test is 140 or above, a 3-hour GTT is done.

24. (3) Pelvic ultrasound is an easy, inexpensive, and relatively noninvasive test that assists the WHNP/midwife with confirming the diagnosis of ectopic pregnancy. It can be obtained quickly and is often available rapidly. Abdominopelvic CT will also show an ectopic pregnancy but is neither cost-effective nor noninvasive. Barium enema and flat plate of the abdomen are not useful in this patient.

25. (1) The biophysical profile includes amniotic fluid volume (index [AVI]), fetal breathing movements (FBMs), fetal movements, and fetal tone determined by ultrasound and fetal heart rate (FHR) reactivity determined by means of the NST. Each parameter is given a score of 0 or 2; the scores from all parameters are then added together, the normal is 8 to 10. Alpha-fetoprotein screening, amniocentesis, and a contraction stress test are not part of the biophysical profile.

26. (3) The most common reason for a nonreactive NST is fetal sleep or inactivity. The fetal sleep-wake cycle ranges from 20 to 40 minutes. If reactivity is not demonstrated in 20 minutes, continuing to 40 minutes usually accommodates the sleep-wake cycles. Fetal hypoxia and maternal smoking and drug use certainly affect fetal heart rate but are not the most common causes. Infants with a congenital heart defect do not exhibit a significant incidence of nonreactive NSTs.

27. (3) Serum beta HCG levels are highly accurate with early pregnancies. There tends to be a surge of the levels around day 8 postimplantation at the time of the luteinizing hormone surge. During the first 6 weeks of pregnancy, beta HCG levels continue to rise and plateaus around 100,000 IU/L. With ectopic pregnancies or nonintrauterine pregnancies, the doubling does not occur, and the level of beta HCG is much lower.

28. (2) The US Preventative Services Task Force and the ACOG both recommend screening for gestational diabetes between 24 and 28 weeks for all women and at the initial prenatal visit for those deemed high risk.

29. (4) For a fetus greater than 32 weeks gestation, there must be 2 accelerations that are 15 beats above the baseline and that each last at least 15 seconds within a 20-minute time period. For a fetus less than 32 weeks gestation, there must be 2 accelerations at least 10 beats above the baseline lasting at least 10 seconds over a 20-minute time period.

30. (4) Hyperemesis gravidarum is not, by itself, an indication for close fetal surveillance if other signs of fetal distress are not present. Diabetes, intrauterine growth restriction, and maternal concern are indications for closer fetal surveillance.

Urinary

31. (1) The optimal patients for urodynamic studies include those who have not had prior incontinence surgery or who have clear symptoms of stress or urge incontinence. Urodynamic testing is a group of tests that examine how well the bladder, sphincters, and urethra are storing and releasing urine. Most urodynamic tests focus on the bladder's ability to hold urine and empty steadily and completely. Urodynamic tests can also show whether the bladder is having involuntary contractions that cause urine leakage. Postvoid residual volume may be seen in an older adult woman.

32. (1) The primary concern in the patient is the elevated serum creatinine level of 4.2 mg/dL. All the other blood chemistry values are WNL. The patient should be referred to a nephrologist immediately because of the elevated creatinine level. The WHNP/midwife in addition to completing a history and physical should order a parathyroid hormone level, liver function tests, lipid and renal panels, CBC, and magnesium/calcium levels. Having these laboratory tests completed will assist the nephrologist in determining the cause of the patient's renal failure. A review of the patient's medications should be initiated to determine whether she is taking any medications that are nephrotoxic, including angiotensin-converting enzyme inhibitors. Nephrotoxic medications should be discontinued. The patient's family history may be reviewed to rule out familial kidney disorders (e.g., Alport syndrome, polycystic kidney disease).

33. (1) The findings of a urine for culture and sensitivity are as follows: negative reports less than 10,000 CFU/mL, and positive reports are greater than 100,000 CFU/mL. Transport the specimen to the laboratory immediately (within 30 minutes). If this is not possible, the specimen may be refrigerated for up to 2 hours; however, it is preferable to not refrigerate the specimen or to place the specimen on ice. In symptomatic patients, a smaller number of bacteria (between 100 and 10,000 CFU/mL of midstream urine) are recognized as an infection.

34. (2) Normal specific gravity for an adult is 1.005 to 1.030, usually with a range of 1.010 to 1.025. A few hyaline casts are normally present, especially after strenuous exercise. Too numerous to count numbers of hyaline casts are associated with proteinuria. The presence of occasional epithelial cells are not remarkable; however, large numbers are abnormal. Tubular (epithelial) casts are often seen with renal tubular disease or toxicity. A few WBCs (≤5) and RBCs (≤2) are considered normal. The presence of five or more WBCs in the urine indicates a urinary tract infection involving the bladder or kidneys, or both. Patients with more than three RBCs per high-power field in two out of three properly collected urine specimens should be considered to have microhematuria, and hence should be evaluated for possible pathologic causes.

Cardiac

35. (2) An 8- to 12-hour fast is recommended because of the influence of intake on cholesterol levels, which may increase. A normal diet for the 7 days before drawing the lipid profile is recommended so that an accurate picture of the patient's normal life is obtained. Alcohol should not be consumed for 48 hours before the test because it may increase cholesterol, high-density lipoprotein, low-density lipoprotein, and triglyceride levels. If possible, all medications should be withheld until the blood test is drawn, especially corticosteroids, diuretics, beta blockers, oral contraceptives, and estrogens.

36. (3) The Adult Treatment Panel (i.e., ATP IV) cholesterol guidelines no longer recommend treatment adjusted to a specific target lipid value. The patient's 10-year arteriosclerotic cardiovascular disease risk should be calculated, and determination should be made whether the patient falls into a pharmacologic treatment benefit group. A heart-healthy diet, lifestyle modifications, and regular aerobic physical activity should always be included in the treatment regimen. Referral to a cardiologist is not appropriate at this time.

Respiratory

37. (2) Diagnostic studies used to detect group A β-hemolytic streptococci infection include a throat culture and a rapid antigen detection test (RADT). Throat culture has been considered the gold standard method to establish

the microbial cause of acute pharyngitis. RADT is often used because it is rapid and convenient; however, RADT is less sensitive (true positive) than a throat culture. A positive monospot test result reveals heterophile antibodies. The monospot test is highly specific and sensitive. *Candida albicans* and rhinovirus are not diagnosed by bacterial cultures. Rhinovirus is one of the most common viral causes of pharyngitis. Oral candidiasis, a fungal infection, can be diagnosed with a KOH smear showing mycelia (hyphae) or pseudomycelia (pseudohyphae) yeast forms.

38. (2) Although a tuberculin skin test is sufficient to test for latent TB infection, the interferon-gamma release assay is preferred when the patient has received the bacillus Calmette-Guerin vaccine. Nursing programs require proof of absence of infection regardless of vaccination, and there is not a test available to measure a TB titer.

39. (3) Positive interpretation of purified protein derivative skin test results are as follows, based on the criteria from the Centers for Disease Control and Prevention:

Induration	Positive Purified Protein Derivative Skin Test Result
≥5 mm	Individuals with HIV infection
	Individuals in recent close contact with persons who have active tuberculosis (TB)
	Individuals with chest x-ray indicating healed TB
≥10 mm	Medically underserved individuals
	Intravenous drug users
	Residents in long-term care facilities and health care workers
≥15 mm	All individuals

40. (2) Fibrin D-dimer is normally less than 500 ng/mL and is elevated when plasmin crosslinks fibrin and creates degradation products in the blood. Unless the suspicion of a pulmonary embolism is high, a D-dimer level of less than 500 can be used to rule out pulmonary embolism. D-dimer is sensitive but not specific and cannot be used to diagnose pulmonary embolism.

41. (3, 4, 5) The presence of clubbing is an abnormal finding indicating compromise in perfusion that can originate from the pulmonary or cardiovascular system. Therefore obtaining a pulse oximetry reading would provide evidence of a patient's current perfusion. An electrocardiogram could provide evidence of cardiac status in terms of rate and rhythm. A chest x-ray would provide evidence of the cardiac silhouette, as well as lung fields, thus allowing for an overview of the patient's cardiac and respiratory status. Imaging studies of the hands would not necessarily reveal pathology unless the practitioner suspected structural deformities. There is no evidence to support ordering orthostatic blood pressures in a patient who presents with clubbing unless there is evidence of dizziness or fainting episodes.

HEENT (Head, Eyes, Ears, Nose, and Throat)

42. (4) Xanthelasma is a soft or hard yellow plaque on the inside corners of the eyelids (near the inner canthus). It is made up of cholesterol and is found more often on the upper lid than the lower lid. Xanthelasma is a type of xanthoma and is associated with hyperlipidemias, so a lipid profile would be an appropriate test to order.

43. (2) The Rinne test is positive (or normal) when air conduction is greater than bone conduction. If the patient hears the tuning fork better by bone conduction, the Rinne test is negative, which suggests a conductive hearing loss.

Endocrine

44. (3) Naturally occurring insulin has a C-peptide bond, which is removed during the processing of exogenous insulin as a drug. The level of C-peptide in the blood can show how much insulin is being made by the pancreas. Classically, a patient with type 1 diabetes has no C-peptide bonds because all circulating insulin is from exogenous sources. In comparison, a patient with type 2 diabetes is expected to have some innate insulin production, so C-peptides should be present. The hemoglobin A1C or glycosylated fructose can be used for either patient group. The Apo A and B levels deal with lipid values, not sugars. It should be noted that newer research shows that some patients with type 1 diabetes actually produce a bit of natural insulin, especially after the initial period, so the C-peptide laboratory is not the absolute determinant of disease status.

45. (2) The increased bone turnover related to abnormal parathyroid hormone levels is linked with increased calcium levels. Changes in other lab values can be associated with bone loss, but the link is stronger with calcium changes.

46. (3) The American Diabetes Association (ADA) recommends an A1C level of <7% as an important treatment goal to decrease the risk of long-term complications. A lab test result of >6.5% A1C is an indication that action needs to be taken, either by a change in medication or a reinforcement of education. Counseling should be provided for prediabetes patients with A1C >5.7%. In some

older patients, those with multiple comorbidities, or limited life expectancy, a goal of <8% may be used.

47. (4) The low-dose dexamethasone suppression test is the best screening test, and the 24-hour urine test for free cortisol is the best confirmatory test to use for Cushing disease. Late-night salivary cortisol is a screening test that would be elevated. TSH and T_4 may also be appropriate to rule out a thyroid condition because some of the patient's signs and symptoms are consistent with thyroid dysfunction. ANA and rheumatoid factor are ordered when rheumatoid arthritis or systemic lupus erythematosus is suspected; however, the patient's clinical picture is not consistent with these conditions. The RBC count would be done to rule out anemia, a potential problem for this patient based on the history of fatigue, but the rest of the clinical picture indicates more than anemia. No clinical findings support a calcium level being drawn.

48. (2) TSH levels should be decreased in a patient with Graves disease because thyroid-stimulating immunoglobulins bind to TSH receptors, which increase T_4 and triiodothyronine synthesis and release, subsequently suppressing TSH levels.

49. (1) An A1C of >8.0% indicates poor glucose control over the past few months. According to the ADA, an A1C of >8.0% is equal to an average daily blood glucose of 355 mg/dL. The normal serum glucose for adults ranges from 70 to 120 mg/dL. Diabetic acidosis is not of concern until the glucose level is >300 mg/dL.

50. (3) The ADA has defined the diagnostic criteria for diabetes to include any one of the three following methods, which must be confirmed on a subsequent day:
    - Random plasma glucose ≥200 mg/dL and acute symptoms (polyuria, polydipsia, polyphagia).
    - Fasting plasma glucose ≥126 mg/dL.
    - Plasma glucose ≥200 mg/dL during an oral GTT.
    - Hemoglobin A1C >6.5%.

51. (1) The woman is likely experiencing the life-threatening syndrome that can occur in decompensated hyperthyroidism. The clues are her symptom presentation and progression, the new "antidrug," and upcoming throat surgery, which suggest that the patient is likely on propylthiouracil (PTU) or methimazole and has thyroid cancer. Although other possible causes of delirium are eventually considered, the WHNP/midwife needs to go with the probabilities of occurrence within the given context.

52. (3) Hypothyroidism often follows this treatment, with 50% of patients requiring replacement therapy in the first year and almost 100% requiring therapy in 10 years. For this reason, regular monitoring of TSH and T_4 levels should be performed. Patients emit a small amount of radioactivity after receiving the dose used to treat this condition and do not require isolation for 7 days. Radioactive iodine is perceived to be safe, without an increased risk of chromosomal abnormalities; therefore no contraindication exists to becoming pregnant after therapy, although patients are counseled to avoid pregnancy during treatment and to avoid children and pregnant women after receiving the oral ablation dose. This therapy is recommended for patients who have cardiac disease associated with their thyroid condition.

Musculoskeletal

53. (3) ESR provides a general indicator that inflammation is occurring within the musculoskeletal system. Serum amyloid A proteins are apolipoproteins that are rapidly associated with high-density lipoprotein and can influence cholesterol metabolism. Antinuclear antibodies provide specific information related to immunologic diseases. Hemoglobin A1C provides information related to glycemic control.

54. (2) The World Health Organization defines osteoporosis as a DEXA T-score below −2.5 SD, and osteopenia as a T-score between −1 and −2.5. The woman has early signs of osteopenia. She is not a candidate for HRT (estrogen + medroxyprogesterone acetate) because of her past cardiovascular history. Raloxifene has been shown to prevent the progression of osteoporosis and, as a selective estrogen-receptor modulator, may be a good alternative to HRT. The other two lifestyle modifications are important counseling issues to reduce the risk of developing osteoporosis.

55. (2) The clinical assessments point to a chronic inflammatory process, such as rheumatoid arthritis. The dizziness, fatigue, lightheadedness, and weakness may be a problem with anemia. The anemia of chronic disease is either a microcytic or normocytic anemia. The value that differentiates the anemia of chronic disease from other anemias is the serum ferritin (iron stores). The value will be either normal or high. An MCV of 104 indicates a macrocytic anemia, which would not include the anemia of chronic disease. Low serum ferritin would not be considered a possibility with this disorder. The uric acid level would be elevated in gout. The WBC count does not address the signs of anemia.

56. (3) The T-score is a comparison of a person's bone density with that of a healthy 30-year-old of the same sex. Osteoporosis is defined as having a T-score of −2.5 or less. The greater the negative number, the more severe the osteoporosis. Osteopenia (low bone density) is a T-score between −1.0 and −2.5. A T-score between +1 and −1 is considered normal or healthy.

57. (1) Recommendations made by the US Preventative Services Task Force with regard to screening intervals to establish better risk fracture prediction suggest that intervals longer than the minimum of 2 years are suggested.

Gastrointestinal and Liver

58. (2) Screening for colorectal cancer includes annual fecal occult blood screening for individuals over age 50 years. Avoiding medications that can cause gastrointestinal irritation and bleeding can help avoid false-positive results. Rare meat and vegetables that are high in peroxidase will cause false-positive results, whereas vitamin C can cause false-negative results.

59. (3) Positive HBV surface antigen indicates active infection present. A positive core antibody can indicate infection, immunity, or an unclear interpretation, depending on other results. Negative surface antigen and positive core or surface antibody indicates immunity. Negative core and surface antibodies together indicate there is no immunity.

60. (4) The current guidelines for those who have had prior negative screening (especially with colonoscopy) may have screening discontinued when they reach age 75 years or have less than a 10-year life expectancy. However, if someone has not had prior screening then it is recommended that testing be considered up to age 85 years, depending on the age and comorbidities. Because she is healthy, a colonoscopy would be the most appropriate option. CT colonography is not recommended as a first-line screening. She needs a colonoscopy regardless of an FOBT, so this is not needed.

61. (4) Vitamin D level is **not** needed for a workup of elevated transaminases. Some of the differential diagnoses for elevated liver function tests include hemochromatosis (iron studies), chronic HB and HC (chronic hepatitis panel), and autoimmune hepatitis (ANA and smooth muscle antibodies). Additional differentials to test for include thrombocytopenia indicative of cirrhosis, celiac sprue (celiac panel), and fatty liver disease (lipids and abdominal ultrasound).

62. (1) The antibody test for total anti-HAV measures both IgG anti-HAV and immunoglobulin M (IgM) anti-HAV. The presence of IgM anti-HAV is found in the blood during an acute HAV infection. Persons who are total anti-HAV positive and IgM anti-HAV negative have serologic markers indicating immunity consistent with either past infection or vaccination. IgG anti-HAV appears in the convalescent phase of HAV infection, remains present in serum for the lifetime of the person, and confers lifelong protection against disease.

Hematology

63. (3) Iron deficiency anemia is a hypochromic, microcytic anemia. Decreased iron stores (serum ferritin) are the hallmark of iron deficiency anemia along with increased transferrin. The liver compensates by increasing production of transferrin, which also increases TIBC. Because iron stores are depleted, the percent of transferrin saturated with iron (percent transferrin saturation) is decreased. Normal to increased iron stores (serum ferritin) with concurrent low-serum iron is the hallmark finding of anemia of chronic disease. Serum iron is decreased along with TIBC. Decreased iron, increased TIBC, and decreased serum ferritin contains the findings for iron deficiency anemia.

64. (3) The serum ferritin correlates with total body iron stores because it is the major iron storage protein. Its value is reduced in iron deficiency anemia. Direct Coombs measures in vivo RBC coating by immunoglobulins and is positive in autoimmune hemolytic anemia, blood transfusion reactions, and drug-induced hemolysis. Serum folate measures the folic acid level in the blood. Ferritin levels less than 15 mcg/L diagnoses iron deficiency anemia (levels <30 mcg/L likely diagnoses). Levels greater than 100 mcg/L rules out iron deficiency.

65. (4) It is important to determine the type of macrocytic anemia so that the appropriate therapy can be ordered. Therefore the vitamin B_{12} and RBC/folate levels would be ordered. These tests would determine whether the patient has a pernicious anemia (the most common type) or a folate deficiency (also common in older adult patients). Serum iron and TIBC would be ordered if an iron deficiency anemia was suspected. There is no indication for a colonoscopy. It would be premature to order a bone marrow biopsy without performing initial testing and potentially overlooking an easily treated condition (e.g., pernicious anemia, folate-deficiency anemia). Measurement of certain metabolites of vitamin B_{12}, methylmalonic acid, and homocysteine, provide additional information to help identify the cause of the anemia.

66. (1) DIC is a complication of infection, malignancy, blood transfusions, liver disease, complications of pregnancy, and sometimes trauma. DIC is the inappropriate accelerated systemic activation of the coagulation cascade, resulting in simultaneous hemorrhage and thrombosis. Laboratory results would show increased PT and decreased platelet count and fibrinogen in response to the hemorrhage and clotting. There is an increase in fibrin degradation product and positive D-dimer.

67. (1) An FOBT or guaiac testing would identify blood loss from the gastrointestinal tract—the most common cause of iron deficiency anemia, along with menorrhagia in female patients. The other tests should be done if the FOBT results are positive. Finding the cause of the iron deficiency is paramount, and the FOBT is an easy, noninvasive method of ruling out gastrointestinal bleeding as the cause.

68. (3) Normal and abnormal hemoglobin can be detected by electrophoresis, which matches hemolyzed RBC material against standard bands for the various known hemoglobins, including hemoglobin S, the abnormal hemoglobin associated with sickle cell anemia. CBC with peripheral smear and hemoglobin/hematocrit would not yield enough information to diagnose sickle cell anemia. Low hemoglobin, normal to increased MCV, increased mean corpuscular hemoglobin concentration, chronic reticulocytosis, mild-to-moderate anisocytosis, and poikilocytosis with numerous sickle cells and Howell-Jolly bodies would be noted on the CBC and differential. A bone marrow biopsy would not be necessary and would not indicate the presence of hemoglobin S.

69. (4) The WHNP/midwife needs to distinguish iron deficiency anemia from thalassemia in this patient. It is important to note that the anemia was not improved with iron supplementation. The gold standard diagnostic test is the hemoglobin electrophoresis. The test is normal with iron deficiency anemia and in beta-thalassemia it is abnormal, as noted by a variable increase in the amount of hemoglobin A2 and possibly increased hemoglobin F for beta-thalassemia and presence of hemoglobin H in hemoglobin H disease. The Sickledex is a screening blood test for sickle cell anemia.

70. (2) Based on the MCV, anemias are classified as microcytic (MCV <80 fL), normocytic (MCV 80–99 fL), or macrocytic (MCV >100 fL). If the MCV is above 100 fL, then order vitamin B_{12} and folate tests to evaluate for deficiencies. The tests should be ordered even if there are no neurologic signs (tingling, numbness). If the MCV is below 80 fL, then a TIBC, ferritin, and serum iron would be ordered, not a platelet count. The reticulocyte count evaluates bone marrow production of RBCs. Any value higher than 100,000/μL is considered a marrow that is responding normally to anemic conditions. Reticulocyte count values below 75,000/μL are considered consistent with impaired (decreased) RBC production and should be referred to a hematologist. Consultation with a physician (not necessarily a hematologist) is recommended for hemoglobin values less than 10 g/dL.

71. (4) The following tests would be ordered to evaluate for a bleeding disorder: PT and aPTT, CBC (including platelet count and peripheral blood smear), thrombin time, fibrinogen level, and platelet function analyzer 100. Hemoglobin electrophoresis would be used to diagnosis sickle cell disease, thalassemia, and other hemoglobinopathies that identifies and quantifies abnormal forms of hemoglobin.

PART 2 Gynecology and Family Planning Tests

4

Gynecology

Anatomy and Physiology of Reproduction

1. The endometrial cycle is often described in three phases. Select the correct phases:
   1. Follicular, menstrual, and luteal.
   2. Proliferative, luteal, and menstrual.
   3. Follicular, secretory, and menstrual.
   4. Proliferative, secretory, and menstrual.

2. The WHNP/midwife understands that premenstrual syndrome (PMS) occurs with greatest frequency and severity in the:
   1. Late luteal phase.
   2. Follicular phase.
   3. Proliferative phase.
   4. Ovulatory phase.

3. What is the primary function of follicle stimulating hormone (FSH)?
   1. Stimulation of maturation of ovarian follicles.
   2. Milk secretion.
   3. Triggering ovulation.
   4. Inhibiting release of luteinizing hormone (LH) from the pituitary gland.

4. What is the best definition of menopause?
   1. Cessation of ability for natural reproduction.
   2. Completion of 12 months of amenorrhea after last menstrual period (LMP).
   3. Follicle stimulating hormone (FSH) level of 30 and estradiol level of 30.
   4. Last menstrual period.

5. In the ovarian cycle, what phase begins with ovulation and ends with the onset of menses?
   1. Follicular phase.
   2. Ovulation.
   3. Proliferative phase.
   4. Luteal phase.

6. Which of the following clinical symptoms would occur in response to vaginal changes during menopause?
   1. Increase in acidity causing pelvic discomfort.
   2. Increased vaginal discharge because of increased lubrication.
   3. Hypertrophy of vaginal tissue leading to pelvic discomfort.
   4. Increased likelihood to develop urinary tract infections (UTIs) due to change in vaginal flora.

7. What function do the Bartholin glands have in reproduction?
   1. Prevent vaginitis by maintaining adequate pH.
   2. Prepare the mucous plug that occurs during early pregnancy.
   3. Produce an alkaline secretion that enhances sperm viability.
   4. Produce small amounts of hormones necessary for ovulation.

Family Planning

8. Which statement is true regarding the diaphragm?
   1. May be inserted up to 24 hours before intercourse.
   2. May be inserted any time up to 6 hours before intercourse.
   3. Should be removed within 1 hour after intercourse.
   4. Should not be left in place longer than 24 hours.

9. A contraceptive method associated with an increase in urinary tract infections (UTIs) is the:
   1. Intrauterine device (IUD).
   2. Diaphragm.
   3. Norplant.
   4. Oral contraception (OC).

10. An adult female patient is seen in the family planning clinic for a consultation on contraception with the WHNP/midwife. She is using oral contraceptives (OCs) but forgets to take them because her work schedule changes every week; she is looking for an effective method that will be easy to remember. She has been married for 14 years, is G2 T2 P0 A0 L2, and is a nonsmoker. She has a negative past history for major diseases and a negative gynecologic history for abnormalities. She has never been treated for a sexually transmitted disease (STD) and is in a mutually monogamous relationship. She is needle phobic and faints when she has to have blood drawn. What contraceptive method would be the best choice for the patient?
    1. Depo-Provera injection every 3 months.
    2. Implantation system for 5 years.
    3. Intrauterine device (IUD).
    4. Diaphragm.

11. A young woman is seen at the family planning clinic by the WHNP/midwife. The patient wants birth control pills but has heard that OCs are "dangerous to one's health." When asked for clarification, she lists weight gain, ovarian cancer, heavy or irregular periods, and infertility. After saying, "I can see that you are concerned about your health," what would be the most appropriate for the WHNP/midwife to tell the patient?
    1. "There are a lot of fallacies about birth control pills. They actually are thought to reduce the risk of ovarian cancers and to help regulate the bleeding, and they are not associated with causing infertility. There can be a minor increase in body weight of 3 to 5 pounds."
    2. "Perhaps you would be better off trying the implantation system or Depo-Provera."
    3. "What you have heard is true. They can be dangerous to your health, and many women experience these problems."
    4. "There are a lot of fallacies about birth control pills. Ovarian cancer and infertility are risks when taking the pills, but they do not cause weight gain or bleeding changes during periods. Papanicolaou (Pap) smears done every year will detect such problems as ovarian cancer."

12. An adult female patient is taking oral contraceptives (OCs). She calls into the clinic with complaints of bleeding through the first 2 weeks of every package of pills. She has been taking this pill for 4 months at the same time every day. Her present OC is a low-dose monophasic pill. She is not taking any other medications and denies any adverse effects from the OCs. She would prefer to keep taking the OCs if possible. The WHNP/midwife's advice should include:
    1. Discontinue the pills and do not restart them. Use an alternative contraceptive method.
    2. Change to a higher dosage, and higher progestational agent.
    3. Try taking the pills early in the morning on an empty stomach to improve their metabolism.
    4. There is no cause for concern; breakthrough bleeding is a normal side effect of OCs.

13. An adult female patient is seen by the WHNP/midwife at the family planning clinic. The patient notes heavy, irregular menses and an increase in facial acne and facial/abdominal hair growth over the past few years. She is G1 T1 P0 A0 L1 and is not planning future pregnancies. After a normal pelvic exam, she decides she wants oral contraceptives (OCs). What is the best medication choice for this patient?
    1. Loestrin 1/20.
    2. Triphasil.
    3. Demulen 1/35.
    4. OCs are inappropriate for this patient.

14. A 41-year-old patient is seen for her 6-week postpartum exam by the WHNP/midwife. She is breastfeeding without difficulty and plans to continue for a year. She wants to begin using a contraceptive and plans no further pregnancies. Which of the following is an *inappropriate* choice for this patient?
    1. Depo-Provera 150 mg IM every 3 months.
    2. Intrauterine device (IUD).
    3. Progestin-only oral contraceptive.
    4. Combination oral contraceptive.

15. A 38-year-old patient is seen for her 6-week postpartum exam by the WHNP/midwife. The patient was breastfeeding for a short time but discontinued 4 weeks ago. Her menses have resumed. She is contemplating another pregnancy in approximately 2 years, but if she became pregnant before then, she "wouldn't mind." She is seeking contraception. She smokes one pack per day. Her exam is normal, with the uterus well involuted. Which of the following is contraindicated in this patient?
    1. Progestasert IUD.
    2. Combined oral contraceptive.
    3. Depo-Provera injection.
    4. Condoms and spermicide.

16. A single woman presents for contraceptive counseling, expressing preference for a diaphragm. Which factor in her history would make a diaphragm a poor choice?
    1. Three UTIs in the past year.
    2. Strong desire to avoid pregnancy.
    3. Last two Pap smears showing atypical cells.
    4. Nulliparous cervix.

17. Combination oral contraceptives (OCs) prevent pregnancy primarily by:
    1. Decreasing fallopian tube motility.
    2. Thinning of cervical mucus.
    3. Suppressing ovulation.
    4. Causing inflammation of the endometrium.

18. What is a unique advantage of a hormonal intrauterine device (IUD)?
    1. Lowest failure rate of IUDs.
    2. May be left in place for up to 10 years.
    3. Decreases menstrual blood loss and dysmenorrhea.
    4. Must be replaced annually.

19. Which statement about progestin-only pills is true?
    1. Women who are breastfeeding should not use progestin-only pills.
    2. Ovulation suppression is as effective with progestin-only pills as with combination OCs.
    3. There is an increased incidence of functional ovarian cysts.
    4. The risk of ectopic pregnancy is lower for women using progestin-only pills.

20. The most common side effect associated with depot medroxyprogesterone acetate (DMPA; Depo-Provera) is:
    1. Nausea.
    2. Acne.
    3. Menstrual cycle changes.
    4. Increased menstrual cramps.

21. A young woman who is taking a low-dose oral contraceptive (OC) calls the clinic in a panic, stating that she forgot her pill 2 days ago. She is taking phenytoin (Dilantin) for seizure activity and has been seizure free for over a year. She asks, "What should I do about my pills?" What would be the WHNP/midwife's most appropriate response?
    1. "Take the forgotten dose today along with the regular dose."
    2. "See your physician for advice about the phenytoin."
    3. "Continue the pills but use another contraceptive through the rest of this cycle."
    4. "Come to the clinic for a 'morning-after' pill."

22. On Monday morning a patient calls to tell you her vaginal contraceptive ring (NuvaRing) was out of her vagina for 2 hours this past weekend. She is not due to change the ring for another 2 weeks. She is worried about pregnancy and wants to know what she should do. What should the patient be told?
    1. "You are at risk for pregnancy and should not have intercourse for the remainder of this cycle."
    2. "Please schedule an appointment today so we can talk about a different method of contraception that is easier for you to use."
    3. "You are at risk for pregnancy. Restart the ring and use a back-up method of birth control for the next 7 days."
    4. "There is no increased risk of pregnancy if the ring has been out of the vagina for less than 3 hours."

23. Women who use the subdermal implant for contraception may experience:
    1. Increased side effects if their body mass index (BMI) is less than 19 kg/m^2.
    2. Thyroid function abnormalities.
    3. Irregular bleeding or spotting.
    4. A delayed return to fertility after discontinuation.

24. A patient is requesting contraception and has no contraindications to any method. She is also considering a pregnancy in the next year. Which of the following methods are not a good choice for her to use?
    1. Combined oral contraceptive pills.
    2. Condoms.
    3. DMPA (Depo-Provera) injection.
    4. Vaginal contraceptive ring.

25. A progesterone-releasing IUD is a better choice than a copper IUD for women who:
    1. Do not want to have any more children.
    2. Are currently breastfeeding.
    3. Have never been pregnant.
    4. Have heavy menstrual periods and dysmenorrhea.

26. When providing contraceptive counseling to adolescents (ages 13–17 years), the WHNP/Midwife knows that long-acting reversible contraception (LARC), which includes IUDs and the contraceptive implant:
    1. Is unsafe to use by the adolescent population.
    2. Can be considered for all adolescents.
    3. Is not acceptable to adolescent patients.
    4. Does not represent the most effective methods for adolescents.

27. An absolute contraindication to the use of combined (estrogen and progesterone) hormonal contraception is:
    1. Migraine with aura.
    2. Dyslipidemia.
    3. Type I diabetes for 10 years without complication.
    4. Previous pelvic inflammatory disease (PID).

28. A 25-year-old patient has been using DMPA (Depo-Provera) for 1 year. The patient is at the clinic for her annual exam. Considering what you know about DMPA, what dietary information should you include in your counseling?
    1. You should decrease empty calories and increase your exercise to avoid weight gain.
    2. You should decrease your consumption of foods high in sodium.
    3. You should increase your consumption of iron-rich foods.
    4. You should make sure you are getting adequate calcium and vitamin D in your diet.

29. The WHNP/midwife is seeing a patient for contraception counseling. She is interested in fertility awareness-based methods. What information from her history is a possible reason for not adhering strictly to any type of fertility awareness method?
    1. Busy lifestyle, erratic schedule, frequent travel.
    2. Regular, 29-day menstrual cycles.
    3. Partner supportive, also interested in nonhormonal birth control.
    4. Detail oriented, organized.

30. Which of the following women is the best candidate for progesterone-only pills as a method of contraception?
    1. An 18-year-old woman who has trouble remembering to take her prescribed medications.
    2. A 32-year-old woman with well-controlled hypertension.
    3. A 28-year-old woman who is homeless and has a history of intravenous drug abuse.
    4. A 42-year-old woman who wants to regulate her menstrual cycle.

Disorders

31. The WHNP/midwife understands that the following are US Preventive Services Task Force (USPSTF) recommendations regarding the effectiveness of specific preventive care services for patients without obvious related signs or symptoms of breast cancer.
    1. The USPSTF recommends prescribing risk-reducing medications, such as tamoxifen, raloxifene, or aromatase inhibitors, to women who are at increased risk for breast cancer and at low risk for adverse medication effects.
    2. Women 65 years and older having a history of breast cancer should not take risk-reducing medications.
    3. The USPSTF recommends the routine use of risk-reducing medications, such as tamoxifen, raloxifene, or aromatase inhibitors, in women who are not at increased risk for breast cancer.
    4. Women who have atypical ductal or lobular hyperplasia and lobular carcinoma in situ should not take risk-reducing medication therapy.

32. Which is *not* a risk factor for heart disease in the postmenopausal woman?
    1. Regular exercise.
    2. Cigarette smoking.
    3. Hormone replacement therapy (HRT).
    4. Diabetes mellitus.

33. An adult patient's last menstrual period (LMP) was 2 months ago. She has had an intrauterine device (IUD) in place for the last 4 months. She is complaining of nausea, fatigue, breast tenderness, and abdominal bloating. Physical exam reveals the following:
    - Abdomen: no abnormalities noted.
    - Pelvic: cervix—positive Chadwick sign, IUD strings protruding from cervical os.
    - Uterus: enlarged and nontender.
    - Adnexa: nontender, without mass and no cervical motion tenderness.

    What should the WHNP/midwife identify as the most likely diagnosis?
    1. Uterine fibroid.
    2. Ovarian cancer.
    3. Dislodged IUD.
    4. Pregnancy.

34. Which is *not* a risk factor for osteoporosis?
    1. Cigarette smoker.
    2. White race.
    3. Alcohol consumption.
    4. Obesity.

35. A young woman complains to the WHNP/midwife that she is experiencing headaches, irritability, decreased appetite, and fatigue approximately 1 week before menses. Appropriate management includes which of the following?
    1. Treat premenstrual syndrome (PMS) with increased protein and salt in the diet.
    2. Incorporate daily aerobic exercise and dietary changes into her lifestyle.
    3. Order complete blood count (CBC), comprehensive metabolic panel, and urinalysis.
    4. Supplement her diet with an additional 1 to 2 g of vitamin C.

36. A middle-aged woman presents with abnormal uterine bleeding. A hormonal profile reveals increased follicle stimulating hormone (FSH) and luteinizing hormone (LH) levels. What is the most likely cause for these findings?
    1. Hypothalamic disorder.
    2. Onset of climacteric.
    3. Premature ovarian failure.
    4. Anterior pituitary disorder.

37. Which physical finding would be present in a patient with a clinical diagnosis of uterine fibroids?
    1. Diarrhea.
    2. Shoulder pain.
    3. Increased blood flow during menses.
    4. Amenorrhea.

38. Menopause occurs at a mean age of 51 years. Which of the following factors has been linked to influencing the age at which menopause occurs?
    1. Use of oral contraceptives.
    2. Socioeconomic status.
    3. Age at menarche.
    4. Smoking.

39. A female patient presents to the clinic with complaints of pelvic pressure and discomfort. When questioned about her menstrual cycle, the patient relates a history of heavy bleeding recently. Age of menarche was 16. Pelvic exam of the uterus reveals a bicornuate uterus. The WHNP/midwife suspects that the patient may have:
    1. Premenstrual syndrome (PMS).
    2. Secondary dysmenorrhea.
    3. Pelvic inflammatory disease (PID).
    4. Dyspareunia.

40. A WHNP/midwife is discussing therapeutic management with a patient who is being actively treated for polycystic ovarian syndrome. Which finding would indicate that the disease has progressed?
    1. Positive pregnancy test.
    2. Hemoglobin A1c level is 5.4%.
    3. Blood pressure reading 150/92 mm Hg.
    4. Menstrual period lasts between 5 and 7 days.

41. During a yearly physical exam, a WHNP/midwife asks a woman if she has any problems or questions about sexual function or activity. Initially the patient hesitates, but with further questioning and discussion, she states that she is unsure if she has ever experienced an orgasm. The WHNP/midwife suspects:
    1. Vaginismus.
    2. Primary orgasmic dysfunction.
    3. Secondary orgasmic dysfunction.
    4. Dyspareunia.

42. The WHNP/midwife is talking with a young woman who has been diagnosed with herpes simplex virus type 2. In discussing her care, it would be important for the WHNP/midwife to include what information?
    1. The initial lesions are usually worse than lesions that occur with outbreaks at a later time.
    2. Her sexual partner will not contract it if she does not have sex when the lesions are present.
    3. This condition can be treated and cured if she takes all of the antibiotics for 2 weeks.
    4. If she becomes pregnant in the future, she will need to have a cesarean delivery.

43. The definition of bacterial vaginosis (BV) is:
    1. A syndrome resulting from homeostatic disruption in the vagina.
    2. Vaginitis caused by a flagellated protozoan.
    3. A bacterial sexually transmitted infection that can be symptomatic or asymptomatic.
    4. A virus characterized by recurrent outbreaks and remissions.

44. A 22-year-old married patient complains of severe dysmenorrhea. Her gynecologic exam is normal. Which management protocol is preferred?
    1. Assess for contraceptive interest and, if interested, suggest use of oral contraceptives (OCs).
    2. Suggest use of a prostaglandin synthetase inhibitor.
    3. Suggest use of over-the-counter ibuprofen.
    4. Assess exercise patterns and use of relaxation techniques.

45. Which is *not* a criterion for the diagnosis of bacterial vaginosis (BV)?
    1. Positive amine test (whiff test).
    2. Presence of clue cells.
    3. Vaginal pH greater than 4.5.
    4. Presence of pseudohyphae.

46. A WHNP/midwife is reviewing information about a patient with a history of dilation and curettage (D&C) after a first-trimester spontaneous abortion leading to subsequent amenorrhea. Which working diagnosis should the nurse suspect?
    1. Polycystic ovarian syndrome.
    2. Asherman syndrome.
    3. Hypogonadism.
    4. Premature ovarian failure.

47. The LH/FSH ratio in polycystic ovarian syndrome (Stein-Leventhal syndrome) is:
    1. 1.5:1.
    2. 3:1.
    3. 6:1.
    4. 1:3.

48. What are common findings in a patient with polycystic ovarian syndrome?
    1. Weight loss, dental caries, and amenorrhea.
    2. Hyperprolactinemia and galactorrhea.
    3. Dysmenorrhea, nodules palpated on bimanual exam, and infertility.
    4. Chronic irregular menses, hirsutism, and increased abdominal girth.

49. What is the **most** common cause of dysfunctional uterine bleeding?
    1. Thyroid disorder.
    2. Blood dyscrasia.
    3. Anovulation.
    4. Uterine tumor.

50. A 30-year-old patient presents with scant pubic hair, minimal breast development, absent cervix, and uterus with a 46 XY karyotype. Which diagnosis should the WHNP/midwife suspect?
    1. Turner syndrome.
    2. Müllerian agenesis.
    3. Testicular feminization.
    4. Gonadal dysgenesis.

51. The most common cause of a breast mass in patients ages 15 to 25 years is:
    1. Fibroadenoma.
    2. Intraductal papilloma.
    3. Infiltrating lobular carcinoma.
    4. Fibrocystic breast syndrome.

52. An effective treatment for primary dysmenorrhea is:
    1. Nonsteroidal antiinflammatory drugs.
    2. Tranquilizers.
    3. Progestins.
    4. Steroids.

53. What is a cause of secondary amenorrhea?
    1. Testicular feminization.
    2. Hypogonadotropic hypogonadism.
    3. Congenital absence of uterus.
    4. Extreme exercise.

54. A young woman comes into the clinic for a well-woman checkup. She states that approximately 3 weeks ago, she had a sore on her labia that went away. It was not particularly painful, did not itch, and apparently caused no residual problems. The WHNP/midwife would treat this patient by:
    1. Ordering the treponemal-specific test (i.e., FTA-ABS).
    2. Swabbing the area of the lesion for a viral culture.
    3. Advising her to notify her sexual contacts to determine if they have had any symptoms.
    4. Ordering nystatin (Mycostatin) cream to be applied to the area three or four times a day.

55. Which is *not* a risk factor for the development of cervical cancer?
    1. Human papillomavirus (HPV).
    2. Virginal status.
    3. Multiple sexual partners.
    4. Previous high-grade squamous intraepithelial lesion.

56. A young woman is complaining of tenderness and burning of her vulva. On exam, the vulva is edematous and excoriated. The WHNP/midwife performs a wet mount preparation of the vaginal secretions. It reveals pseudohyphae and spores. The diagnosis for this patient is:
    1. Vulvovaginal candidiasis.
    2. Chlamydial infection.
    3. Bacterial vaginosis (BV).
    4. Gonorrhea.

57. Which type of genital cancer has the highest rate of death?
    1. Ovarian cancer.
    2. Endometrial cancer.
    3. Cervical cancer.
    4. Vulvar/vaginal cancer.

58. A young woman presents with complaints of an irritation in the vaginal area. This is the first time it has occurred. On vaginal exam, the cervix is inflamed and friable. Flagellated protozoa are seen on the wet mount. The most likely diagnosis is:
    1. Trichomoniasis.
    2. Cervicitis.
    3. Chlamydial infection.
    4. Bacterial vaginosis.

59. A 26-year-old female patient presents to the emergency department complaining of gradual onset of abdominal pain. The pain started in the periumbilical region and is now in the right lower quadrant, accompanied by nausea, anorexia, constipation, and low-grade fever. Physical exam confirms the diagnosis of acute appendicitis. What diagnostic studies are least useful in confirming this diagnosis?
    1. CBC with differential.
    2. Flat plate of abdomen, kidneys-ureter-bladder.
    3. Pelvic ultrasound.
    4. Pregnancy test.

60. Which is *not* a risk factor for endometrial cancer?
    1. Obesity.
    2. Oral contraceptive use.
    3. Unopposed estrogen use.
    4. Advancing age, older than 50 years.

61. Which is *not* a risk factor for ovarian cancer?
    1. Family history of ovarian cancer.
    2. Advancing age, older than 50 years.
    3. Oral contraceptive use.
    4. Positive *BRCA-2* gene.

62. What is the most commonly occurring female genital malignancy, excluding the breast?
    1. Ovary.
    2. Endometrium.
    3. Cervix.
    4. Vulva/vagina.

63. A 20-year-old college student presents to urgent care with new onset of painful sores in the vulva. These erupted yesterday and are associated with exquisite pain, fever, and flu-like symptoms of headache, general body aches, and mild dysuria. She has a new sexual partner. The exam reveals vesicular lesions covering the labia, extreme tenderness of external genitalia to palpation, normal Bartholin glands, and normal vaginal inspection with mild leukorrhea, normal cervical mucosa, and slightly tender, minimally enlarged inguinal lymph nodes bilaterally. What is the most likely diagnosis?
    1. Gonorrhea.
    2. Chlamydial infection.
    3. Herpes simplex virus type 2.
    4. Lymphogranuloma venereum.

64. A 21-year-old patient is seen for her annual gynecologic exam. She is sexually active, rarely uses condoms for sexually transmitted infection (STI) prevention, and has multiple sexual partners. She smokes one pack of cigarettes per day, admits to a sedentary lifestyle, and eats two meals per day, most often at fast-food restaurants. Her exam is negative for any abnormalities. Her family history and personal medical history are negative for major disease. She has no menstrual abnormalities; her last menstrual period (LMP) was 1 week ago. The WHNP/midwife obtains a Pap smear. Which action would *not* be appropriate for this patient?
    1. Obtaining cultures for gonorrhea and chlamydia.
    2. Laboratory testing of glucose, cardiac risk profile, and thyroid stimulating hormone.
    3. HIV titer and rapid plasma reagin.
    4. Counseling on safe sex practice and contraceptive information.

65. The initial workup for abnormal uterine bleeding should include:
    1. Referral for diagnostic dilatation and curettage.
    2. Referral for endometrial biopsy to rule out cancer.
    3. CBC, pregnancy test, and endocrine studies.
    4. Coagulation studies and sexually transmitted infection (STI) cultures.

66. Which is *not* a risk factor for breast cancer?
    1. History of maternal breast cancer, premenopausal onset.
    2. First pregnancy after age 35.
    3. Late menopause, after age 54.
    4. Fibrocystic breast disease.

67. A 21-year-old female patient presents for her first well-woman exam. She has never been sexually active. Her family history and past medical history are negative for any gynecologic diseases. Her menses occur every 28 days, lasting 5 days, with a relatively moderate flow and no significant abdominal cramps. Her physical exam/visit today should include which tests?
    1. Pap smear.
    2. Cultures for gonorrhea and chlamydia.
    3. Stool hemoccult.
    4. Baseline mammogram.

68. What is the leading cause of death for women in the United States?
    1. Breast cancer.
    2. Colon cancer.
    3. Heart disease.
    4. Stroke.

69. Reactive cellular changes noted on a Pap smear are most often associated with:
    1. Inflammation.
    2. Use of estrogen vaginal cream.
    3. Drying artifact.
    4. Use of OCs.

70. Risk factors for cervical cancer include:
    1. Pregnancy after age 35.
    2. Human papillomavirus (HPV) exposure.
    3. Low parity.
    4. Prolonged contraceptive use.

71. What is the most common cancer in women in the United States?
    1. Breast cancer.
    2. Colon cancer.
    3. Malignant melanoma.
    4. Lung cancer.

72. A 48-year-old patient presents to the clinic complaining of hot flashes, no menses for 14 months, insomnia, crying spells, irritability, decreased libido, and fatigue. At the end of her history and physical, she begins to cry and tells the WHNP/midwife that she "thinks she's going crazy." She then begs the WHNP/midwife to tell her what is wrong. Which action is *inappropriate* for the WHNP/midwife to do at this point?
    1. Obtain laboratory tests, including follicle stimulating hormone (FSH) and luteinizing hormone (LH levels).
    2. Discuss hormone replacement therapy (HRT), including risks and benefits and short- and long-term treatment strategies.
    3. Provide antidepressant therapy and a referral for counseling sessions for depression.
    4. Provide written information regarding menopause and options for treatment of symptoms.

73. Care for a patient with chancroid should include:
    1. Screening for HIV and syphilis.
    2. Mandatory notification and treatment of all sexual partners.
    3. Screening for lymphogranuloma venereum.
    4. Culture for gonorrhea.

74. During her annual exam, a 35-year-old patient complains of recent breast changes. She states that her breasts are painful and frequently feel "lumpy." Because of this, she has stopped doing monthly breast self-exam (BSE), believing BSE is a "waste of time." What would be the most appropriate advice for the WHNP/midwife to give to this patient?
    1. Stress the importance of the woman knowing the normal look and feel of her breasts and to report any changes.
    2. Suggest she at least do BSE every 2 months.
    3. Suggest she start having mammograms to establish some baseline data about her breasts.
    4. Determine when her breasts are nontender and least "lumpy," and change her BSE schedule.

75. During a breast exam on a young woman, palpation reveals a painless, 2-cm lobular mass in the right breast that is firm and freely mobile. Appropriate management includes:
    1. Continued observation and rechecking in 3 months.
    2. Ordering a mammogram.
    3. Referral for probable surgical excision.
    4. Detailed family history to determine breast cancer risk.

76. A woman with bilateral breast implants asks if it is really necessary to do monthly breast self-exam (BSE) because she "does not know what to feel for." How should the WHNP/midwife respond?
    1. Suggest she involve her sexual partner in assessing her breasts on a regular basis.
    2. Review the steps in BSE until she feels comfortable with the process.
    3. Acknowledge the difficulty of doing BSE after implant surgery.
    4. Explain the usefulness of regular mammograms for implant patients.

77. An adult patient comes to the clinic complaining of abnormal vaginal discharge (dark watery brown) along with postcoital bleeding. The WHNP/midwife suspects the possibility of cancer of the cervix. During the vaginal exam, suspicious physical results for cervical cancer would be:
    1. Soft, sill-shaped cervix.
    2. Very firm cervix with an ulcer.
    3. Vague lower abdominal discomfort.
    4. Tender, enlarged cervical lymph nodes.

78. A postmenopausal patient is worried about pain in the upper outer quadrant of her left breast. What action should the WHNP/midwife take?
    1. Do a breast exam and order a mammogram.
    2. Explain that the pain is related to hormone fluctuations, and order laboratory studies.
    3. Reassure the patient that pain is not a presenting symptom of breast cancer, and check for proper fit of the brassiere.
    4. Teach the patient breast self-exam (BSE).

79. A 22-year-old female patient comes to the WHNP/midwife's office with a complaint of 1 day of fever of 102°F (38.9°C), a diffuse macular rash, vomiting, headache, and decreased urine output. Which information obtained in the patient's history would be most significant given the patient's clinical presentation?
    1. Whether the patient's immunizations are up to date.
    2. If the patient is currently menstruating.
    3. If the patient has a history of tuberculosis.
    4. What type of contraception the patient uses.

80. A young female patient presents to the WHNP/midwife's office with a complaint of abdominal pain. Which differential diagnosis should be ruled out given that the patient is of child-bearing age and could lead to increased morbidity and mortality if not treated promptly?
    1. Irritable bowel syndrome.
    2. Cholelithiasis.
    3. Pyelonephritis.
    4. Ectopic pregnancy.

81. A young adult patient presents with a history of vaginal itching and heavy white discharge. The patient gives a history of no sexual activity. On exam, the WHNP/midwife finds a red, edematous vulva and white patches on the vaginal walls. The discharge has no odor. What finding should the WHNP/midwife expect in the patient's history?
    1. Vegetarian diet.
    2. Recent diarrhea.
    3. Early menopause.
    4. Recent antibiotic use.

82. A 22-year-old female patient presents to the urgent care department and is seen by the WHNP/midwife. She is complaining of abdominal pain, low-grade fever, and mucopurulent vaginal discharge. Her symptoms began 3 days ago and are worsening. She has a new sexual partner and has not yet used condoms with him. Her menses just ended; she is taking oral contraceptives (OCs). She denies nausea, vomiting, or anorexia. Her exam reveals findings consistent with PID. Cultures are taken for gonorrhea and chlamydia. Which of the following represents an **inappropriate** treatment plan for the WHNP/midwife to follow?
    1. Ceftriaxone (Rocephin) 250 mg IM.
    2. Doxycycline (Vibratabs) 100 mg PO bid for 10 days.
    3. CBC, erythrocyte sedimentation rate.
    4. Hospitalization.

83. What is the primary role of progestins in prescribing postmenopausal HRT?
    1. Reduce side effects of estrogen-related breast tenderness.
    2. Provide endometrial protection against hyperplasia.
    3. Stabilize mood swings and reduce hot flashes.
    4. Reduce occurrence of breakthrough bleeding.

84. An older female patient is seen by the WHNP/midwife for her annual exam. She has been on hormone replacement therapy (HRT) for 6 months, having started herself on the pills left over by her deceased mother. She brings the pills, which she wants to keep taking, and requests a prescription for Estrace 1 mg daily. She has an intact uterus, is in excellent health, and denies any complaints. She does not have any contraindications to the use of HRT. Her exam is normal. Which represents an incorrect and potentially dangerous plan for the WHNP/midwife to follow?
    1. Endometrial biopsy.
    2. Prescription for Estrace 1 mg daily plus medroxyprogesterone acetate (Provera) 2.5 mg daily.
    3. Prescription for Estrace 1 mg daily.
    4. Instruct patient on the risks and benefits of HRT.

85. Which is *not* a contraindication to the use of hormone replacement therapy (HRT) in the postmenopausal woman?
    1. Recent deep vein thrombosis.
    2. Chronic active hepatitis.
    3. Controlled hypertension.
    4. Undiagnosed abnormal genital bleeding.

86. Posttreatment for cervical cancer, the following suggestions are given to patients:
    1. Reduce use of lubricants to avoid infections.
    2. Use of HRT to help with postmenopausal symptoms that may present posttreatment.
    3. Do not use dilators because of risk of tearing posttreatment.
    4. Do not use HRT because of risk of exogenous estrogen.

87. A postmenopausal patient presents to your clinic with abdominal bloating, early satiety, and edema of the lower extremities. The workup should include:
    1. Ca125 laboratory test, abdominal/pelvic computed tomography.
    2. Upper gastrointestinal (GI) and colonoscopy.
    3. Barium swallow and CBC.
    4. Guaiac stool cards and basic metabolic panel.

88. A 55-year-old patient presents to the clinic and has not been seen for 2 years. At her last visit, the patient described her periods as irregular and approximately 45 days apart. She states that after the last clinic visit, she did not get her period for approximately 14 months, until 1 month ago, at which time she began to have vaginal bleeding. She states that she is surprised her menstrual cycle has restarted because she thought she was done menstruating. What is the most likely diagnosis?
    1. Ovarian cancer.
    2. Miscarriage.
    3. Uterine polyp.
    4. Uterine cancer.

89. A 39-year-old new patient presents to the office and indicated that she would like to discuss her risk of cancer because she found out her sister, who is 45 years old, has been diagnosed with breast cancer. Her mother has a history of postmenopausal ovarian cancer. What is appropriate to include in the workup?
    1. Whole-breast ultrasound.
    2. Breast exam and referral to genetics for testing.
    3. Baseline mammogram in 1 year, when she turns 40.
    4. Breast magnetic resonance imaging (MRI).

90. A 20-year-old patient has been diagnosed with external genital warts. She has not been vaccinated for HPV and is asking about the vaccine. The patient should be told:
    1. She already is infected with HPV, so she is not eligible for the vaccine.
    2. The HPV vaccine may cause the external genital warts to get worse.
    3. She should strongly consider getting the HPV vaccine.
    4. She is too old to receive the HPV vaccine.

91. Classic “strawberry spots” on the cervix are often diagnostic of:
    1. Trichomoniasis.
    2. Bacterial vaginosis (BV).
    3. Chlamydia.
    4. Herpes simplex virus.

92. The WHNP/Midwife suspects a diagnosis of primary syphilis when a patient presents with:
    1. A maculopapular rash on the trunk.
    2. A cluster of fleshy growths on the vulva.
    3. Tender vesicles and papules on the vulva.
    4. An indurated, painless ulcer on the vaginal wall.

93. When performing a wet prep on a patient with increased vaginal discharge, an abundance of clue cells are noted. What condition is this associated with?
    1. Candidiasis (yeast).
    2. Chlamydia.
    3. Trichomoniasis.
    4. Bacterial vaginosis.

94. A 19-year-old patient thinks she has a UTI and is reporting symptoms of dysuria and lower abdominal discomfort. She has a new partner of 1 month and is engaging in frequent sexual activity. In addition to a urine culture, which of the following tests should be ordered?
    1. CBC.
    2. Rapid plasma reagin (RPR).
    3. Chlamydia.
    4. Serum herpes antibodies.

95. A patient comes to the office complaining of fatigue, breast tenderness, abdominal bloating, fluid retention, and irritability approximately 1 week before onset of her menses. This has been occurring for the past 4 months. What is the most important information for the WHNP/midwife to obtain to assist in determining the diagnosis of premenstrual syndrome (PMS)?
    1. Point in menstrual cycle when symptoms occur.
    2. Severity of symptoms.
    3. Number and frequency of symptoms over past 4 months.
    4. Presence or absence of anxiety or depression.

Male Issues Affecting Women's Health

96. Which of the following is true about male hypogonadism?
    1. Usually presents with decreased libido.
    2. May cause an increase in muscle mass.
    3. It causes an increase in body hair.
    4. Does not contribute to infertility.

97. Which of the following is a common cause of erectile dysfunction (ED)?
    1. The use of antihypertensives.
    2. Dietary supplements.
    3. Masturbation.
    4. It is a natural part of aging.

98. A 47-year-old man presents with pain of his right knee and discomfort when grasping objects with his hands for 14 days. He reports a low-grade fever of 100.4°F (38°C) for the last 5 days, and dysuria 5 days ago. He is sexually active with multiple partners and does not use barrier protection. For which of the following organisms should the WHNP/midwife begin immediate treatment?
    1. *Treponema pallidum.*
    2. *Neisseria gonorrhoeae.*
    3. *Staphylococcus aureus.*
    4. *Chlamydia trachomatis.*

99. Which statement is correct concerning circumcision?
    1. Circumcision is helpful in preventing phimosis.
    2. Circumcision is a cause of paraphimosis.
    3. Balanoposthitis is the direct result of circumcision in older men.
    4. Circumcision increases the incidence of cancer of the penis.

100. A 31-year-old man presents with his fifth diagnosis of gonorrhea in the past 3 years and affirms he completed all treatment regimens as prescribed. His wife concurs with his explanation. Which of the following is an appropriate next step by the WHNP/midwife to evaluate the cause of recurrent infections?
    1. Safe sex education.
    2. Screening for complement deficiency.
    3. Intravenous treatment of the resistant gonococcal infection.
    4. Behavioral therapy for sex addiction.

101. Acute epididymitis is characterized by:
    1. Absence of dysuria.
    2. Nonenlarged scrotum.
    3. Tenderness over epididymis.
    4. Lack of abdominal pain.

102. A 65-year-old man presents with a history of well-controlled hypertension and diabetes mellitus. He is a nonsmoker. He has been married for 35 years, is monogamous, and reports that his relationship with his wife is good. He complains of new onset erectile dysfunction (ED). First-line therapy for ED includes:
    1. Relationship counseling.
    2. Oral phosphodiesterase-5 inhibitors.
    3. Intraurethral injections of alprostadil (Caverject).
    4. Use of a vacuum device.

103. Which action is true about the prostate?
    1. Secretes fluid that is acidic.
    2. Secretes fluid that is alkaline.
    3. Secretes androgens.
    4. Produces sperm.

104. A middle-aged patient complains of a tight band causing a dorsal curvature of the penis and shortening of the penis both with and without an erection. What is the most likely diagnosis?
    1. Phimosis.
    2. Lateral phimosis.
    3. Lateral paraphimosis.
    4. Peyronie disease.

105. What organism is the most common cause of nongonococcal urethritis (NGU) in men?
    1. *Chlamydia trachomatis.*
    2. *Neisseria gonorrhoeae.*
    3. *Escherichia coli.*
    4. *Streptococcus faecalis.*

106. A male patient is diagnosed with balanitis. The most likely cause is:
    1. Candidiasis.
    2. Herpes genitalis.
    3. Lichen planus.
    4. Psoriasis.

107. A male patient presents with a complaint of sexual dysfunction. The WHNP/midwife understands that sexual dysfunction is impairment of:
    1. Erection only.
    2. Emission only.
    3. Ejaculation only.
    4. Erection, emission, or ejaculation.

108. The WHNP/midwife knows that erectile dysfunction is:
    1. Primarily psychological in origin.
    2. Unusual in older men.
    3. The persistent inability to achieve and maintain an erection adequate for sexual intercourse.
    4. The physiologic dysfunction when smooth muscle contracts, causing a lack of adequate amount of blood in the penis to render a rigid, larger penis.

109. Priapism is classified as which type of sexual dysfunction:
    1. Erection.
    2. Emission.
    3. Ejaculation.
    4. Priapic.

110. A male patient complains of erectile dysfunction. Which of the following may be a contributing factor?
    1. Antihypertensive drugs.
    2. Sexual intercourse.
    3. Rheumatoid arthritis.
    4. Frequent masturbation.

111. A patient has nongonococcal urethritis (NGU). The WHNP/midwife understands that:
    1. No related problems occur if NGU is untreated.
    2. Patients with NGU are often asymptomatic.
    3. NGU is easily differentiated from gonococcal urethritis on physical exam.
    4. There is a very purulent discharge with a foul odor.

112. The WHNP/midwife is speaking with a group of male teenagers who are most concerned about symptoms associated with gonorrhea. Which of the following would the WHNP/midwife include in the discussion?
    1. Reddish lesions may appear on the palms of the hands and soles of the feet.
    2. Men may observe a rash over the body of the penis.
    3. Urinary dribbling may result from irritation of the urinary tract.
    4. Painful urination results from inflammation of the urethra.

113. What is considered a major contributing factor in erectile dysfunction?
    1. Diet high in vitamin C.
    2. Diabetes mellitus.
    3. Allergies.
    4. Low-sodium diet.

114. A 30-year-old man presents with a macular-papular rash on his body, including the soles of his feet and his palms. He is also complaining of fatigue, fever, malaise, and swollen lymph nodes. On further questioning, it is revealed that the illness began several weeks ago with several papules on his penis. The WHNP/midwife suspects:
    1. Herpes simplex.
    2. Granuloma inguinale.
    3. Gonorrhea.
    4. Syphilis.

115. Which of the following sexually transmitted infections often begins with a prodrome of headaches, fever, malaise, and myalgia?
    1. Genital herpes.
    2. Granuloma inguinale.
    3. Gonorrhea.
    4. Syphilis.

116. Which of the following clinical presentations are commonly associated with genital herpes in the male patient?
    1. Vesicular lesions on an erythematous base.
    2. Chancres on the penis.
    3. Purulent urethral discharge.
    4. Small, flattened papules and larger verrucous lesions.

117. Which of the following is correct regarding short-acting phosphodiesterase-5 inhibitors, such as sildenafil (Viagra) or vardenafil (Levitra)?
    1. They work best in combination with a large, fatty meal.
    2. They should be taken 30 minutes to 1 hour before intercourse.
    3. They are the only class of medications that are effective for treating ED.
    4. They work in all men.

118. Common side effects of phosphodiesterase-5 inhibitors include:
    1. Erections lasting longer than 4 hours.
    2. Headaches, flushing, and dyspepsia.
    3. Nausea and vomiting.
    4. Rash, itching, and loss of appetite.

119. An important contraindication to phosphodiesterase-5 inhibitors is:
    1. Selective serotonin reuptake inhibitors.
    2. Beta blockers.
    3. Nitrates.
    4. Thiazide diuretics.

Pharmacology

120. A female patient has received treatment for *Trichomonas vaginalis* and completed the course of therapy, but the patient remains symptomatic. Which two findings might prompt the WHNP/midwife that the patient has not been compliant with treatment?
    1. Patient states that she had a few alcoholic drinks during the course of therapy.
    2. Uses cotton underwear as an undergarment.
    3. Did not douche during the course of therapy.
    4. Took 2-g dose of metronidazole (Flagyl) as a single dose as opposed to 500 mg twice a day dosage for 7 days.
    5. Patient reports that she has not abstained from sexual intercourse.

121. An older adult patient is seen for follow-up to discuss her hormone replacement therapy (HRT) that she began 3 months ago. She needs a refill on her HRT but is not sure "if it is working right." She continues to feel hot flashes, moodiness, and decreased libido, and has many sleep disturbances. She is taking Premarin 0.625 mg daily and Provera 2.5 mg daily. She denies any vaginal bleeding. Which is **not** an acceptable choice for the patient?
   1. Premarin 0.9 mg 1 tab PO qd and Provera 5 mg 1 tab PO qd on days 1 to 12.
   2. Premarin 0.9 mg 1 tab PO qd and Provera 5 mg 1 tab PO qd on days 16 to 25.
   3. Premarin 0.3 mg 1 tab PO qd and Provera 2.5 mg 1 tab PO qd.
   4. Premarin 1.25 mg 1 tab PO qd and Provera 10 mg 1 tab PO qd on days 1 to 12.

122 A young adult patient presents to the clinic with complaints of a malodorous, yellowish vaginal discharge and vulvovaginal itching. She has never had a gynecologic exam and is extremely apprehensive. She is sexually active and has had a new sexual partner for 2 months. She states that they use condoms "most of the time" and are not interested in alternate forms of contraception at this time. Her last menstrual period (LMP) was 1 week ago. Her wet mount with KOH shows few clue cells, moderate lactobacilli, few WBCs, no yeast, and too numerous to count mobile trichomonads. Appropriate treatment for this patient would include:
   1. Metronidazole (Flagyl) 2 g PO single dose.
   2. Metronidazole (Metrogel) vaginal cream 1 applicator at bedtime for 5 days.
   3. Fluconazole (Diflucan) 150 mg PO single dose.
   4. Terconazole (Terazol) vaginal cream 1 applicator at bedtime for 7 days.

123. Which dose of conjugated equine estrogen (Premarin) is the minimal effective dose to prevent osteoporosis?
   1. 0.3 mg.
   2. 0.625 mg.
   3. 0.9 mg.
   4. Premarin is inappropriate.

124. The results of the Women's Health Initiative provided evidence-based data that have led to new guidelines in assessing the risk/benefit ratio for initiation of hormone replacement therapy (HRT) in postmenopausal women. Which statement is *not* correct?
   1. HRT is indicated for the treatment of menopausal symptoms, such as vasomotor and urogenital symptoms.
   2. HRT should be continued for primary prevention of coronary heart disease.
   3. HRT can be continued for the prevention of postmenopausal fractures due to osteoporosis.
   4. HRT should be limited to the shortest duration consistent with treatment goals and benefits in consideration with risks in the individual woman.

125. A 46-year-old female patient is being seen in the clinic by the WHNP/midwife. She was last seen 2 weeks ago for an upper respiratory tract infection and was treated with amoxicillin (Amoxil) 250 mg PO tid for 10 days. She completed her medication last week, but now is aware of vaginal itching and has cottage cheese–like vaginal discharge. She states that she has never experienced such intense itching. She is in a mutually monogamous relationship. Her LMP was 2 weeks ago. Her partner had a vasectomy 2 years ago. Wet mount with KOH shows negative whiff test, rare clue cells, positive lactobacilli, positive hyphae and spores, few WBCs, and no trichomonads. She is leaving tomorrow for a week-long cruise. She is not taking any medications and has no known drug allergies. The WHNP/midwife knows that the best treatment for this problem is:
   1. Metronidazole (Flagyl) 500 mg PO bid for 7 days.
   2. Clindamycin (Cleocin) vaginal cream one applicator-full vaginally at bedtime for 7 days.
   3. Fluconazole (Diflucan) 150-mg tab PO one time.
   4. Hydrocortisone (Cortaid) 1% cream sparingly bid for 7 days.

126. A 25-year-old patient presents with complaints of a malodorous vaginal discharge, which is described as white and watery. She douches with vinegar and water every 2 weeks. She uses a diaphragm for contraception. She and her boyfriend have been sexually active for 2 years, using condoms for sexually transmitted infection (STI) prevention with every act of coitus. She denies any dyspareunia. Her LMP was 1 week ago, and there are no noted changes in her normal menstrual pattern. Her wet mount with KOH results show a positive whiff test, too numerous to count clue cells/high-power field, no lactobacilli, no hyphae or spores, no trichomonads, and few WBCs. What is the diagnosis and treatment for this patient?
   1. Chlamydia; doxycycline (Vibratabs) 100 mg PO bid for 10 days.
   2. *Candida albicans*; terconazole (Terazol 7) vaginal cream 1 applicator at bedtime for 7 days.
   3. Herpes simplex type 2; acyclovir (Zovirax) 200 mg PO q4h for 5 days.
   4. BV; metronidazole (Metrogel) vaginal gel 1 applicator at bedtime for 5 days.

127. A 55-year-old patient, G2 T2 P0 A0 L2, is being seen in the clinic for her annual exam. She went through a natural menopause 5 years ago and has never been interested in hormone replacement therapy (HRT). She smokes one pack of cigarettes per day and does no formal exercise. Her family history is positive for osteoporosis in her mother, positive for myocardial infarction in her father, and negative for cancer. She has a normal physical exam today and had a negative mammogram yesterday. She is now interested in HRT but wants to know her alternatives. Which choice has **not** been clinically proven for prevention of osteoporosis?
   1. Estradiol (Estrace) 0.5 mg 1 tab PO qd and micronized progesterone (Prometrium) 100 mg 1 tablet PO qd.
   2. Weight-bearing exercise three times weekly.
   3. Discontinue cigarette smoking.
   4. Wild Mexican yam cream applied to skin tid.

128. A young woman is seen in the clinic. She noticed some itchy bumps in the vulvar area and is concerned that they could be cancer. On careful inspection, the WHNP/midwife notes five cauliflower-like, warty, pinkish lesions in the lower introitus. Two smaller lesions nestled anterior to hymeneal ring of vagina and cervix fail to reveal any abnormalities. Wet mount with KOH is negative. Culture for gonorrhea and chlamydia was obtained, Pap smear done, and HIV titer and rapid plasma reagin (RPR) drawn. Which is *not* an appropriate treatment for this patient?
   1. Podophyllin (Podoben) application; wash off in 6 hours with soap and water.
   2. Trichloroacetic acid application; do not wash off.
   3. Cryotherapy with liquid nitrogen to lesions.
   4. Benzathine penicillin 2.4 mu IM weekly for 3 weeks.

129. A young adult complaining of vaginal itching, thick yellow mucous discharge, and urinary discomfort is seen in the urgent care unit by the WHNP/midwife. She is sexually active and uses condoms with only one of her two partners. On physical exam, the abdomen is negative; pelvic exam reveals the Bartholin glands within normal limits, cervix with mucopurulent discharge from the os, and mucosa friable to palpation; bimanual exam is negative. Cultures were taken but are not yet available. Wet mount with KOH reveals a negative whiff test, few clue cells, too numerous to count WBCs/high-power field, no yeast, and no trichomonads. What is the most likely diagnosis and appropriate treatment?
   1. Chlamydia; azithromycin (Zithromax) 1 g PO single dose.
   2. Chlamydia; ceftriaxone (Rocephin) 125 mg IM.
   3. Herpes simplex virus; acyclovir (Zovirax) 200 mg 1 capsule PO q4h for 5 days.
   4. Trichomoniasis; metronidazole (Flagyl) 2 g PO single dose.

130. A 52-year-old woman presents for her annual gynecologic exam from her primary care provider. She received a hysterectomy with ovarian conservation at age 40 years for uterine fibroids and dysfunctional uterine bleeding. She has been taking oral estrogen (conjugated equine estrogen 0.625 mg) hormone replacement therapy (HRT) for 1 year. Although HRT has definitely reduced the discomfort of hot flashes, vaginal dryness, and mood swings from insomnia, she still experiences hot flashes and some night sweats. Her diagnostic lipid panel shows total cholesterol 180; low-density lipoprotein 112; high-density lipoprotein 52; and triglycerides 325. What, if any, change should the WHNP/midwife consider in her medication regimen?
   1. No change should be considered at this time.
   2. Decrease estrogen dosage to 0.3 mg daily.
   3. Recommend stopping estrogen therapy.
   4. Suggest changing route of administration to transdermal.

131. An older female patient is seen by the WHNP/midwife for her annual exam and needs a refill on her hormone replacement therapy (HRT). She is feeling well and has not voiced concerns. The patient had a total abdominal hysterectomy and bilateral salpingo-oophorectomy 2 years ago for benign fibroids. Her exam is normal. She takes conjugated estrogen (Premarin) 0.625 mg days 1 to 25, and medroxyprogesterone acetate (Provera) 10 mg from days 16 to 25. What changes would be appropriate for the WHNP/midwife to make in the HRT regimen?
   1. No changes needed; the patient is doing well on the present regimen.
   2. Premarin 0.625 mg daily and discontinue the Provera.
   3. Premarin 0.625 mg daily and Provera 2.5 mg daily.
   4. Premarin 0.625 mg days 1 to 25, and Provera 5 mg days 16 to 25.

132. Before prescribing hormone replacement therapy (HRT) to a patient with no risk factors, which clinical approach should have the highest priority?
   1. The decision about use should rest primarily with the patient after providing appropriate education and counseling.
   2. For most women the benefits of HRT far outweigh any possible side effects, so HRT should be actively encouraged.
   3. Involving the sexual partner in the counseling session is likely to lead to a higher compliance rate for HRT.
   4. Education regarding HRT should include a thorough review of risk factors and possible side effects to avoid liability issues.

133. The addition of a progesterone to an estrogen regimen in a postmenopausal woman with a uterus reduces the risk of:
    1. Endometrial cancer.
    2. Cervical cancer.
    3. Gallbladder disease.
    4. Breast cancer.

134. The single-dose treatment of choice for trichomoniasis is:
    1. Azithromycin (Zithromax) 1 g PO.
    2. Ofloxacin (Floxin) 500 mg PO.
    3. Metronidazole (Flagyl) 2 g PO.
    4. Clindamycin (Cleocin) 300 mg PO.

135. A 25-year-old woman comes into the office with complaints of profuse malodorous discharge. The WHNP/midwife makes a diagnosis of bacterial vaginosis, and then would:
    1. Advise the patient to notify her sexual contacts regarding the diagnosis.
    2. Treat the problem with metronidazole (Flagyl) 2 g for one dose.
    3. Initiate treatment with doxycycline (Vibramycin) 100 mg PO bid for 7 days.
    4. Determine the presence of pregnancy before initiating a course of treatment.

136. A vaginal culture has confirmed the presence of a chancroid in a homeless woman who presented with a painful genital ulcer. The treatment regimen of choice should be:
    1. Ceftriaxone (Rocephin) 250 mg IM single dose.
    2. Erythromycin (E-Mycin) 500 mg PO qid for 7 days.
    3. Metronidazole (Flagyl) 2 mg PO single dose.
    4. Clindamycin (Cleocin) 2% vaginal cream 1 applicator for 5 days.

137. You are counseling a 49-year-old woman who had her last menstrual period (LMP) 10 months ago. She is experiencing some hot flashes and night sweats and is not sleeping well. These symptoms are affecting her ability to work effectively because she finds herself tired and "cranky." She does not want hormone replacement therapy (HRT). Which of the following evidence-based alternative measures is most accurately described?
    1. Venlafaxine (Effexor SR) has been effective in reducing hot flashes in randomized controlled trials.
    2. Raloxifene (Evista) has demonstrated a significant reduction in hot flashes compared with placebo in clinical trials.
    3. Black cohosh (*Cimicifuga racemosa*) has been reported as efficacious in treating menopausal symptoms in many large, controlled trials.
    4. Isoflavones, specifically soy, have been shown in studies to be significantly more effective than placebo in reducing hot flashes.

138. Which information about hormone replacement therapy (HRT) should the WHNP/midwife understand when discussing short-term HRT with patients?
    1. Estrogen replacement delays the onset of menopause.
    2. Estrogen and progesterone cause vasomotor symptoms.
    3. Estrogen decreases the risk of osteoporosis.
    4. Estrogen replacement with progesterone increases risk of ovarian cancer.

139. A patient has been prescribed tranexamic acid (Lysteda) tablets for menorrhagia. Which statement is accurate regarding the medication?
    1. Normal dosing is only 1 tablet per day during the first 3 days of the menses.
    2. Oral contraceptives improve the effectiveness of the medication.
    3. Blood clots can occur with taking the medication.
    4. Common side effects are nausea, vomiting, and constipation.

140. A patient is prescribed oral metronidazole (Flagyl) with a diagnosis of bacterial vaginosis (BV). She has no known drug allergies. Which of the following should be included in medication teaching?
    1. Avoid drinking alcohol for the duration of medication use and for 24 hours after you have finished the medication.
    2. Once your symptoms resolve you can stop the medication.
    3. You should take the medication on an empty stomach.
    4. Your partner will also need to be treated.

141. A 25-year-old woman presents with complaints of clumpy, white vaginal discharge, itching and irritation after finishing a course of antibiotics. On speculum exam, the cervix is red, and clumpy white discharge is present on the cervix and vaginal walls. Based on a presumptive diagnosis, what will be ordered for her medication therapy?
    1. Clindamycin (Cleocin) vaginal cream nightly for 7 nights.
    2. Metronidazole (Metrogel) vaginal gel nightly for 5 nights.
    3. Terconazole (Terazol) vaginal cream nightly for 7 nights.
    4. Azithromycin (Zithromax) 1 g orally in a single dose.

142. A patient is pregnant and has tested positive for chlamydia. An appropriate treatment is:
    1. Doxycycline 100 mg PO bid for 7 days.
    2. Azithromycin (Zithromax) 1 g PO in a single dose.
    3. Ceftriaxone (Rocephin) 250 mg IM in a single dose.
    4. Metronidazole (Flagyl) 500 mg PO bid for 7 days.

4 Answers and Rationales

Anatomy and Physiology of Reproduction

1. (4) The uterine lining first proliferates, and then prepares for implantation. During the secretory phase, glandular epithelium develops, further enhancing the lining. If no fertilized egg arrives for implantation, the lining sloughs off; this is the menstrual phase.

2. (1) Premenstrual syndrome (PMS) occurs approximately 5 to 11 days before onset of menses (late luteal phase) and subsides within 1 to 2 days of menses onset. This phase is progesterone dominant. The follicular phase is estrogen dominant.

3. (1) Follicle stimulating hormone (FSH) stimulates the maturation of ovarian follicles, resulting in a dominant follicle. Milk secretion depends on prolactin. The production and release of LH is regulated by estrogen. LH is responsible for ovulation.

4. (2) Menopause is one point in time and is defined after 12 months of amenorrhea, following the final menstrual period. In post menopause, follicle stimulating hormone (FSH) levels rise 10- to 15-fold with marked reductions in estradiol, but other menstrual irregularities can create a variation in these levels. Therefore these levels are not considered the best definition for menopause.

5. (4) The ovarian cycle is divided into three phases. The follicular phase begins on the first day of menses and continues until day 14, when ovulation usually occurs. Immediately after ovulation, the empty follicle begins to enlarge and develops into a corpus luteum, which releases increasing amounts of progesterone. If implantation does not occur, the corpus luteum regresses, causing the onset of menses. This phase, from ovulation to menses, is the luteal phase.

6. (4) During menopause, vaginal flora changes leading to an increased likelihood for pathogenic growth and urinary symptoms. Vaginal tissue becomes more alkaline, drier (decreased lubrication), and thinner (atrophy).

7. (3) Maintaining an alkaline pH is important to promote viability of sperm that are deposited into the vaginal vault.

Family Planning

8. (4) The diaphragm may be inserted up to 2 hours before intercourse and should be removed no sooner than 6 hours after intercourse has ended. It should not be left in place longer than 24 hours.

9. (2) Urethral discomfort and recurrent urinary tract infections (UTIs) are associated with diaphragm use and are the most common reasons for discontinuing use and changing birth control methods.

10. (3) The IUD would be a good choice for this patient because it is extremely effective (>99%). Maintenance is minimal, and no injections are involved for insertion or removal. The Depo-Provera injections, although extremely effective as well (>99%), require an injection every 3 months, which could lead to decreased patient compliance. The system of implants are also very effective (>99%) but also requires injections for insertion and removal, which this patient is trying to avoid. The diaphragm is a noninvasive contraceptive that is effective (88%) but requires her to be more active in its use. None of these methods is contraindicated for this patient, but an attempt should be made to help her choose one with which she is likely to be comfortable.

11. (1) The WHNP/midwife should try to determine what the patient has heard and dispel the fallacies if possible. Recent research supports the protective benefit of OCs against ovarian cancer, as well as endometrial cancer. Amount of menstrual bleeding is usually decreased, and the cycle regulated. Minimal weight fluctuations are reported. Infertility is not associated with OC use. To suggest either implantation system or Depo-Provera injections to someone who voices concerns about irregular menses or weight gain is sure to lead to an unhappy patient because these are common side effects of both methods. Pap smears do not screen for ovarian cancer.

12. (2) Changing to a pill with a stronger progestational agent or changing to a different progestational agent often will resolve the problem of bleeding irregularities with OCs. Many choices are available regarding the dose or strength of an OC, and her problem likely can be resolved with a different pill. Taking the pills at a different time of day or on an empty stomach will do nothing to resolve the stated problem, which is not breakthrough bleeding, but rather prolonged bleeding, probably secondary to poor endometrial support. If a change is not made in the pills, the patient will continue to bleed and may eventually develop anemia.

13. (3) An OC, such as Demulen 1/35, is a good choice for women with more androgenic characteristics because of its strong estrogenic effect with moderate progestational effect. Loestrin 1/20 is a poor choice; the weaker dose of estrogen and progestin may not adequately support her endometrium and will not have a positive effect on this patient's androgenic characteristics. Triphasil is a triphasic pill and does have a positive progestational effect that should support the endometrium, but the progestin in this OC tends to be slightly more androgenic, which is undesirable in this patient.

14. (4) Combination oral contraceptives (OCs) are not recommended for breastfeeding mothers because of the potential effect on decreasing milk quantity and quality. Progestin-only OCs are approved for nursing mothers because no deleterious effect on milk quantity or quality have been shown. Depo-Provera and the IUD are also accepted contraceptive methods for lactating women.

15. (2) OCs are contraindicated in a cigarette smoker age 35 years or older. No contraindication exists to the use of Depo-Provera injection in the cigarette smoker. The Progestasert IUD would probably be a good IUD choice for this patient because it is only approved for 1-year use and is safe in a cigarette smoker. The only contraindication to condoms and spermicide is allergy to either substance.

16. (1) The diaphragm predisposes many women to UTIs. Some women are sensitive to the contraceptive cream or jelly. The diaphragm has been associated with toxic shock syndrome, so its use should be avoided during menses, and it should not be left in place longer than 24 hours.

17. (3) The primary mechanism of action of oral contraceptives (OCs) is suppression of ovulation. Ovulation is suppressed in 95% to 98% of patients. Should ovulation occur, the other mechanisms of action likely to prevent conception are thickening of cervical mucus, causing the endometrium to become atrophic and making the uterine environment unfavorable for implantation.

18. (3) A hormonal IUD acts to decrease blood loss and cramping. Hormonal IUDs thicken the cervical mucus, thicken the endometrium, and inhibit ovulation. Copper-containing IUDs can increase bleeding and dysmenorrhea. There are two hormonal IUDs available: one works for 3 years and the other for 5 years. The copper IUD can stay in place for up to 10 years.

19. (3) The progestin-only pill does not consistently suppress ovulation. This suppression only occurs in 40% to 60% of cycles, which makes the progestin-only pill less effective than combination OCs. Mechanisms of action that contribute to the progestin-only pill's effectiveness include creating an atrophic endometrium and possibly altering tubal physiology by decreasing ovum transport. Progestin-only pills contain no estrogen and are a good choice for the breastfeeding woman. There is an increased incidence of functional ovarian cyst.

20. (3) Depo-Provera is frequently associated with menstrual cycle changes and weight gain. In fact, this irregular bleeding is the most frequently cited reason for discontinuation. These menstrual changes range from heavy, irregular bleeding to spotting and even amenorrhea. Nausea and acne are usually effects of estrogen and are not seen with Depo-Provera.

21. (3) This patient requires added protection through this cycle because of the low-dose oral contraceptive (OC). Phenytoin may also decrease the effectiveness of OCs, especially low-dose forms.

22. (4) The contraceptive ring can be out of the vagina for 3 hours without any need for an additional form of contraception. Based on the information given, this woman is not at risk for pregnancy, does not need a back-up method of contraception, and does not need to abstain from intercourse. She is using the method appropriately.

23. (3) The subdermal implant is a progesterone-only method of contraception and can cause irregular bleeding and spotting, which may not resolve completely during use. There is no delay in return to fertility once removed. The implant does not cause thyroid abnormalities and women with a low BMI do not experience more side effects than women with a BMI in other categories.

24. (3) DMPA has a longer return to fertility than the other methods listed and should not be recommended for a woman that wants to become pregnant within 1 year. Barrier methods and short-acting methods, such as pills and the vaginal ring, are all appropriate.

25. (4) Progestin IUDs reduce menstrual bleeding and dysmenorrhea. Copper IUDs can increase bleeding and cramping and are not the best choice for women who already have heavy, painful periods. Both methods can be used during breastfeeding and by women who have never been pregnant.

26. (2) LARCs can be considered for all adolescents if they are interested in a long-acting method. They are safe for this population and are listed as a category 2 recommen-

dation by the Centers for Disease Control and Prevention's US Medical Eligibility Criteria for Contraceptive Use. LARCs are some of the most effective methods and are generally acceptable to adolescents.

27. (1) Migraine with vascular symptoms, such as aura, is an absolute contraindication to estrogen for women of any age. For other conditions, benefits generally outweigh the risks.

28. (4) Women using DMPA are at risk for bone loss and should be counseled about adequate calcium intake. Decreasing salt and calories may help with weight gain but are not the most important counseling points. The WHNP/midwife needs to be responsive to the black box warning for bone loss. Although overall bleeding days may increase with DMPA, the bleeding is usually light and does not cause anemia.

29. (1) Women who use fertility awareness-based methods as their contraceptive method should have regular menstrual cycles, partner support and cooperation, and be able to keep good records of their cycles. Women with busy and erratic schedules may have more difficulty tracking their cycles and determining fertile and nonfertile days.

30. (2) Progesterone-only pills (POPs) contain no estrogen, so they are a good choice for women with a preexisting history of hypertension. POPs must be taken every day at the same time and are not a good choice for women who cannot remember to take medication or may have a lifestyle that interferes with their ability to maintain a regular schedule. Breakthrough bleeding and spotting are common with progestin-only methods; therefore they are not a good choice for women who want a regular menstrual cycle.

Disorders

31. (1) The USPSTF recommends that clinicians offer to prescribe risk-reducing medications, such as tamoxifen, raloxifene, or aromatase inhibitors, to women who are at increased risk for breast cancer and at low risk for adverse medication effects. This recommendation applies to asymptomatic women 35 years and older, including women with previous benign breast lesions on biopsy (such as atypical ductal or lobular hyperplasia and lobular carcinoma in situ). The USPSTF recommends *against* the routine use of risk-reducing medications, such as tamoxifen, raloxifene, or aromatase inhibitors, in women who are not at increased risk for breast cancer.

32. (1) Regular exercise and a healthy diet reduce the risk for heart disease in postmenopausal women. As many as 30% of all coronary events are associated with tobacco use. Hormone replacement therapy (HRT) increases the risk of cardiovascular disease. Diabetes increases the mortality from cardiovascular disease two to four times compared with nondiabetic patients.

33. (4) Pregnancy is the most likely diagnosis in this patient, given the list of symptoms and physical findings. She could have a uterine fibroid, but it is not contributing to the symptoms listed. Ovarian cancer could present with nausea, fatigue, and abdominal bloating, but would not cause the enlarged uterus or the positive Chadwick sign. A dislodged IUD will usually change the position of the IUD, decreasing visibility of the strings or causing the IUD itself to be expelled into the vagina or endocervical canal.

34. (4) Obesity is not a risk factor for osteoporosis. Cigarette use, white race, and alcohol consumption, among others, are considered risk factors for osteoporosis.

35. (2) Conservative management for PMS includes daily exercise, stress reduction, dietary changes, and reassurance that her symptoms are valid should help the patient gain more control. A low-salt diet is encouraged; when necessary, a diuretic may be used for fluid retention. The use of vitamins B_6, A, and E may be helpful as well. Laboratory studies are not indicated here but might be helpful if the symptoms were sustained throughout the menstrual cycle.

36. (2) As the function of the ovaries declines and the amount of circulating estrogen begins to fall, the middle-aged woman may begin to experience the symptoms typically associated with menopause. The body's feedback system will attempt to stimulate the ovaries and increase the estrogen level. FSH and LH levels rise in response to these efforts.

37. (3) Uterine fibroids are associated with heavy menstrual blood flow, which can be prolonged. Constipation, pelvic, leg, and back pain are also associated with uterine fibroids.

38. (4) The age of menopause has fluctuated little over the past several centuries, even though life expectancy has increased. Of the options, only smoking has been found to cause an earlier menopause. Research shows a direct correlation among number of cigarettes smoked, number of years of smoking, and age at menopause. Nulliparity and epilepsy have also been associated with an earlier age at menopause.

39. (2) Secondary dysmenorrhea is associated with clinical symptoms that are due to anatomic abnormalities in the pelvis. Premenstrual syndrome (PMS) presents with both physical and psychological clinical symptoms, which typically occur prior to menses. Pelvic inflammatory disease (PID) is an infectious process that affects uterine and pelvic structures that can impact fertility. Dyspareunia is pain experienced during intercourse.

40. (3) Complications associated with polycystic ovarian syndrome include hypertension, increased glucose levels, and infertility. Hemoglobin A1c level between 4% and 5.6% is within normal range, as is a menstrual period lasting between 5 and 7 days.

41. (2) Dyspareunia is painful intercourse, and vaginismus is painful vaginal spasms on penetration. Primary orgasmic disorder is when an individual has never achieved orgasm, usually a lifelong problem. Secondary orgasmic dysfunction refers to an acquired problem of loss of orgasmic function after an individual has experienced orgasm.

42. (1) The initial outbreak is usually the worst. It can be transmitted even when there is no lesion present, and it cannot be cured. Vaginal delivery is allowed if there are no genital lesions at the time of labor.

43. (1) Bacterial vaginosis (BV) results when the normal environment in the vagina is disrupted. The normal vaginal lactobacilli are decreased or absent, and there is an overgrowth of many different types of anaerobic bacteria. Trichomoniasis is caused by a flagellated protozoan, and gonorrhea is caused by a bacterium and may be asymptomatic. The virus that causes recurrent outbreaks of genital lesions is herpes simplex virus type 2 (HSV-2).

44. (1) Oral contraceptives (OCs) will reduce prostaglandin production, which is thought to be the primary cause of dysmenorrhea.

45. (4) The criteria for the diagnosis of bacterial vaginosis (BV) are characteristic milky homogeneous discharge, pH greater than 4.5, amine odor (positive whiff test) with addition of potassium hydroxide (KOH), and presence of epithelial cells studded with coccobacilli that obscure the borders (clue cells). Pseudohyphae are present in candidiasis.

46. (2) In Asherman syndrome, a normally functioning uterus has been damaged and scarred secondary to surgical intervention with resultant trauma, primarily following a dilation and curettage. Ovulation may be occurring normally, but no endometrium is built up, and therefore no endometrium is shed (menstruation does not occur). Pregnancy, as well as the other diseases listed, should be ruled out in this patient.

47. (2) The LH/FSH ratio in polycystic ovarian syndrome is 3:1. The normal LH/FSH ratio is 5:1.

48. (4) The criteria for the diagnosis of polycystic ovarian syndrome include menstrual irregularity, increased body weight, hirsutism, and androgen excess evidenced by laboratory studies and physical findings, chronic anovulation, and multiple bilateral ovarian cysts. Weight loss, dental caries, and amenorrhea would be more common in anorexia nervosa/bulimia. Hyperprolactinemia and galactorrhea are found with a prolactin-secreting pituitary tumor. Dysmenorrhea, nodules palpated on bimanual exam, and infertility are associated with endometriosis.

49. (3) Anovulation causes 90% of dysfunctional uterine bleeding. The lack of progesterone allows for asynchronous, excessive proliferation of the endometrium to take place. This tissue is fragile, and the normal hemostatic mechanism is altered. Thyroid disease, blood dyscrasias, and uterine tumors can mimic dysfunctional uterine bleeding and must be excluded.

50. (3) A female-appearing person with a 46 XY karyotype has androgen insensitivity syndrome, or testicular feminization. This maternal X-linked recessive disorder accounts for approximately 10% of all cases of amenorrhea, and these persons appear normal until puberty. These patients present with amenorrhea, scant or absent pubic hair, and abnormal or no breast development. Persons with Müllerian abnormalities have a normal XX karyotype with abnormalities of fallopian tubes, uterus, and upper vagina occurring in fetal development. In Turner syndrome, congenital absence of ovaries results from loss of one X chromosome (XO karyotype).

51. (1) The most common breast mass in young women less than 30 years old is the fibroadenoma. This benign breast mass is the third most common breast mass after fibrocystic changes and carcinoma. Fibrocystic breast changes are seen most commonly in women 30 to 50 years old. Intraductal papilloma is a wart-like growth located in the mammary duct and occurs in women 40 to 50 years old. Malignant breast neoplasms occur most frequently in women over 40 years and are rarely seen in women 15 to 25 years old.

52. (1) Nonsteroidal antiinflammatory drugs (NSAIDs) inhibit prostaglandin synthesis and are effective agents in primary dysmenorrhea. The other agents listed have not demonstrated effectiveness in primary dysmenorrhea. Other measures to decrease discomfort are exercise, relaxation techniques, heat application, and low-dose OCs.

53. (4) Secondary amenorrhea is defined as no menses for three-cycle lengths or 6 months in a woman with previously established menses. Exercise can cause an increase in estrogen and endorphin levels, which influences the release of gonadotropin-releasing hormone. Without appropriate gonadotropin-releasing hormone release, follicle stimulating hormone (FSH) and luteinizing hormone (LH) are not released adequately, resulting in anovulation, which may lead to amenorrhea. The other conditions listed are causes of primary amenorrhea.

54. (1) This has the characteristics of a syphilitic lesion and needs to be evaluated. Only after determining the presence or type of sexually transmitted infection can it be treated effectively. The herpes viral culture should be done while the lesion is present and the fluid from the vesicles can be obtained.

55. (2) A person who has never engaged in coital activity is not considered at risk for cervical cancer because exposure to human papillomavirus (HPV) is unlikely. In addition to other factors not listed, the presence of HPV, multiple sexual partners, and previous high-grade squamous intraepithelial lesion are considered to be risk factors in the development of cervical cancer.

56. (1) The pseudohyphae and spores on the wet mount with KOH are diagnostic for *Candida* infection. *Chlamydia trachomatis* is diagnosed by direct immunofluorescent assay or by chlamydial culture. Gonorrhea is diagnosed by cervical culture, and BV has microscopic findings of clue cells and positive amine odor.

57. (1) Cancer of the ovary is the leading cause of death from female genital cancer, excluding the breast, in the United States.

58. (1) Flagellated protozoan confirms the diagnosis of trichomoniasis. Chlamydial infection is best diagnosed by direct immunofluorescent assay or culture. Bacterial vaginosis is diagnosed by wet mount revealing clue cells and positive amine test. Inflammatory cervicitis is generally asymptomatic and will not cause vaginal irritation.

59. (3) The pelvic ultrasound is not a useful test for appendicitis because it does not allow for adequate exam of the appendix. The CBC with differential is useful because of the expected rise in white blood cells (WBCs) seen in this inflammatory state. The flat plate of the abdomen and kidney-ureters-bladder are helpful to determine the extent of the problem and to rule out other diagnoses. Because pregnancy can cause these symptoms if complicated by an ectopic state, the practitioner should consider it as part of the differential diagnosis.

60. (2) Oral contraceptives (OCs) have been shown to reduce the risk of endometrial cancer. Obesity, unopposed estrogen use, and advanced age, in addition to others not listed here are considered to be risk factors for developing endometrial cancer.

61. (3) OC use has been shown to reduce the risk of ovarian cancer. Family history of ovarian cancer, advancing age, and positive *BRCA-2* gene are considered risk factors for developing ovarian cancer.

62. (2) Endometrial cancer is the most common female genital cancer, with ovarian cancer causing the most deaths annually. Endometrial cancer is more common than ovarian cancer and is easier to cure with just surgery alone. Because ovarian cancer is usually diagnosed in a later stage, the condition is more difficult to cure.

63. (3) Herpes simplex virus type 2 typically presents dramatically in the newly infected primary outbreak. Gonorrhea generally is associated with a mucopurulent vaginal discharge and is not accompanied by vesicular lesions. Chlamydial infection may be associated with dysuria, and unless accompanied by PID is not generally accompanied by fever or body aches and is not associated with vesicular lesions. Lymphogranuloma venereum is a rare disease classically accompanied by pustular enlargement of the lymph nodes, particularly the inguinal nodes. It is associated not with vesicles, but buboes.

64. (2) Screening blood studies for glucose, cardiac risk profile, and thyroid stimulating hormone in this age group without any stated risk factors is not cost effective and is of little value. The patient can be better served with a discussion regarding diet and exercise. Because this patient is at risk for sexually transmitted infections, counseling and testing for these is a reasonable approach. Contraceptive information educates the patient and allows her to make wiser choices in her family planning.

65. (3) Baseline laboratory work should be obtained to determine the presence of anemia, possible pregnancy, and endocrine dysfunction. It is likely that the other listed tests will be completed after the initial workup is completed.

66. (4) Fibrocystic breast disease is not a risk factor for breast cancer. In addition to others, those listed in the other options are considered to be risk factors for breast cancer.

67. (1) The recommended age for a female to begin screening Pap smears is at the onset of sexual activity or at 21 years of age. Because this patient is 21 years old and has not yet had her first Pap smear, this would be the most appropriate test to perform. It is not necessary to

perform STI screening on patients who have not been sexually active. Stool guaiac (hemoccult) testing and mammography are not recommended as screening procedures in the young adult.

68. (3) Heart disease remains the leading cause of death for women in the United States.

69. (1) Reactive cellular changes are most often associated with inflammation, including typical repair. Other causes include atrophy with inflammation (atrophic vaginitis), IUD use, radiation, and diethylstilbestrol exposure in utero. OCs do not cause reactive changes, and estrogen vaginal cream may be used to improve atrophy.

70. (2) Cervical cancer has been directly linked with high-risk types of human papillomavirus (HPV). Pregnancy after age 35, low parity, and prolonged contraceptive use are not risk factors for cervical cancer.

71. (1) Breast cancer is the most common cancer in women in the United States. Lung cancer mortality is higher than that for breast cancer.

72. (3) These symptoms are classic for menopausal syndrome, although some depressive symptoms are listed. Antidepressant therapy and counseling for depression at this stage of treatment is not appropriate. Testing, teaching, and treatment in this case should be aimed at the menopause. The depressive symptoms will undoubtedly improve with greater understanding and treatment of the menopausal symptoms.

73. (1) Chancroid is well established as a cofactor for HIV transmission. Chancroid is a sexually transmitted infection of the genitals that is caused by the bacteria *Haemophilus ducreyi*. It is characterized by an open sore or ulcer and can be transmitted from skin-to-skin contact with an infected person. It should be noted that it is rarely seen in the United States but occurs more in third-world countries.

74. (1) According to the American Cancer Society, women should be advised of the benefits and limitations of monthly breast self-exam (BSE) and should be aware of how their breasts normally look and feel and to report any new breast changes.

75. (2) Symptoms are most likely indicative of benign fibroadenoma. Mammography is indicated. Surgical excision is unlikely for a young woman.

76. (2) This patient needs to become more knowledgeable about the normal feel of implants, as well as her own breast tissue. Mammography is not a substitute for breast self-exam (BSE).

77. (2) A very firm cervix along with a cervical lesion/ulcer is suspicious for cancer of the cervix, which can be confirmed with a Pap smear.

78. (1) This complaint is an indication for clinical breast exam and mammography. Although uncommon, breast pain can be a presenting symptom for breast cancer. Teaching breast self-exam (BSE) is important, but not the most important action at this point. Hormonal fluctuations can explain breast pain, as can excessive caffeine intake, but should be a diagnosis of exclusion after ruling out malignancy.

79. (2) Toxic shock syndrome occurs primarily in menstruating women ages 12 to 24 who use tampons. The diagnosis is made with the presence of fever over 102°F (38.9°C), macular rash, hypotension, and involvement of three or more organ systems.

80. (4) Ectopic pregnancies, if not diagnosed and treated promptly, can lead to increased morbidity and mortality accounting for up to 4% of all pregnancy-related deaths.

81. (4) Almost half of all vaginal infections are caused by candidiasis. The majority of women who develop the infection have recently taken antibiotics. It is not a sexually transmitted infection.

82. (4) It is not necessary to hospitalize the patient with acute PID who is not vomiting or pregnant. If she does not respond well to outpatient treatment, hospitalization may be recommended. The medications listed are the accepted treatment of choice for outpatient management of PID and should be started before laboratory results are available, based on the patient's clinical presentation. The CBC and erythrocyte sedimentation rate are helpful to track the WBC count and inflammatory response of the body.

83. (2) Unopposed estrogen in a woman with an intact uterus increases her risk of endometrial hyperplasia and progression to endometrial cancer. Women who have taken unopposed estrogen for more than 3 years have a five-fold increased risk of endometrial cancer compared with women not on this regimen. The addition of progesterone to the regimen provides uterine protection. However, the progestin component of HRT is responsible for the breakthrough bleeding, a chief complaint at the initiation of therapy that may lead to discontinuance of the drug. Some women also are intolerant of progestins, which have been linked to irritability.

84. (3) The use of unopposed estrogen in the patient with an intact uterus could put her at risk for endometrial hyperplasia or cancer. The addition of a progestin protects the endometrium adequately. The patient is an excellent candidate for endometrial biopsy to document the status of the endometrium. This patient also needs to be educated on the risks and benefits of HRT.

85. (3) Well-controlled hypertension is not a contraindication to the use of HRT.

86. (2) Patients who undergo surgery and radiation therapy for cervical cancer need to use lubrication for reduced vaginal secretions, use dilators to keep the vaginal canal stretched, and HRT to help with the possibility of postmenopausal symptoms. Cervical cancer is most common in women ages 35 to 44 years of age, and therefore it is important to address issues about sexual intercourse and sexuality, as it could impact the patient for many years.

87. (1) The patient most likely is presenting with ovarian cancer; therefore Ca125 cancer marker along with imaging of the abdomen and pelvis is most relevant. It is important to distinguish from GI symptoms that can be present along with shortness of breath and edema of the lower extremities, which then makes a primary GI problem less likely.

88. (4) The most important sign or symptom of endometrial cancer in the postmenopausal patient is bleeding. Patients often have complaints of a single episode of postmenopausal bleeding or a fullness or pressure in the pelvis. Uterine polyps can cause bleeding during pre- or postmenopausal status. Miscarriage is only possible in a patient who has been proven to be ovulating. Ovarian cancer should be suspected in women with persistent bloating, upper abdominal discomfort, or GI symptoms of unknown etiology.

89. (2) The patient might be in the high-risk category with a sister with premenopausal breast cancer, and a mother with an ovarian cancer diagnosis. The patient should undergo genetic testing. If she has a *BRCA* mutation, she will become eligible for high-risk screening, including magnetic resonance imaging (MRI) and mammograms every 6 months. Additionally, if she is found to have a greater than 20% risk of developing breast cancer in her lifetime or has dense breast tissue, she would be eligible for high-risk screening. Because she is under 40 years of age, whole-breast ultrasound to replace mammogram until she reaches 40 is an option.

90. (3) The HPV vaccine is US Food and Drug Administration–approved for men and women through age 45, and the Advisory Committee on Immunization Practices recommends routine vaccination through age 26, so she is eligible for vaccination and should consider receiving the HPV vaccine series. Current or prior HPV infection is not a contraindication to vaccination, and there is no evidence that vaccination makes an existing HPV infection worse.

91. (1) Strawberry spots on the cervix are characteristic of trichomoniasis. Infection with *Trichomonas vaginalis* can cause an erythematous cervix with petechiae, which results in the strawberry appearance. Bacterial vaginosis, chlamydia, and herpes do not present in this manner.

92. (4) A chancre is a painless, indurated lesion that is seen with primary syphilis. A maculopapular rash is characteristic of the secondary stage of syphilis. Fleshy growths are seen with external genital warts, and painful vesicles are associated with herpes simplex virus.

93. (4) Clue cells seen with microscopy are associated with bacterial vaginosis. Pseudohyphae are present with candidiasis. An increase in WBCs can be seen with chlamydia, and mobile or immobile trichomonads are present with trichomoniasis.

94. (3) Symptoms of chlamydia for young women can be similar to those of a UTI and include dysuria. Nucleic acid amplification testing for chlamydia can be performed from a urine sample. This women's age and history of a new sexual partner are risk factors for chlamydia. Her history is not consistent with syphilis or herpes and there is no indication that a CBC would be helpful at this time.

95. (1) The occurrence of the symptoms during the luteal phase of the cycle (following ovulation) will assist the family nurse practitioner in making the diagnosis of premenstrual syndrome (PMS). Having the patient keep a calendar to track her symptoms for three cycles is helpful in making the diagnosis and measuring successful treatment. Severity of symptoms, although important, is not the most important information.

Male Issues Affecting Women's Health

96. (1) A man with primary hypogonadism will often present with low energy and decreased libido. These same men will often have gynecomastia because of the low or absent production of gonadotropin. Men with hypogonadism often have decreased body hair, which may result in decreased need for shaving. Males with Klinefelter syndrome (chromosomal abnormality with karyotype of 47,XXY–47,XXXXY) is the most common genetic cause of male hypogonadism, with failure of both spermatic function and virilization.

97. (1) Erectile dysfunction can be commonly caused by antihypertensives, particularly thiazide diuretics and beta-blockers. Other causes of impotence are diabetes, trauma, vascular disorders, behavioral health disorders, and relationship problems.

98. (2) A high suspicion of disseminated gonococcal infection (DGI) resulting from an untreated infection by the bacteria *Neisseria gonorrhoeae* should be treated. DGI presents rarely in patients and includes a triad of tenosynovitis, arthritis, and dermatitis. Variable symptoms of DGI include dysuria, penile discharge, and low-grade fever. Treatment includes ceftriaxone and azithromycin or doxycycline, and evaluation for other sexually transmitted infections.

99. (1) Circumcision can be helpful in preventing chronic or severe phimosis and paraphimosis because both are a retraction dysfunction of the prepuce. In phimosis, the foreskin is too tight to be retracted backward over the glans penis. In paraphimosis, once the foreskin has been retracted behind the glans penis it is too constricted to return to a position of covering the glans penis. Balanoposthitis is inflammation of the foreskin in an uncircumcised male.

100. (3) Patients with recurrent or systemic, disseminated *Neisseria* infections should be evaluated for a deficiency of the complement system. Late components of the complement pathway (C5–C9) place patients at high risk of contracting infections by *Neisseria* organisms, especially meningitis. Other reasons for recurrent infections include failure to treat the patient's partner and continued high-risk sexual activity. Safe sex education is indicated in all patients.

101. (3) Acute epididymitis is characterized by an acute scrotal pain, dysuria, and enlarged unilateral scrotum with abdominal pain. Scrotal pain is relieved when the involved testicle is elevated.

102. (2) Oral phosphodiesterase-5 inhibitors are a safe, effective, and reasonable first-line therapy for ED. The class includes commonly known drugs such as sildenafil (Viagra), vardenafil (Levitra), tadalafil (Cialis), and avanafil (Stendra). Patients should be educated on side effects and proper use prior to first administration. Relationship issues can compound or cause ED and should be investigated as a part of the initial evaluation. Second-line therapies for the treatment of ED include intraurethral suppositories, intracavernous injections, and vacuum pump devices. If the patient has only difficulty in maintaining an erection, a constriction band or a vacuum device are the least invasive and least expensive of the current treatment options for this condition.

103. (2) The prostate secretes an alkaline fluid that helps sperm survive in the acidic environment of the female reproductive tract. Androgens are produced by Leydig cells of the testes. Sperm are produced in the seminiferous tubules of the testes.

104. (4) Peyronie disease is a fibrotic condition that causes a lateral curvature of the penis during erection. Most patients simply require reassurance. Some patients with more severe symptoms may require surgical intervention.

105. (1) *Chlamydia trachomatis* is the most common organism in male patients with NGU.

106. (1) Candidiasis is the usual cause of balanitis and is often found in men with poorly controlled diabetes.

107. (4) In sexual dysfunction, erection, emission, or ejaculation may not be functioning because of multifactorial causes, such as medications, vascular disorders, neuropathy, and trauma. Peyronie disease and priapism are examples of erection dysfunction.

108. (3) This is the correct definition of erectile dysfunction (ED). The incidence of ED increases significantly in men as they age, particularly at age 60 and over. It involves a dysfunction in the hemodynamic mechanism of smooth muscle relaxation that increases blood flow in the penis and ultimately causes venous trapping (compression of subtunical venules) and rigidity. Patients who present with vascular ED are at a higher risk for cardiovascular events.

109. (1) Priapism is a condition of prolonged penile erection related to venous obstruction and unrelated to sexual arousal. Although rare, men with sickle cell disease are at greatest risk. Men with erections lasting longer than 4 hours are at increased risk for impotence and should be evaluated immediately by a urologist.

110. (1) Antihypertensive drugs, such as thiazide diuretics and beta-blockers, can cause impotence. Other common causes include cardiovascular disease, diabetes, smoking, prostate surgeries, antidepressants, relationship problems, and depression.

111. (2) Nongonococcal urethritis (NGU) does not always present with dysuria and is difficult to diagnose. NGU typically has a clear discharge and is usually caused by chlamydia. Gonococcal urethritis produces a yellow, purulent discharge. If there is a discharge, NGU is difficult to differentiate from gonorrhea without a culture. Epididymitis and reactive arthritis are also associated with untreated chlamydial infection of the urogenital tract.

112. (4) Dysuria is one of the most common complaints of young men with gonorrhea. No lesions, rash, or urinary dribbling accompanies the yellow discharge.

113. (2) Diabetes is a common contributor to erectile dysfunction because of the impaired circulation.

114. (4) This patient has classic symptoms of secondary syphilis. Granuloma inguinale also presents with ulcerative lesions on the penis and lymphadenopathy but lacks the maculopapular rash and the systemic symptoms associated with syphilis. In this stage, syphilis is particularly infectious.

115. (1) Many patients with genital herpes experience a prodrome of constitutional symptoms with their primary infection. In syphilis, systemic symptoms appear weeks to months after the genital lesions. Gonorrhea and granuloma inguinale are not typically associated with constitutional symptoms.

116. (1) Vesicular lesions on an erythematous base are typical of genital herpes. Later in the course of the outbreak, the blisters break and leave a painful sore. Chancres on the penis are associated with syphilis. Purulent urethral discharge is found in those with gonorrhea or chlamydial infection. Small, flattened papules are associated with genital warts.

117. (2) Phosphodiesterase-5 inhibitors should be taken 30 to 60 minutes prior to intercourse. Large, fatty meals interfere with absorption and should be avoided. Although this class of medications works best for treating erectile dysfunction, there are other medications that can be prescribed by a urologist should they not prove to be effective.

118. (2) Common side effects of phosphodiesterase-5 inhibitors include headaches and flushing owing to vasodilation. Erectile dysfunction lasting longer than 4 hours is rare but should be promptly evaluated in an emergency room or by a urologist.

119. (3) Patients who are on phosphodiesterase-5 inhibitors cannot concurrently take nitrates due to dangerous effects of synergistic vasodilation. Patients who are on selective serotonin reuptake inhibitors, beta blockers, and thiazide diuretics often find that phosphodiesterase-5 inhibitors are effective for treating erectile dysfunction.

Pharmacology

120. (1, 5) Recommended treatment for *Trichomonas vaginalis* is metronidazole (Flagyl), which can be delivered as a single dose (2 g) or as 500-g dose, twice a day for 7 days. During the course of therapy, both alcohol and sexual activity avoidance are recommended. As the patient relates drinking and sexual activity, this is indicative of noncompliance with treatment therapy. Use of cotton underwear and avoiding douching are part of the treatment plan.

121. (3) Lowering the dose of the estrogen would not help this patient's symptoms. The other dosage regimens listed are all acceptable choices for this patient, proving that there are many effective ways to utilize HRT, allowing for individualization of the regimen to the patient.

122. (1) Metronidazole 2 g PO in a single dose is the treatment of choice for trichomoniasis. Metronidazole vaginal cream does not effectively treat vaginal trichomoniasis. Fluconazole and terconazole are treatments for vaginal candidiasis.

123. (1) A dose of 0.3 mg of conjugated equine estrogen (Premarin) is the minimal effective dose to prevent osteoporosis. Hormone replacement therapy (HRT) helps maintain bones, but this effect only lasts as long as HRT is taken. Because of the risks for cardiovascular disease from using HRT, it is no longer recommended for osteoporosis prevention. Other methods of osteoporosis prevention include regular exercise, smoking cessation, and sufficient calcium (1200–1500 mg of elemental calcium) and vitamin D (400–800 IU) daily.

124. (2) The Women's Health Initiative study was stopped early because after 5.2 years, in the opinion of the Safety/Data Monitoring Board, the health risks for the women on the study (mean age 63 years) taking estrogen plus progestin exceeded the benefits. Women taking estrogen/progestin were at higher risk for developing myocardial infarction, strokes, thromboemboli, and breast cancer than women taking placebo. However, women taking HRT were less likely to have a fracture caused by osteoporosis and less likely to develop colorectal cancer. The study did not address the shorter term use of HRT for treatment of menopausal symptoms, the primary indication for initiating the therapy. This landmark study stresses the need for providers to discuss the risks/benefits of initiating or continuing HRT with postmenopausal women.

125. (3) Fluconazole is for a single-dose oral treatment of uncomplicated vulvovaginal candidiasis. It is the most convenient approach for this patient, who is unlikely to be compliant with vaginal creams, given the upcoming travel. She does not have contraindications to its use. Metronidazole and clindamycin are for bacterial vaginosis, not *Candida* infections. Hydrocortisone is a topical steroid used for inflammatory dermatologic conditions, and although it may help the itching, it would not treat the candidiasis.

126. (4) Metronidazole vaginal gel is the treatment of choice for bacterial vaginosis in the nonpregnant woman. The presence of clue cells, and the associated malodorous discharge and absence of lactobacilli, are markers for the diagnosis of bacterial vaginosis.

127. (4) Although some authors may recommend herbal treatments for menopausal symptoms, more controlled studies need to be done to provide recommendations that they are effective toward disease prevention. Traditional allopathic Western medicine supports the use of HRT for the prevention of osteoporosis. Weight-bearing exercise and increased calcium intake have been shown to help maintain bone health. Cigarette smoking increases the risk for bone loss. This patient can reduce her risk by quitting smoking.

128. (4) Benzathine penicillin 2.4 mu IM is the treatment of choice for syphilis, but this patient has condyloma acuminatum, not condyloma latum. Topical use of podophyllin, trichloroacetic acid, and cryotherapy are all accepted treatment modalities for condyloma acuminatum.

129. (1) Chlamydia often presents this way (dysuria, mucopurulent discharge, and cervical friability). The treatment of choice in ambulatory care settings is single-dose azithromycin 1 g PO. Another treatment dose regime would be 250 mg IM of ceftriaxone for a chlamydial infection, not 125 mg, plus doxycycline 100 mg PO for 14 days with or without metronidazole 500 mg PO bid for 14 days. Herpes simplex virus will present with painful vesicles in the vulvovaginal region and is treated with acyclovir 200 mg 1 capsule PO q4h for 5 days for recurrences. Trichomoniasis can present this way, but trichomonads on the wet mount are absent. Therapy for trichomoniasis is single-dose metronidazole 2 g PO.

130. (4) A hepatic effect because of the first-pass metabolism in the liver occurs with oral estrogen products. A 25% increase in triglycerides has been associated with this route of administration. Because transdermal estrogen is not dependent on GI absorption or affected by the first-pass metabolic effect, this option should be considered. A discussion regarding risks/benefits of continuing HRT is appropriate from the primary provider. Because the patient is only 52 years old and is still experiencing menopausal symptoms, reducing the most common dosage, or stopping the medication, unless significant risks are apparent, is probably not the most therapeutic option.

131. (2) The patient no longer requires Provera to protect the endometrium from the potential effects of estrogen; therefore the progestin can be discontinued, and the patient given continuous estrogen therapy without concern. The other dosage regimens listed are appropriate for an HRT patient with an intact uterus.

132. (1) Informed consent is essential. The pros and cons of hormone replacement therapy (HRT) should be explained, but the choice is up to the patient.

133. (1) Women with a uterus taking unopposed exogenous estrogen have an increased risk of endometrial cancer. The addition of progesterone decreases this risk. The addition of progesterone may prompt bleeding, which many women view unfavorably. Progesterone does not affect cervical cancer, breast cancer, or gallbladder disease.

134. (3) Metronidazole in a single 2-g dose is the treatment of choice for trichomoniasis. An alternative is giving the 2 g in divided doses the same day to reduce nausea and improve compliance.

135. (4) Metronidazole is the treatment of choice for BV. Currently there is no evidence to suggest that metronidazole places a pregnancy at risk at any stage; however, it is important to know if the patient is pregnant. BV is associated with preterm birth and also increases the likelihood of other infections. The sexual partners do not require treatment, and doxycycline is not the drug of choice.

136. (1) Because of the patient's homeless status, the WHNP/midwife needs to use a single-dose treatment. Erythromycin, although a correct medication, is a poor dosing choice for this patient.

137. (1) The most accurate answer is venlafaxine. This combination serotonin and norepinephrine reuptake inhibitor has been found to reduce hot flashes at doses of 25 to 150 mg/day in several clinical trials. Although many individuals consider the "natural" over-the-counter products to be safer than prescription drugs, these products can have pharmacologic effects and side effects. Use of these drugs by patients should be questioned at the time of the exam. Critics argue that the trials studying black cohosh (*Cimicifuga racemosa*) have been too small, uncontrolled, and not randomized to provide evidence-based information on the herb's efficacy and safety. Soy has been found to be moderately effective in reducing hot flashes, but comparable results have been seen in the placebo groups as well. A side effect of raloxifene, used to prevent postmenopausal osteoporosis, is hot flashes.

138. (3) Hormone replacement therapy (HRT) may be considered for short-term use (3–4 years) to alleviate menopausal symptoms and the risk of osteoporosis in high-risk patients. The ovarian cancer risk may increase for women using estrogen alone for 10 years or longer. Current data are insufficient to know if combination HRT has the same risk. HRT reduces colorectal cancer risk.

139. (3) Tranexamic acid is used to treat heavy menstrual bleeding in women. Tranexamic acid is an antifibrinolytic agent and works by blocking the breakdown of blood clots, which prevents bleeding. The greatest concern with tranexamic acid is venous or arterial thrombosis. The normal dosing is two tablets (650 mg per tablet) three times a day. The tablets should not be taken more than 5 days in a row for each monthly period. The medication should not be taken if the patient is using oral contraceptives because it may increase the chance of having a blood clot, heart attack, or stroke. Back pain and muscle cramps are known side effects.

140. (1) Drinking alcohol while taking metronidazole can cause a severe nausea and vomiting reaction (e.g., disulfiram-type reaction). Alcohol should be avoided for the duration of treatment and for 24 hours after the medication is finished. Partner treatment for bacterial vaginosis is not recommended. Taking metronidazole with food will help decrease stomach upset and it is important to finish all medication.

141. (3) This woman is reporting classic symptoms of a candidiasis (yeast) infection and her exam is consistent with candidiasis. Yeast can overgrow after taking antibiotics. Appropriate treatment is terconazole. The other choices are not antifungals.

142. (2) First-line treatment for confirmed or suspected chlamydia is a single 1-g dose of azithromycin, which is appropriate for use during pregnancy. Although doxycycline is effective for the treatment of chlamydia, it is contraindicated during pregnancy owing to staining of the fetal teeth. Ceftriaxone is used to treat gonorrhea, and metronidazole for bacterial vaginosis and trichomoniasis.

PART 3 Obstetrics

5

Antepartum

Physiology of Pregnancy

1. Normal cardiovascular physiologic responses to pregnancy include:
   1. Increased heart rate, increased cardiac output, decreased blood volume, and systolic murmur.
   2. Increased heart rate, decreased cardiac output, increased blood volume, and systolic murmur.
   3. Increased heart rate, increased cardiac output, increased blood volume, and systolic murmur.
   4. Decreased heart rate, increased cardiac output, increased blood volume, and diastolic murmur.

2. How does progesterone affect the gastrointestinal (GI) system during pregnancy?
   1. Causes nausea and vomiting early in pregnancy.
   2. Causes hypertrophy and bleeding of gums.
   3. Delays gastric emptying time and decreases intestinal peristalsis.
   4. Causes diarrhea due to increased intestinal peristalsis.

3. A pregnant patient has a hemoglobin value of 11.7g/dL. Which factor explains this finding?
   1. Presence of iron-deficiency anemia.
   2. Nausea and vomiting.
   3. Physiologic anemia of pregnancy.
   4. Anemia of chronic disease.

4. Several physiologic changes in pregnancy may mimic heart disease. Which of the following is an abnormal finding in pregnancy?
   1. Third heart sound.
   2. Leg edema.
   3. Systolic murmur.
   4. Diastolic murmur.

5. For obese women with a body mass index (BMI) of greater than or equal to 30, the Institute of Medicine recommends a total weight gain of how many pounds in pregnancy?
   1. 25 to 35 lbs.
   2. 20 to 30 lbs.
   3. 11 to 20 lbs.
   4. 11 to 25 lbs.

6. What are three common urinary system findings during pregnancy?
   1. Physiologic hydronephrosis.
   2. Increased glomerular filtration rate.
   3. Increased urinary frequency.
   4. Moderate proteinuria.
   5. Decreased renal plasma blood flow.

7. Which laboratory finding remains unchanged during pregnancy?
   1. White blood cell count.
   2. RBC volume.
   3. Fibrinogen level.
   4. Prothrombin level.

8. During pregnancy, estrogen is responsible for:
   1. Hyperpigmentation.
   2. Facilitating implantation.
   3. Reducing smooth muscle tone.
   4. Decreased uterine contractility.

9. Which is not a placental hormone?
   1. Human chorionic gonadotropin (hCG).
   2. Estrogen.
   3. Relaxin.
   4. Cortisol.

10. What is the function of the placental hormone relaxin?
    1. Causes changes in endometrium and relaxes smooth muscle.
    2. Stimulates development of the ductal system of the breasts and causes hypertrophy and hyperplasia of the uterus.
    3. Aids in softening smooth muscle and connective tissue.
    4. Involved with metabolizing certain nutrients and aids in the growth of breasts and other maternal tissues.

11. The WHNP/midwife understands that at 12 weeks of fetal development:
    1. Quickening is felt.
    2. Fetal heart tones should be heard with Doppler ultrasound.
    3. Fetal heart tones are heard with the stethoscope.
    4. Respiratory movements occur.

12. A positive sign of pregnancy is:
    1. Softening of the cervix.
    2. Fetal heartbeat.
    3. Enlargement of the uterus and abdomen.
    4. Mother's perception of fetal movement.

13. The bluish discoloration of the cervix and vagina is known as:
    1. Goodell sign.
    2. Chadwick sign.
    3. Hegar sign.
    4. Braxton Hicks sign.

14. What is the MacDonald method of abdominal measurement in the pregnant woman?
    1. With the woman on her back and knees slightly flexed, the top of the fundus is palpated, and a measuring tape is stretched from the top of the symphysis pubis over the abdomen to the top of the fundus.
    2. Midline of abdomen is determined, and a measuring tape is placed around the abdomen and measured at the point where the fundus is determined to be at midline.
    3. Distance from the xiphoid process to the symphysis pubis is measured, and dimensions of abdominal curve or fundus is calculated.
    4. With the woman on her back and knees flexed, the bony pelvis is determined, ischial tuberosities are identified, and distance from tuberosities to top of the fundus is measured.

15. During the regular prenatal visits, what assessment data other than vital signs and weight are determined with each visit?
    1. Fundal height, fetal heart rate (FHR), urine dip for protein and glucose, and presence of edema.
    2. Urinalysis, glucose screen, fundal height, and FHR.
    3. Presence of/changes in Chadwick sign, complete blood count, and blood glucose screening.
    4. Pelvic measurements, fundal height, urinalysis, and complete blood count.

16. A 25-year-old patient is 5 weeks pregnant and comes in for a visit to discuss her weight during her pregnancy. She has always struggled with her weight and currently has a BMI of 27. She has been feeling great and feels like she should start "eating for two." The WHNP/midwife reminds her she should gain weight within a range based on her BMI, which is:
    1. 11–20 lbs.
    2. 28–40 lbs.
    3. 15–25 lbs.
    4. 23–25 lbs.

17. Which of the following statements is true regarding obesity in pregnancy?
    1. Surgical intervention for weight loss prior to pregnancy does not improve pregnancy outcomes.
    2. The ideal weight gain for an obese woman is less than 10 lbs., according to the Institute of Medicine.
    3. Obese woman are at risk for stillbirth up to 40% more than nonobese woman.
    4. Obese women have similar breastfeeding continuation rates as normal-weight women.

Antepartum Care

18. A patient is pregnant for the fifth time and is in her 7th month. She had two spontaneous abortions in the first trimester. She has a son and daughter, both full-term pregnancies. What is her calculation of gravida and para using the TPAL (Term, Pre-term, Abortion, Living children) acronym?
    1. Gravida 2, para 5, T1, P1, A2, L4.
    2. Gravida 5, para 2, T2, P0, A2, L2.
    3. Gravida 2, para 4, T0, P2, A0, L2.
    4. Gravida 5, para 2, T0, P2, A2, L2.

19. A patient comes in for her first prenatal visit. Her last menstrual period was on June 15, 2021. Using the Nagele rule, the WHNP/midwife computes the estimated date of delivery as:
    1. March 22, 2022.
    2. April 20, 2022.
    3. February 15, 2022.
    4. April 3, 2022.

20. Dietary changes to reduce nausea and vomiting in pregnancy include:
    1. Consuming small, frequent, low-fat meals and avoiding spicy foods.
    2. Avoiding carbonated beverages.
    3. Avoiding eating when awakening in the morning.
    4. Increasing iron and prenatal vitamins to twice daily.

21. The pregnant woman requires an average of how many extra calories per day?
    1. 100.
    2. 300.
    3. 500.
    4. 800.

22. A pregnant patient at 22 weeks' gestation is planning a prolonged car trip. The WHNP/midwife's recommendations would not include:
    1. Support stockings.
    2. Frequent (every 1–2 hours) walking.
    3. Wearing a seat belt.
    4. Knee-high stockings.

23. The recommended office visit interval for a low-risk patient at 28 weeks of pregnancy is every:
    1. 4 weeks.
    2. 1 week.
    3. 2 weeks.
    4. 6 weeks.

24. At 20 weeks' gestation, the WHNP/midwife would expect to palpate the fundus at:
    1. The symphysis pubis.
    2. The umbilicus.
    3. Halfway between the symphysis pubis and umbilicus.
    4. The xiphoid.

25. Which of the following conditions does not have a higher incidence in women over 35 years of age?
    1. Spontaneous abortion.
    2. Preeclampsia.
    3. Gestational diabetes mellitus (GDM).
    4. Anemia.

26. Patients at highest risk for having a child with Tay-Sachs disease are:
    1. Black.
    2. Jewish.
    3. Asian.
    4. 35 years or older at conception.

27. The WHNP/midwife teaches a prenatal patient that a significant food source that is a significant risk for toxoplasmosis is:
    1. Rare hamburger.
    2. Fresh fruits.
    3. Raw oysters.
    4. Raw vegetables.

28. What would be appropriate management for a primigravida at term who experiences rupture of the membranes?
    1. Begin timing contractions.
    2. Begin pushing.
    3. Take a warm bath.
    4. Immediately go to the emergency department.

29. A woman who has missed her period for 5 weeks states that she has been having nausea with some vomiting in the morning hours. The woman also states that she may have a urinary tract infection due to frequency and fatigue. The WHNP/midwife would recognize these symptoms to be:
    1. A possible systemic infection.
    2. Positive signs of pregnancy.
    3. Presumptive signs of pregnancy.
    4. Probable signs of pregnancy.

30. An adult patient presents with her spouse for a prenatal visit. During the exam, the WHNP/midwife notices bruises on her abdomen and back. The spouse does most of the talking during the history. What is the best approach for the WHNP/midwife to take in this situation?
    1. Ask the spouse to leave the room so the nurse can do a pelvic exam.
    2. Ask the woman to accompany the nurse to the laboratory for blood work and ask about bruises.
    3. Ask the woman about the bruises during the exam.
    4. Do nothing; domestic violence is beyond the scope of the nurse's practice.

31. A pregnant employee who works at a daycare center is concerned about a recent outbreak of "fifth disease." The WHNP/midwife understands that:
    1. Most parvovirus B19 infections in utero are associated with an increased number of congenital anomalies.
    2. There are no isoimmunization-associated problems for the mother exposed to a young child with fifth disease.
    3. Parvovirus B19 has caused hydrops fetalis and death in some fetuses infected in utero.
    4. Mortality risk for a fetus is extremely high, especially if the mother has never had fifth disease.

32. Which statement is true about smoking during pregnancy?
    1. The rate of spontaneous abortion among smokers is the same as in nonsmokers.
    2. Risks of complications increase with the number of cigarettes smoked.
    3. Discontinuation of smoking during pregnancy has no effect on pregnancy outcome.
    4. No relationship exists between smoking during pregnancy and sudden infant death syndrome (SIDS).

33. Chlamydial infections during pregnancy may be associated with:
    1. Transplacental transmission to fetus.
    2. Congenital anomalies of the eyes.
    3. Premature rupture of membranes.
    4. Fetal hydrops.

34. Which is not a normal cervical finding in the second trimester?
    1. Cervix firm.
    2. Cervical dilation.
    3. Cervix 3 cm long.
    4. Cervix posterior.

35. During pregnancy, sexual relations are contraindicated:
    1. During the first trimester when patient has a history of spontaneous abortion.
    2. After 36 weeks' gestation.
    3. With the diagnosis of placenta previa.
    4. With excessive maternal weight gain.

36. Which is an abnormal complaint in the first trimester of pregnancy?
    1. Nausea and vomiting.
    2. Fatigue.
    3. Vaginal bleeding.
    4. Low backache.

37. A pregnant patient requests further information regarding exercise guidelines. She runs on the treadmill 4 mph for 30 minutes daily, and then does 30 additional minutes of free weight and lower leg exercises at the gym. General guidelines should include all *except*:
    1. Keep the heart rate less than 140 beats/min.
    2. Limit free weight for upper body to less than 10 lbs. each.
    3. Limit exercise time to 30 minutes total.
    4. Avoid breathlessness and excessive heat.

38. Testing for gestational diabetes mellitus (GDM) should be done in which of the following patients?
    1. Patient with a previous macrosomic infant.
    2. Obese patients.
    3. All pregnant patients.
    4. Patient with glycosuria.

39. A young adult patient, G2 P1 A0 L1, 10 weeks' gestation with intrauterine pregnancy (IUP), is seen for her first obstetric intake history and physical. She knows when she conceived and denies any vaginal bleeding or abdominal pain. The patient has a soft, nontender fundus that measures 14 cm; adnexal exam negative for mass or tenderness; no fetal heart rate (FHR) audible with doptone. What is the most likely diagnosis seen on ultrasound?
    1. Multiple gestations.
    2. Fibroid uterus.
    3. Ectopic pregnancy.
    4. 14-week viable IUP.

40. A healthy patient is at 36 weeks' gestation. On her regular clinical visit, the fundus is measured at the level of the xiphoid process. At the 40-week gestational visit, the fundus is measured at just below the xiphoid process. What is the most likely interpretation of this observation?
    1. Fetus has stopped growing.
    2. Fetal head has descended into pelvic cavity.
    3. Labor will probably begin within 24 hours.
    4. Amount of amniotic fluid is decreased.

41. On her first prenatal visit, a patient's blood work indicates that she is Rh negative. This is her first pregnancy, and she has no history of abortions. What will the WHNP/midwife explain to the patient regarding this information?
    1. To prevent complications of future pregnancies, the patient will receive an injection of rho(D) immune globulin (RhoGAM) at approximately 28 weeks' gestation and after the birth of an Rh-positive infant.
    2. Her husband needs to be tested to determine if his blood type is Rh-positive and if there is a problem.
    3. The patient needs to receive RhoGAM at approximately 20 weeks' gestation and after the birth of the first child to prevent hemolytic disease.
    4. There could be a problem with the mother's blood sensitizing the infant's blood to the Rh factor; the mother will receive RhoGAM after the birth of each child.

42. In discussing the timing of contractions with a patient, the WHNP/midwife explains "frequency" as the interval from the:
    1. Beginning of one contraction to the beginning of the next.
    2. Beginning of one contraction to the end of that contraction.
    3. End of one contraction to the start of the next.
    4. End of one contraction to the end of the next.

43. A predisposing factor in preterm labor is:
    1. Obesity.
    2. Previous spontaneous abortions.
    3. Prior preterm delivery.
    4. White race.

44. The ability of amniotic fluid to produce a ferning pattern when dried may be altered by:
    1. Meconium.
    2. Changes in vaginal pH.
    3. Presence of cervical mucus.
    4. Heavy contamination with blood.

45. Ten weeks into her pregnancy, a patient begins to experience light vaginal bleeding. Her human chorionic gonadotropin (hCG) levels remain elevated. The WHNP/midwife would instruct the patient to report which of the following symptoms?
    1. Nausea and vomiting.
    2. Abdominal pain or severe cramping.
    3. Urinary frequency.
    4. Fatigue.

46. Which statement is true regarding the course of pruritic urticarial papules and plaques of pregnancy?
    1. Perinatal mortality is increased.
    2. Pruritus is increased postpartum.
    3. Lesions first appear on the abdomen.
    4. Onset is usually in the first trimester.

47. A 32-year-old female patient, G2 T1 P1 A0 L2, is seen in the clinic by the WHNP/midwife for her annual exam and is requesting information on preconception counseling. She has been taking oral contraceptives for 3 years without complications. During the past year, she has started an exercise program at a health club 5 days a week and is eating three nutritionally sound meals daily. She has lost 33 lbs. and is now at her ideal body weight. She quit her job as a postal worker and now stays home with her children. As part of her preconception care, what should the WHNP/midwife recommend?
    1. Start prenatal vitamins with folic acid.
    2. Discontinue exercise.
    3. Update measles-mumps-rubella (MMR) vaccine.
    4. Start genetic counseling due to advanced maternal age.

48. Regardless of planned mode of birth, all pregnant women should undergo antepartum screening for Group B *Streptococcus* (GBS). When is the appropriate gestational week interval for GBS screening?
    1. 35 0/7 to 37 0/7.
    2. 34 1/7 to 36 6/7.
    3. 35 1/7 to 36 5/7.
    4. 36 0/7 to 37 6/7.

49. The fundus should be at the umbilicus at what gestational age?
    1. 14 weeks.
    2. 16 weeks.
    3. 18 weeks.
    4. 20 weeks.

50. The correct procedure to measure fundal height is:
    1. Position the woman in the supine or semirecumbent position; walk the hands up the sides of the uterus until the hands meet at the top of the uterus. Place the "zero" mark of the tape at the superior border of the symphysis; measure in a straight line upward over the midline of the uterus to the top of the fundus; record the measurement in centimeters.
    2. Position the woman in the left tilt position; walk the hands up the sides of the uterus until the hands meet at the top of the uterus. Place the "zero" mark of the tape at the superior border of the symphysis; measure in a straight line upward over the midline of the uterus to the top of the fundus; record the measurement in centimeters.
    3. Position the woman in the supine or semirecumbent position; walk the hands up the midline of the abdomen to the fundal crest. Place the "zero" mark of the tape at the superior border of the symphysis; measure in a straight line upward over the midline of the uterus to the top of the fundus; record the measurement in centimeters.
    4. Position the woman in the left tilt position; walk the hands up the sides of the uterus until the hands meet at the fundal crest. Place the "zero" mark of the tape at the superior border of the symphysis; measure in a straight line upward over the midline of the uterus to the fundal crest; record the measurement in centimeters.

51. When performing Leopold maneuvers, the first maneuver determines the fetal lie. Fetal lie refers to:
    1. Position of the fetal head in relation to the maternal pelvis.
    2. Position of the fetal long axis in relation to the maternal long axis.
    3. Relation of fetal parts to each other (flexion or extension).
    4. Relationship of the presenting part to the maternal pelvis.

52. Which clinical sign would indicate a need for intervention for the woman with nausea and vomiting?
    1. Loss of 2% body weight.
    2. Ketonuria.
    3. Dry mucous membranes.
    4. Patient complaint of hunger.

Complications

53. The WHNP/midwife would note which finding as a possible sign of preeclampsia?
    1. Urgency to urinate at night.
    2. Edema in extremities and puffy face.
    3. Stomach cramps.
    4. Clear fluid discharge from nipple.

54. A multigravida who is at 30 weeks gestation calls the WHNP/midwife complaining of vaginal bleeding, abdominal pain, and uterine contractions. On physical exam, no watery discharge is noted, and the uterus feels hard. The WHNP/midwife suspects:
    1. Placental abruption.
    2. Placenta previa.
    3. Molar pregnancy.
    4. Ectopic pregnancy.

55. Which finding would the WHNP/midwife assess in a patient with a ruptured tubal pregnancy?
    1. Sharp, stabbing pain localized to left lower quadrant with blood pressure (BP) of 90/58 mm Hg.
    2. Board-like rigidity of the uterus with abdominal distention.
    3. Dilation of the cervix and rapidly falling BP and pulse.
    4. Serosanguineous vaginal fluid with grape-like vesicles.

56. A pregnant patient at 20 weeks' gestation comes into the clinic with complaints of vaginal bleeding for the past 6 hours, and abdominal cramping before the bleeding started. Vaginal exam reveals a decrease in the uterine size, loss of pregnancy symptoms, and a closed, firm cervix. The most likely diagnosis for this patient is:
    1. Threatened abortion.
    2. Braxton Hicks contractions.
    3. Placenta previa.
    4. Missed abortion.

57. Which is an abnormal complaint in the second trimester of pregnancy?
    1. Frequent uterine contractions.
    2. Frequent fetal movement.
    3. Calf cramps.
    4. Heartburn.

58. Which would be incorrect for the treatment of preeclampsia without severe features?
    1. Modified bed rest.
    2. Monitor BP, weight, and urinary protein.
    3. Methyldopa (Aldomet) 250 mg PO tid.
    4. Daily urine dipstick for protein.

59. What would be incorrect advice to a nonlaboring pregnant patient with a second-trimester diagnosis of marginal placenta previa?
    1. Pelvic rest.
    2. Report any bright-red bleeding.
    3. Planned cesarean section.
    4. Follow-up ultrasound at 32 weeks' gestation.

60. Which is not true about an ectopic pregnancy?
    1. 90% occur in the fallopian tube.
    2. Ectopic pregnancies account for approximately 5% of maternal deaths.
    3. Prior history of pelvic inflammatory disease is reported in 50% of patients.
    4. Previous ectopic pregnancy does not increase the risk of another ectopic pregnancy.

61. Which is an abnormal complaint of the third trimester of pregnancy?
    1. Leukorrhea.
    2. Headache with blurred vision.
    3. Urinary frequency.
    4. Uterine contractions.

62. Which is not a predisposing factor of preeclampsia?
    1. Primigravida.
    2. Age older than 35 years.
    3. Multiple gestations.
    4. Hyperthyroidism.

63. For a pregnant patient at 32 weeks' gestation with a BP of 140/92 mm Hg, weight gain the past 2 weeks of 6 lbs., 2+ protein on urine dip, 1+ pitting edema in the feet and nondependent edema of the face and hands, and 2+ reflexes, the probable diagnosis would be:
    1. Preeclampsia without severe features.
    2. Preeclampsia with severe features.
    3. Eclampsia.
    4. HELLP syndrome.

64. The WHNP/midwife is assessing a patient who has a positive pregnancy test. Laboratory data indicate that the mother's blood group is O positive and the father's is AB negative. What risk is associated with this pregnancy?
    1. The mother may build up antibodies to the infant's blood if the infant is type B positive, which will be significant in future pregnancies.
    2. The mother is Rh-positive; if the infant is Rh-negative, there is an increased incidence of the infant building up Rh antibodies.
    3. Because the mother is O and the father is AB, there is an increased risk for the development of an ABO incompatibility.
    4. Type O blood is the dominant characteristic; the infant's blood will be in the O group, with no complications.

65. Which is not an expected complication of the pregnant adolescent age 17 years or younger?
    1. Premature labor and birth.
    2. Anemia.
    3. Gestational diabetes mellitus (GDM).
    4. Gestational hypertension.

66. Which is least likely to be found in a patient presenting with an ectopic pregnancy?
    1. Pain.
    2. Missed menses.
    3. Vaginal bleeding.
    4. Abdominal mass.

67. A patient presents to the clinic with a diagnosis of threatened abortion. The WHNP/midwife describes this as:
    1. Vaginal bleeding with or without cramping and no cervical change.
    2. Vaginal bleeding with cramping and cervical change.
    3. Loss of pregnancy symptoms, decrease in uterine size, and cervix closed and firm.
    4. Cramping, bleeding, and incomplete expulsion of products of conception.

68. The WHNP/midwife knows that delivery is the cure for preeclampsia. What is the pathophysiological basis for early delivery of a mother with severe preeclampsia?
    1. Diffuse microvesicular fatty infiltration of the liver due to long-chain 3-hydroxyacyl-coenzyme A dehydrogenase deficiency.
    2. A high level of estrogen, increasing the saturation of cholesterol in bile.
    3. Widespread vasoconstriction leading to systemic hypertension, increased coagulation, and worsening placental ischemia.
    4. Thrombocytopenia, depletion of plasma coagulation factors and fibrinogen, and bleeding leading to multiple organ failure.

69. Which of the following are possible complications for mothers with preexisting diabetes but not for those with gestational diabetes?
    1. Congenital cardiac anomalies, fetal macrosomia, polyhydramnios.
    2. Neonatal hypoglycemia, stillbirth, birth trauma.
    3. Obesity/diabetes in the baby later in life, cesarean section, shoulder dystocia.
    4. Miscarriage, neonatal hypoglycemia, stillbirth.

70. The obese pregnant woman is more likely to experience:
    1. Obstructive sleep apnea, stillbirth, and glucose intolerance.
    2. Congenital anomalies, intrauterine growth restriction, and postoperative infections.
    3. Venous thromboembolism, cesarean delivery, and inadequate pregnancy weight gain.
    4. Preeclampsia, thyroid storm, and pregnancy loss.

71. The woman with hydatidiform molar pregnancy may present with:
    1. Hyperemesis, hypertension, tachycardia.
    2. Small for dates uterine growth, nonreactive nonstress test, bradycardia.
    3. Low B-hCG levels, toxemia before 24 weeks.
    4. Blood clots, hypertension, clinical hypothyroidism.

Pharmacology

72. Which immunization is contraindicated in pregnancy?
    1. Polio vaccine.
    2. Hepatitis B vaccine.
    3. MMR.
    4. Tetanus.

73. Which medication is helpful in preventing preterm labor?
    1. Glucocorticoids.
    2. Nifedipine.
    3. Hydroxyprogesterone.
    4. Terbutaline.

74. **QSEN** The WHNP/midwife is discussing intrapartum prophylaxis regimen for a patient without drug allergies and a positive Group B *Streptococcus* (GBS) screening. The American College of Obstetricians and Gynecologists (ACOG) recommendation should include in your discussion which *preferred medication* and route of administration?
    1. Intravenous penicillin (Penicillin G).
    2. Intramuscular amoxicillin (Amoxil).
    3. Intravenous first-generation cephalosporin, cefazolin (Ancef).
    4. Intramuscular clindamycin (Cleocin).

75. The current recommendation for antepartum treatment of Rh-negative pregnant women with Rh_0(D) immune globulin (RhoGAM) includes:
    1. Administration of 300 mcg at 28 and 36 weeks' gestation.
    2. Administration of 300 mcg at 28 weeks' gestation.
    3. Administration of 300 mcg in each trimester.
    4. No administration is needed until postpartum.

76. The patient comes in for her first prenatal visit. She is healthy and has no history that would contribute to complications during the pregnancy. She asks the WHNP/midwife what she can take for her occasional headaches caused by eyestrain and allergies. Which of the following would the WHNP/midwife recommend for the patient?
    1. Ibuprofen (Advil) 200 mg every 4 to 6 hours, not to exceed 600 mg over 24 hours.
    2. Naproxen (Aleve) 220 mg every 8 to 12 hours.
    3. Aspirin (ASA) 60 mg every 6 hours, not to exceed 300 mg over 24 hours.
    4. Acetaminophen (Tylenol) 650 mg every 4 to 6 hours, not to exceed 650 mg over 24 hours.

77. Which medication would be considered safe to use in all trimesters of pregnancy?
    1. Metronidazole (Flagyl).
    2. Tetracycline (Achromycin).
    3. Isotretinoin (Accutane).
    4. Angiotensin-converting enzyme inhibitors.

78. The use of misoprostol (Cytotec) is the least expensive agent for cervical ripening and can be given vaginally or orally. Vaginal misoprostol (Cytotec) may be selected as the preferred route for which patient:
    1. Vaginal bleeding.
    2. Prolonged rupture of membranes.
    3. Maternal fever with unknown membrane status.
    4. Late term induction for preeclampsia.

79. A pregnant patient in the last trimester complains of a constant backache aggravated by walking, moving, and bending. The pain does not radiate to either leg. In addition to rest, massage, and physiotherapy, which of the following medications is appropriate?
    1. Acetaminophen.
    2. Codeine.
    3. Naproxen.
    4. Aspirin.

80. A 16-week pregnant patient comes into the clinic and complains of an abnormally thick vaginal discharge. She notes increased discomfort when she urinates. On exam she has a copious amount of thick discharge that is on the external labia and also in the vaginal vault. KOH wet prep test is negative. This is most consistent with a candidiasis infection. What is the best option for treatment?
    1. Diflucan 500 mg for 1 dose.
    2. Miconazole 100 mg vaginally for 4 days.
    3. Clotrimazole 100 mg vaginal tablet for 7 days.
    4. Clindamycin 300 mg twice a day for 7 days.

81. A prenatal patient has a history of preterm births. She is going to receive hydroxyprogesterone caproate (Makena). Which statement is accurate about this medication?
    1. Medication is given the last 4 weeks of the pregnancy.
    2. Medication is taken orally starting in week 16 of the pregnancy.
    3. Medication is effective in women with multiple gestations.
    4. Medication should be avoided in women with a history of blood clots.

82. The WHNP/midwife confirms diagnosis of missed abortion at 8 weeks gestation with ultrasonography. After reviewing management options, the patient chose medical management with 800 mcg of misoprostol (Cytotec) vaginally. Follow-up ultrasonography impression reveals area with increased vascularization and evidence of retained products of conception. The WHNP/midwife most appropriate action would be:
    1. Immediately schedule dilatation and evacuation.
    2. Recommend repeat 800 mcg of misoprostol (Cytotec) vaginally.
    3. Schedule follow-up ultrasonography in 1 week.
    4. Administer 400 mcg of misoprostol (Cytotec) by oral route.

83. The WHNP/midwife is discussing cervical ripening and induction agents for trial of labor after previous cesarean section (TOLAC). The patient is 39 4/7 weeks gestation with a Bishop score of 3. The WHNP/midwife is providing education about cervical ripening agents. The WHNP/midwife understands risk associated with TOLAC induction and discusses the following agent is contraindicated:
    1. Oxytocin (Pitocin).
    2. Misoprostol (Cytotec).
    3. Foley balloon catheter with 30 to 40 mL of saline solution.
    4. Lactated Ringers.

84. **QSEN** Misoprostol (Cytotec) is used in the prevention and treatment of gastroesophageal reflux disease and peptic ulcer disease secondary to NSAID use. Misoprostol (Cytotec) is used "off label" in obstetrics. The WHNP/midwife understands that when the medication is used in obstetrics the mechanism of action is:
    1. A synthetic oxytocic.
    2. A synthetic tocolytic.
    3. A synthetic prostaglandin E1.
    4. A synthetic prostaglandin E2.

85. Which of the following may reduce the risk of neural tube defects when taken before conception?
    1. Vitamin A.
    2. Pyridoxine.
    3. Folic acid.
    4. Vitamin C.

5 Answers and Rationales

Physiology of Pregnancy

1. (3) During pregnancy, a hyperdynamic state is caused by an increase in blood volume, which results in a slightly increased heart rate and increased cardiac output. Systolic ejection murmurs are common and caused by increased flow across the pulmonic and aortic valves. Diastolic murmurs are abnormal and require referral.

2. (3) Progesterone affects the GI system by decreasing smooth muscle tone, delaying gastric emptying, and decreasing intestinal peristalsis. Human chorionic gonadotropin (hCG) is associated with nausea and vomiting early in pregnancy. Estrogen causes the gums to become hyperemic, soft, and swollen with a tendency to bleed.

3. (3) The increase in plasma volume combined with a slower rise in red blood cell (RBC) production produces a dilutional anemia. Hemoglobin and hematocrit decrease in relation to plasma volume, reaching the lowest levels during the second trimester. True anemia occurs with hemoglobin less than 11 g/dL and hematocrit less than 35%, although some providers will allow the hemoglobin to drop to 10 g/dL and hematocrit to drop to 33% before treating. Nausea and vomiting will increase hemoglobin and hematocrit.

4. (4) Leg edema is caused by increased venous pressure in the legs. Both components of the first heart sound become louder, with exaggerated splitting, and a third heart sound gallop is common after midpregnancy. Systolic ejection murmurs are common and result from the increased flow across the aortic and pulmonic valves. Diastolic murmurs are an abnormal finding and should always be referred.

5. (3) The Institute of Medicine recommends weight gain of 28 to 40 lbs. for underweight women (BMI <18); 25 to 35 lbs. for normal-weight women (BMI 18.5–24.9); 15 to 25 lbs. for overweight women (BMI 25–29.9), and 11 to 20 lbs. for obese women (BMI ≥ 30).

6. (1, 2, 3) Changes in renal structure are influenced by estrogen, progesterone, increased blood volume, and uterine pressure. Changes in the collection system, such as dilation of the renal pelvis and ureters, cause a physiologic hydronephrosis. The glomerular filtration rate does increase during pregnancy, along with renal plasma flow. Increased urinary frequency is related to the increasing size of the uterus and its pressure on the bladder. Some proteinuria (1+) is common during pregnancy due to increased glomerular filtration rate (GFR) and impaired proximal tubular function. Proteinuria is abnormal when the amount exceeds 300 mg/24 hours or albuminuria is greater than 30 mg/24 hours, except in very concentrated urine or in the first voided specimen on arising. Proteinuria (moderate or large amount) is a warning of impaired kidney function or preeclampsia.

7. (4) RBC volume increases approximately 30%, and white blood cells increase 5000 to 12,000/mm^3. Fibrin, fibrinogen, and plasma levels of factors VII, IX, and X are also increased. Prothrombin levels remain unchanged.

8. (1) During pregnancy, estrogen is responsible for stimulation of melanin-stimulating hormone, resulting in hyperpigmentation. Progesterone from the corpus luteum and later the placenta is responsible for facilitating implantation, decreasing uterine contractility, and reducing smooth muscle tone.

9. (4) There are five placental hormones: hCG, estrogen, progesterone, human placental lactogen, and relaxin. Cortisol is produced in the adrenal glands.

10. (3) Relaxin helps soften smooth muscle and connective tissue in preparation for labor and delivery. Progesterone relaxes smooth muscle and causes changes in the endometrium. Estrogen stimulates the development of the ductal system of the breasts and causes hypertrophy and hyperplasia of the uterus. Human placental lactogen is involved with metabolism of glucose, fatty acids, and amino acids. It also aids in the growth of the breasts and other maternal tissues.

11. (2) Fetal heart rate (FHR) should be heard by 12 weeks' gestation and may be heard as early as 10 weeks, dependent on the maternal adipose tissue and amniotic fluid. Quickening is felt at 16 to 22 weeks. FHR can be heard by stethoscope at 20 weeks. Respiratory movements occur later in fetal development, at approximately 24 weeks.

12. (2) Positive evidence of pregnancy includes fetal heartbeat, palpation of fetal movement by examiner, and visualization of fetus by ultrasonography. Amenorrhea, nausea, emesis, urinary frequency, fatigue, skin changes, and mother's perception of fetal movement are presumptive evidence of pregnancy. Probable evidence of pregnancy includes softening of the cervix, softening of the lower uterine segment, cyanosis of the cervix and vagina, Braxton Hicks contractions, ballottement, palpation of the fetal outline by examiner, and pregnancy tests.

13. (2) The Chadwick sign occurs at 6 to 8 weeks' gestation and is the bluish discoloration of the cervix and vagina. The Goodell sign is the softening of the cervix that is seen as early as 4 weeks' gestation. The Hegar sign is the softening of the lower uterine segment. The Braxton Hicks sign consists of contractions of the uterus that can occur as early as 16 weeks' gestation.

14. (1) The MacDonald measurement is taken at each prenatal visit to estimate uterine size. Fundal height is measured with a tape that is stretched from the top of the fundus to the symphysis pubis. If the fundal height is less or more than expected based on the gestational age, the estimated date of delivery should be reevaluated and confirmed. Further fetal assessment may be necessary.

15. (1) Fundal height, fetal heart rate (FHR), urine dip for protein and glucose, and assessment for edema are determined with each prenatal visit. Urinalysis and complete blood count are done as part of the initial exam and are repeated as necessary. The Chadwick sign is an early indication of pregnancy. Pelvic measurements are done to determine adequacy of the pelvic outlet for delivery.

16. (3) Her current BMI is considered overweight, 25.0–29.9. Therefore the recommendation for weight gain is between 15 and 25 lbs. There are health implications for being overweight going into pregnancy that can lead to medical issues, like diabetes and high blood pressure, which can negatively affect pregnancy.

17. (3) Compared with normal-weight women, obese women are 40% more likely to experience stillbirth. Complications of obesity during pregnancy includes stillbirth and early cessation of breastfeeding. Weight loss prior to pregnancy improves comorbidities, whether by surgical or behavioral means.

Antepartum Care

18. (2) *Gravida* is the number of pregnancies, including the present pregnancy, gravida 5 for this patient. *Para* is the number of pregnancies that have progressed past 20 weeks, para 2. *T* is the number of pregnancies that have progressed to term, T2. *P* is the number of pregnancies with delivery preterm, P0. *A* is number of abortions, A2. *L* is living children, L2.

19. (1) The WHNP/midwife counts back 3 months to March 15 and adds 7 days. This brings the date to March 22 of the next year.

20. (1) Patients should eat frequent small meals to keep some food in the stomach at all times and to avoid stomach distention. Sipping on carbonated beverages may be helpful. Having crackers at the bedside to take before rising in the morning may be a successful preventive measure.

21. (2) The pregnant woman requires approximately 15% more calories per day than the nonpregnant woman. This is approximately 300 calories per day and depends on the patient's weight and activity level. Breastfeeding requires 500 calories per day.

22. (4) Venous stasis occurs with prolonged sitting and may be a risk factor for thrombophlebitis. Support stockings and frequent walking should be encouraged. Knee-high stockings have elastic around the calf that may act as a tourniquet. They should be avoided during pregnancy. Seat belts are recommended.

23. (3) The American College of Obstetricians and Gynecologists (ACOG) recommends visits every 2 weeks starting at 28 weeks until 36 weeks of pregnancy. During the first and second trimester, the recommendation is every 4 weeks, starting as early as the woman realized she may be pregnant. At 36 weeks of pregnancy, visits are weekly until delivery.

24. (2) The expected fundal height at 20 weeks' gestation is at the umbilicus. At 12 weeks' gestation, the fundus can be palpated just above the symphysis pubis, and at 16 weeks' gestation, between the symphysis and umbilicus. The fundus is palpated at the xiphoid process at approximately 36 weeks' gestation.

25. (4) The risk for anemia in pregnancy does not increase with age. The risks for spontaneous abortion, preeclampsia, and gestational diabetes mellitus (GDM) do increase with maternal age.

26. (2) The incidence of the Tay-Sachs gene in the Jewish population is 1 in 30, compared with 1 in 300 for the non-Jewish population.

27. (1) Undercooked red meat is a major source of toxoplasmosis. Pregnant women should be cautioned against eating undercooked meats. Cats are also shown to be hosts. Toxoplasmosis is spread through cat feces. Pregnant women should be warned about cleaning the litter box and about contaminated soil.

28. (1) The patient should begin to count the contractions to determine the progress of beginning labor. Because she is a primagravida, delivery probably is not imminent, so going to the emergency department is not appropriate. She should not try to "push" this early in labor. Without the protective barrier of the amniotic membrane, the mother and fetus are susceptible to infection. Bathing would be a hazard because of the possibility of

contracting an infection from the bath water. The patient should note the time, count the contractions, and call the health care provider.

29. (3) Missed menstrual periods, nausea, vomiting, frequency, and fatigue are presumptive signs (subjective) of pregnancy. Probable signs of pregnancy are objective, such as the Chadwick sign, ballottement, and a positive pregnancy test. Positive signs of pregnancy are fetal heart rate, fetal movement felt by a health care provider, and sonographic evidence.

30. (2) Although asking the spouse to leave the room during a pelvic exam may work, it may also arouse the spouse's suspicion and create a situation. Asking the woman to accompany the nurse to the laboratory and asking about the bruising is best because it gives a legitimate reason to move the woman quickly from the room, offers privacy to inquire about the bruises, and provides an opportunity to move the woman to a safe place, if needed, without creating confrontation.

31. (3) Most fetuses are not affected; however, some undergo isoimmunization, which leads to hydrops fetalis and death. The mortality risk is actually low, and there are usually no associated congenital anomalies.

32. (2) The risk of complications and perinatal loss increases with the number of cigarettes smoked. Discontinuation of or decrease in the amount of cigarettes smoked during pregnancy can reduce the risk of complications, especially for high-risk women.

33. (3) Premature rupture of membranes may be associated with chlamydial infections. Intrauterine transmission of *Chlamydia trachomatis* to the fetus has not been demonstrated. There is no evidence of fetal eye anomalies; without prophylaxis, however, conjunctivitis will develop in 30% to 50% of infants 7 days after birth.

34. (2) It is not considered normal or expected for a woman to have a dilated cervix at any time in the second trimester of pregnancy. The cervix will typically be firm, 2 cm long, and posterior, as well as closed.

35. (3) In placenta previa, the placenta is improperly positioned in the lower uterine segment, covering all or part of the cervical os. There is an increased risk of bleeding. Management includes bed rest, no intercourse, no vaginal exams, instruction on managing bleeding, and close fetal surveillance.

36. (3) Vaginal bleeding could represent a potential problem in the pregnancy during the first trimester. The other symptoms listed are important as well and warrant further discussion to rule out a problem.

37. (3) No reason exists to limit the amount of time for exercise, provided the patient is feeling well. Keeping the heart rate below 140 beats/min reduces the risk of internal overheating and exhaustion. The American College of Obstetricians and Gynecologists (ACOG) suggests limiting free weights to less than 10 lbs. to avoid undue stress and strain on muscles and ligaments. Avoidance of breathlessness and excessive heat allows for better circulation to the fetus.

38. (3) More than one-half of pregnant women who exhibit GDM lack the classic risk factors of family history of diabetes, unexpected stillbirth, prior macrosomic infant, obesity, and advanced maternal age. Glycosuria in pregnancy is not necessarily an indication of gestational diabetes. The best answer is that all women should be screened for gestational diabetes.

39. (1) Multiple gestations will cause the uterus to enlarge faster than normal. Fetal heart rate (FHR) may be inaudible with the doptone at 10 weeks' gestation. A fibroid could cause the uterus to enlarge, but it is generally accompanied by firmness to palpation of the uterus. Ectopic pregnancy could be the cause of an inaudible FHR, but is usually accompanied by adnexal tenderness, a mass, or vaginal bleeding. A 14-week viable intrauterine pregnancy (IUP) should have an audible FHR with the doptone.

40. (2) "Lightening" often occurs at approximately 40 weeks' gestation when the infant's head descends into the pelvic cavity and becomes "engaged." At any other time during pregnancy, a decrease in fundal height would cause concern for the infant's growth. Amniotic fluid amount does not indicate that labor is imminent.

41. (1) The unsensensitized Rh-negative pregnant woman is given RhoGAM at 28 weeks' gestation as a preventive measure. It effectively prevents the formation of active antibodies if there is accidental transport of fetal Rh-positive blood cells into the circulation during the remainder of the pregnancy. At delivery, the infant's blood type is determined. If the infant is Rh-positive, the mother will receive another dose of RhoGAM within 72 hours of delivery. If the infant is Rh-negative, there is no antibody formation and RhoGAM is unnecessary.

42. (1) Frequency of contractions should be timed from the beginning of one contraction to the beginning of the next contraction.

43. (3) History of preterm birth is associated with a 20% to 40% recurrence risk. Low prepregnancy weight and inadequate weight gain, not obesity, are associated with preterm labor. Maternal smoking, drug use (especially cocaine), low socioeconomic status, maternal age younger than 17 years and older than 35 years, and

non-white race are all predisposing factors for preterm labor. Previous spontaneous and elective abortions are not risk factors.

44. (4) Ferning is due to high levels of estrogen and when air-dried, amniotic fluid produces a fern pattern. This microscopic arborization is accurate in confirming rupture of membranes in 90% to 95% of cases. Samples heavily contaminated with blood may not fern.

45. (2) Contractions, cramping, or abdominal pain along with continued bleeding could signify a spontaneous abortion. The other symptoms are common during the first trimester.

46. (3) Pruritic urticarial papules and plaques of pregnancy skin rash typically starts on the abdomen and spreads to the thighs and possibly the buttocks. Onset of lesions is usually in the third trimester and usually resolves postpartum. It is thought to be related to the stretching of the skin. There is no associated adverse perinatal outcome.

47. (1) The use of prenatal vitamins with folic acid before conception has been found to reduce the risk of neural tube defects in the fetus. It is important for the patient to continue her exercise program, although some discussion about the type of exercise and any limitations are important once pregnancy is achieved. Because the patient has had two previous pregnancies, it is likely that her rubella immune status has been determined; if she is found to not be immune to rubella, an MMR vaccination should be recommended. This patient is not of advanced maternal age, and therefore does not require genetic counseling for this reason.

48. (4) The American College of Obstetricians and Gynecologists (ACOG) (2019) updated guideline recommended timing for screening provides a 5-week window for valid GBS culture results that includes births that occur up to a gestational age of at least 41 0/7 weeks.

49. (4) The fundal height should be approximately equal to the weeks of gestation beginning at 20 weeks. At the 20th week, the fundus should be palpable at the umbilicus. At week 12, the fundus may be palpable at the symphysis pubis. At 16 weeks gestation, the fundus is approximately half-way between the symphysis pubis and the umbilicus.

50. (1) The uterus should be palpated to accurately note the top of the fundus for measurement. This is done by walking the hands up the sides of the uterus until they meet at the top of the uterus. The tape measure should be held at the superior border of the symphysis and carried upward over the midline of the uterus to the fundus. To have accurate measurements, the same procedure should be used by each provider at each visit.

51. (2) Fetal lie is the relationship of the fetal long axis to the maternal long axis and is stated as longitudinal, transverse, and oblique. The presenting part is the fetal part that is lowest in the pelvis and is typically the head (cephalic), although the feet, buttocks, or chin may also present. The presenting part is described by the fetal bones in relationship to the planes in the maternal pelvis (as an example, right occiput posterior means the fetal occiput is against the right posterior plane of the maternal pelvis). Flexion and extension describe fetal attitude.

52. (2) Ketonuria indicates muscle wasting due to starvation. Weight loss of 5% or more of prepregnancy weight is another sign of starvation. Dry mucous membranes indicate dehydration but not necessarily starvation. Hunger is an early sign of inadequate nutrition but can be present without starvation.

Complications

53. (2) Classic signs of preeclampsia are hypertension and proteinuria. Generalized edema of the extremities and around the face occurs due to increased permeability and capillary leakage. Stomach cramps could be an indication of early labor or GI upset. Clear nipple fluid would be an early sign of colostrum.

54. (1) Symptoms of placental abruption are bright-red vaginal bleeding, board-like uterus on palpation, uterine contractions, and uterine tenderness and pain. Vaginal bleeding is not always present, that is, concealed abruption. Placenta previa is painless bleeding and occurs in the second and third trimester. Ectopic pregnancy occurs during the first trimester. Molar pregnancy or gestational trophoblastic disease would not progress to 30 weeks gestation.

55. (1) The ruptured fallopian tube causes a sharp, sudden, stabbing pain. Symptoms of shock (decreased BP, increased pulse, and increased respiration) occur, and the patient quickly becomes a surgical emergency. The cervix does not dilate. Board-like abdominal rigidity is often noted with abruptio placentae. Grape-like vesicles are associated with hydatidiform mole, a gestational trophoblastic disease.

56. (4) A missed abortion is characterized by a loss of pregnancy symptoms, vaginal bleeding, and a closed cervix. A threatened abortion has vaginal bleeding and cramping, but the symptoms of pregnancy are still present. Placenta previa is bleeding without pain, and symptoms of pregnancy are present. Braxton Hicks contractions can occur as early as the second trimester but are more commonly experienced in the third trimester. The uterine muscles tighten for 30 to 60 seconds and then relax.

57. (1) Contractions could represent early premature labor and should be monitored to rule out early cervical change. Not all contractions are "Braxton Hicks," and contractions require serious consideration. The other symptoms listed are important to discuss and to rule out other associated symptomatology.

58. (3) The use of medication is no longer thought to be useful in the treatment of preeclampsia without severe features and could be hazardous. The patient is best treated conservatively with modified bed rest on the left side and dietary counseling, along with close monitoring of BP, weight, and urinary protein. Close follow-up with exam for edema or symptomatic change and monitoring of the fetus are also performed.

59. (3) There is no reason to plan a cesarean section on diagnosis of the placenta previa at this stage of the pregnancy because the lower segment of the uterus goes through its final maturation between 28 and 32 weeks of gestation. The placenta could likely resolves by the third trimester, thus allowing for vaginal birth, barring any other unforeseen factors.

60. (4) It is true that 90% of ectopic pregnancies are found in the fallopian tubes. Patients with pelvic inflammatory disease have a seven-fold increase in the rate of ectopic pregnancy. Maternal deaths from ectopic pregnancy have decreased markedly over the last few years as a result of improved diagnostic procedures. A previous ectopic pregnancy is a risk factor and does increase the risk of a subsequent ectopic pregnancy.

61. (2) Headache associated with blurred vision could represent early symptoms of preeclampsia and warrants further workup to rule out a problem. The other symptoms are not of concern if not associated with other symptoms.

62. (4) Predisposing factors in preeclampsia include primigravida, age younger than 20 years or older than 35 years, women with vascular diseases (hypertension, systemic lupus erythematosus, diabetes mellitus, and renal disease), family history, previous history of preeclampsia, and multiple gestations. Hyperthyroidism does not predispose to preeclampsia.

63. (1) Preeclampsia without severe features is consistent with systolic BP >140 mm Hg or systolic rise >30 mm Hg, diastolic >90 mm Hg or diastolic rise >15 mm Hg, weight gain >2 lbs/week, and nondependent edema >1 + with normal reflexes. Severe features of preeclampsia include BP >160/110 mm Hg, proteinuria >2 g/24 hours, serum creatinine >1.2 mg/dL, platelets <100,000, ↑ LDH, ↑ ALT, persistent headache or cerebral/visual disturbances, and persistent epigastric pain. Eclampsia includes the above plus seizures. The hemolysis, elevated liver enzymes, low platelets (HELLP) syndrome includes signs and symptoms of severe preeclampsia, an enlarged and firm liver, and epigastric or right upper quadrant pain.

64. (3) There is an increased incidence of ABO incompatibility if the mother is blood group O and the infant is either blood group A or B. Rh incompatibility occurs only when the mother is Rh-negative and is carrying an Rh-positive infant. In the most common cases of ABO incompatibility, there is production of maternal antibodies against the A or B cells.

65. (3) The pregnant adolescent is at increased risk for premature labor, anemia, and preeclampsia. There is no documentation that the pregnant teen is at greater risk of gestational diabetes.

66. (4) Greater than 90% of patients presenting with ectopic pregnancies will complain of pain and report a missed period. Approximately 80% will describe vaginal bleeding. Only 50% will have a palpable abdominal mass.

67. (1) A threatened abortion progresses to complete spontaneous abortion in 50% of cases. Clinical findings are vaginal bleeding with or without cramping and no cervical change. Vaginal bleeding with cramping and cervical change is an inevitable abortion. An incomplete abortion is demonstrated by vaginal bleeding, cramping, and incomplete expulsion of the products of conception. A missed abortion is diagnosed when products of conception are retained after fetal death. There is a decrease in uterine size, loss of pregnancy symptoms, and often a closed and firm cervix.

68. (3) It is postulated that uteroplacental ischemia results in oxidative and inflammatory stress, with the involvement of secondary mediators leading to endothelial dysfunction, vasospasm, and activation of the coagulation system. Endothelial dysfunction leads to an imbalance between different classes of locally produced vasoconstrictors and vasodilators. The net effect of these processes would be widespread vasoconstriction leading to hypoxic/ischemic damage in different vascular beds, systemic hypertension, activation of the coagulation system, and worsening placental ischemia. Diffuse microvesicular fatty infiltration of the liver due to long-chain 3-hydroxyacyl-coenzyme A dehydrogenase deficiency is seen in acute fatty liver of pregnancy. A high level of estrogen, increasing the saturation of cholesterol in bile, is seen in acute cholecystitis and cholelithiasis. Thrombocytopenia, depletion of plasma coagulation factors and fibrinogen, and bleeding leading to multiple organ failure is seen in disseminated intravascular coagulation.

69. (1) Organogenesis occurs during the first weeks of pregnancy, before insulin resistance affects the pregnancy and vascular system; therefore congenital anomalies are not a factor in the gestational diabetic. However, effects of impaired glucose control on the fetus do occur and can include macrosomia, polyhydramnios, stillbirth, birth trauma, shoulder dystocia, and a higher risk for cesarean section delivery.

70. (1) Obese pregnant women are at risk for obstructive sleep apnea, stillbirth, glucose intolerance, congenital anomalies, large for gestational age, postoperative infections, venous thromboembolism, cesarean delivery, excessive pregnancy weight gain, preeclampsia, hypothyroid, and pregnancy loss.

71. (1) Hyperemesis, hypertension, tachycardia, uterine growth large for dates, high B-hCG levels, toxemia, absent fetal heart tones, and clinical hyperthyroidism are all signs of hydatidiform molar pregnancy.

Pharmacology

72. (3) The measles-mumps-rubella (MMR) is a live virus vaccination and is contraindicated in pregnancy. Polio, tetanus, and hepatitis B vaccine are inactivated bacterial or DNA-based vaccines and are safe when indicated.

73. (3) Hydroxyprogesterone is useful in preventing preterm labor. Antenatal glucocorticoids are given to the mother to accelerate fetal lung maturity by stimulating fetal surfactant production. Tocolytics are medications given to arrest labor after uterine contractions and cervical change have occurred, which are nifedipine and terbutaline.

74. (1) First-line intravenous penicillin remains the agent of choice for intrapartum prophylaxis, with intravenous ampicillin as an acceptable alternative. First-generation cephalosporins (i.e., cefazolin) are recommended for women whose reported penicillin allergy indicates a low risk of anaphylaxis or is of uncertain severity. For women with a high risk of anaphylaxis, clindamycin is the recommended alternative to penicillin only if the GBS isolate is known to be susceptible to clindamycin.

75. (2) Current recommendations for RhoGAM is administration of 300 mcg to all Rh-negative women at 28 weeks of pregnancy. This is considered protective for the remainder of the pregnancy. Infants are tested postpartum and a second dose is given if the infant is Rh-positive.

76. (4) Acetaminophen has some risk as a drug, but problems have not been documented; it should be used with caution. Aspirin may cause bleeding disorders. Nonsteroidal antiinflammatory drugs (NSAIDs) (ibuprofen; naproxen) have been associated with prematurely closing the fetal ductus arteriosus because of antiprostaglandin effects and therefore, it is not used.

77. (1) Metronidazole is safe to use in all trimesters of pregnancy. The other medications are known teratogens and contraindicated in pregnancy.

78. (4) Vaginal misoprostol (Cytotec) can be used for late term induction due to preeclampsia. Vaginal misoprostol should not be used with active vaginal bleeding. Oral misoprostol reduces the need for vaginal exams and thereby decreases risk for uterine infections.

79. (1) Acetaminophen can be safely prescribed to the pregnant patient. Aspirin and NSAIDs are contraindicated in the third trimester. The use of narcotics for the patient is inappropriate.

80. (3) Clotrimazole 100 mg vaginal tablet for 7 days would be an appropriate treatment for candidiasis. Diflucan should be avoided during the first trimester. Miconazole is a good choice for treatment, but it should be for a least 7 days; a 4-day course is too short. Clindamycin is the correct medication and dose for bacterial vaginosis but not for a candida infection.

81. (4) Hydroxyprogesterone caproate (Makena) should not be used in women with any of the following conditions: blood clots or other blood clotting problems, breast cancer or other hormone-sensitive cancers, or history of these conditions; unusual vaginal bleeding not related to the current pregnancy; yellowing of the skin due to liver problems during pregnancy; liver problems, including liver tumors, or uncontrolled high blood pressure. Makena is a progestin indicated to reduce the risk of preterm birth in women with a singleton pregnancy who have a history of singleton spontaneous preterm birth. Treatment is started at 16 weeks and continued with once weekly IM injections until week 37.

82. (2) Misoprostol-based regimens have been extensively studied for the medical management of early pregnancy loss. Most studies suggest that a larger dose of misoprostol is more effective than a smaller dose, and vaginal or sublingual administration is more effective than oral administration; the sublingual route is associated with more cases of diarrhea. The largest randomized controlled trial conducted in the United States demonstrated complete expulsion by day 3 in 71% of women with first-trimester pregnancy loss after one dose of 800 mcg of vaginal misoprostol. The success rate was increased to 84% after a second dose of 800 mcg of vaginal misoprostol.

83. (2) Misoprostol is not utilized for cervical ripening in women with a previous cesarean delivery. ACOG advises that misoprostol (prostaglandin E1) *not* be used for cervical ripening or labor induction in women in the third trimester with prior uterine incisions. Lactated Ringers and isotonic intravenous solution are used for replacing fluids and electrolytes. Foley balloon catheter has been shown as a safe option in many studies to be utilized for TOLAC for mechanical cervical ripening.

84. (3) Misoprostol (Cytotec) is a synthetic prostaglandin E_1 analogue, which binds to myometrial cells to cause strong myometrial contractions. This agent also causes cervical ripening with softening and dilation of the cervix. Misoprostol should not be used for FDA-approved purpose in pregnancy (gastroesophageal reflux disease or peptic ulcer disease) because of this mechanism of action, which may induce unintended miscarriage.

85. (3) Recent studies have confirmed that folic acid taken before conception can reduce the risk of neural tube defect.

6

Intrapartum (Midwifery Only)

Intrapartum Care

1. Which statement regarding a patient in labor is true?
   1. The woman's blood pressure will increase during contractions and quickly decrease to a normal range between contractions.
   2. The use of the Valsalva maneuver is encouraged during the second stage of labor to relieve fetal hypoxia.
   3. Endogenous endorphin released during labor will raise the woman's pain threshold and produce sedation.

2. Which nursing assessment indicates that a woman who is in second-stage labor is almost ready to give birth?
   1. Fetal head is felt at 0 station during the vaginal exam.
   2. Bloody mucous discharge increases.
   3. Vulva bulges and encircles the fetal head.
   4. Membranes rupture during a contraction.

3. Using Leopold maneuvers, the midwife feels a round, firm, and movable fetal part in the fundal portion of the uterus and a long, smooth surface in the mother's left side close to midline. What is the position of the fetus?
   1. Left occiput anterior (LOA).
   2. Left sacrum posterior (LSP).
   3. Left sacrum anterior (LSA).

4. Which statement is accurate regarding how the fetus moves through the birth canal?
   1. Fetal attitude describes the angle at which the fetus exits the uterus.
   2. Of the two primary fetal lies, the horizontal lie is that in which the long axis of the fetus is parallel to the long axis of the mother.
   3. Normal attitude of the fetus is called general flexion.

5. Which statement is correct regarding the mechanism of labor?
   1. Asynclitism is sometimes achieved by means of the Leopold maneuver.
   2. Effects of the forces determining descent are affected by the shape of the woman's pelvis and the size of the fetal head.
   3. At birth, the baby is said to achieve "restitution," which is a return to the C-shape of the womb.

6. What is the primary difference between the labor of a nullipara and that of a multipara?
   1. Total duration of labor.
   2. Level of pain experienced.
   3. Amount of cervical effacement and dilation.

7. The midwife expects which maternal cardiovascular finding during labor?
   1. Increased cardiac output.
   2. Decreased pulse rate.
   3. Decreased blood pressure.

8. Which of the following is not a component evaluated using the Bishop score?
   1. Cervical dilation and effacement.
   2. Station.
   3. Week of gestation.
   4. Cervical position and consistency.

9. Which presentation is accurately described in terms of both the presenting part and the frequency of occurrence?
   1. Breech: sacrum, 15% to 20%.
   2. Cephalic: occiput, at least 96%.
   3. Shoulder: scapula, 10% to 15%.

10. What is the appropriate terminology for the relationship of the fetal body parts to one another?
    1. Lie.
    2. Position.
    3. Attitude.

11. All of the following conditions are indicated for early induction of labor *except*:
    1. Prolapsed cord.
    2. Placenta abruption.
    3. Gestational hypertension.
    4. Premature rupture of the membranes.

12. Which finding is associated with a breech presentation?
    1. Postterm gestation.
    2. Fetal heart rate heard below the umbilicus.
    3. Meconium found during vaginal exam after rupture of membranes.
    4. Presenting part is the occiput.

13. Intrapartum antibiotic prophylaxis for group B *Streptococcus* (GBS) is indicated in which of the following clinical scenarios?
    1. Repeat scheduled cesarean delivery with meconium-stained fluid with history of positive GBS culture with last pregnancy.
    2. Allergy to penicillin with positive *Escherichia coli* with new obstetric urine culture.
    3. History of precipitous labor, 8 cm, GBS-negative with positive GBS culture in all previous pregnancies.
    4. GBS bacteriuria during current pregnancy or history of previous GBS-infected newborn.

14. What correctly describes a frank breech presentation?
    1. Both feet present before the buttocks.
    2. Hips are flexed and knees extended.
    3. Foot is the presenting part.
    4. Hips and knees are flexed.

15. What would be an indication for continuous electronic fetal monitoring?
    1. Term singleton pregnancy.
    2. Reactive nonstress test prior to labor.
    3. Breech presentation.
    4. No history of previous cesarean birth.

16. A patient with an estimated gestational age (EGA) of 39^4 and a normal prenatal course has been admitted in active labor. The midwife is evaluating the fetal heart tracing and notes the rate is 123 beats per minute (bpm) with periodic decelerations and a beat-to-beat variability of 3 to 4 bpm. The midwife understands that initial nonpharmacologic management of this finding is:
    1. Increase intravenous (IV) fluid rate, change in maternal position (lateral recumbent), and maternal oxygen therapy.
    2. Placement of an intrauterine pressure catheter (IUPC) and immediate amnioinfusion of normal saline solution.
    3. Fetal scalp stimulation and continued monitoring.
    4. Tocolytics to stop contractions.

17. Nonpharmacologic pain management techniques, such as hydrotherapy, provide relaxation and thermal stimulation. The midwife recognizes that the following precautions must be observed during hydrotherapy:
    1. Monitor for an increased need for analgesics.
    2. Monitor for maternal fluid shift into the extravascular spaces.
    3. Monitor the mother for hyperventilation during therapy.
    4. Maintain adequate hydration during therapy.

18. The midwife is monitoring a patient with an EGA of 38.6 during active labor. The membranes spontaneously ruptured, and the last sterile vaginal exam (SVE) showed the fetus is vertex, 6 cm/60%/0 station. The patient's history includes late entry to care at 25 weeks of gestation; a 3-hour glucose tolerance test result of 89 mg/dL, 165 mg/dL, 140 mg/dL, and 135 mg/dL; and a positive HIV antibody test. The labor nurse is unable to obtain a fetal heart tracing for longer than 10 seconds at a time. The midwife's next intervention should include:
    1. Contacting the attending to discuss surgical delivery of the fetus.
    2. Applying a fetal scalp electrode to monitor the fetal heart rate without interruption.
    3. Assisting the labor nurse in locating a more consistent fetal heart monitoring location.
    4. Inserting an IUPC and beginning amnioinfusion.

19. During the first stage of labor, the patient, who is low-risk and has an intact bag of waters, prefers to ambulate in the room between contractions. The midwife orders which type of activity and external fetal monitoring?
    1. Bedrest and continuous external fetal monitoring to be evaluated every 30 minutes.
    2. Up ad lib and intermittent external fetal monitoring every 30 minutes.
    3. Up ad lib and intermittent external fetal monitoring every 15 minutes.
    4. Bedrest and continuous external fetal monitoring to be evaluated every 15 minutes.

20. A woman who is G2P1 at 38 weeks gestation is on oxytocin to augment her labor and has just received an epidural for management of her pain. Prior to the epidural, her vaginal exam was 5 cm, 100% effacement, and the fetal head at 0 station. The labor nurse notifies the midwife that the fetal heart tracing for this patient has been in the 80s for the past 2 minutes. Her contractions are every 4 minutes, last for 1 minute, and return to baseline with uterine relaxation between contractions. The patient's vital signs are BP 92/44 mm Hg, pulse 102, respiratory rate is 18, and temp is 36.1°C. The midwife re-examines the patient and notes the cervix is 5 cm dilated and 0 station; there is no vaginal bleeding. What is the most likely cause for the deceleration?
    1. Placental abruption.
    2. Oxytocin administration.
    3. Cord prolapse.
    4. Epidural analgesia.

21. The midwife understands that an effective nonpharmacologic pain management technique to relieve back pain during labor is:
    1. Counterpressure.
    2. Effleurage.
    3. Pattern-paced breathing.
    4. Guided imagery.

22. The midwife is analyzing the fetal monitor of a G3P2 at 41^2 weeks estimated gestational age (EGA) who is having contractions every 2 minutes, and notes the fetal heart rate baseline is 140 bpm with late decelerations with the last 2 contractions. The patient's vital signs are BP 145/87 mm Hg, pulse 100 bpm, respirations 20 breaths per minute, and temperature 37.4°C. The history shows an uncomplicated prenatal course, no medical problems, and a 36-week group B *Streptococcus* (GBS) screen was negative. The patient declined an offered epidural. The midwife knows the most likely cause of late decelerations in this fetus is:
    1. Uterine tachysystole.
    2. Intraamniotic infection.
    3. Postmaturity.
    4. Hypertensive disorder.

23. A patient who is being evaluated in the labor room with the complaint of contractions every 5 minutes suddenly has a large gush of vaginal bleeding and severe abdominal pain. The triage nurse notifies the midwife and states that the baseline for uterine tone has increased from 20 to 35 mm Hg, and the contractions have increased in frequency to every minute and the fetal heart rate is in the 140s with good beat-to-beat variability. The midwife suspects which of the following?
    1. Abruptio placentae.
    2. Uterine rupture.
    3. Fetal bleeding.
    4. Placenta previa.

24. The midwife is notified of an increase in BP of 142/100 mm Hg (previous BPs 138/78, 140/82 mm Hg) and sudden swelling of the face in a laboring woman at an EGA of 38.6. The midwife orders which of the following screening tests to guide her further exploration of this patients' diagnosis?
    1. Urinalysis for proteinuria.
    2. 24-hour urine collection for protein.
    3. A biophysical profile.
    4. A nonstress test.

25. What is the ideal position for a term mother who has a diagnosis of congenital heart disease to labor in?
    1. Lateral decubitus.
    2. Lithotomy.
    3. Reverse Trendelenburg.
    4. Supine.

26. The midwife caring for a pregnant woman does not offer genetic screening for cystic fibrosis to the woman during her pregnancy. The woman gives birth to a child afflicted with cystic fibrosis. Of the following, which statement is true regarding this scenario should the woman desire to seek out an attorney for advice?
    1. A birth injury action is warranted.
    2. A wrongful conception action is warranted.
    3. A wrongful birth action is warranted.
    4. No malpractice action is warranted.

27. A woman who is G2P0010 at 41 weeks has been having regular contractions every 4 to 5 minutes that have increased in intensity over the past 2 hours. She reports a blood-tinged mucoid discharge; no sign that her water has broken. She reports to the labor triage and her cervical exam is 3 cm dilated, 90% effaced, −1 station, vertex presentation in a right occiput posterior (ROP) position. What terminology describes her situation currently?
    1. Active phase of labor.
    2. Dysfunctional labor.
    3. Latent phase of labor.
    4. Prodromal labor.

28. A woman who is G5P3013 at 39 weeks entered labor spontaneously 10 hours ago. She was 6 cm dilated, 100% effaced, 0 station with a cephalic presentation in right occiput anterior (ROA) position on admission 4 hours ago, with an intact bag of water. Contractions were 2 minutes apart and moderate to strong to palpation on admission. Over the past 2 hours, while she has been ambulating, contractions have stretched out to 5 to 6 minutes apart and are now mild to moderate to palpation. She is able to walk and talk through most of the contractions. Cervical exam is now 7 cm, 100% effaced, 0 station, occiput anterior position. Which of the following is indicated at this point?
    1. Discuss amniotomy with the woman.
    2. Encourage her to continue to ambulate.
    3. Recommend that she try to take a nap.
    4. Suggest that she have an epidural placed.

29. A nulliparous woman at 39.0 weeks with an uncomplicated pregnancy, group B *Streptococcus* (GBS) positive presents to the labor triage unit reporting irregular contractions for the past 36 hours. She has been able to nap for short periods. She reports a "slimy" clear vaginal discharge; no large gushes of fluid. Fetal heart rate baseline is 135; there is moderate variability with accelerations present and no decelerations noted. On speculum exam the provider notes no pooling, negative nitrazine, no ferning on sample collected from posterior fornix, and no fluid coming from the cervical os with Valsalva 1. Cervical exam reveals that she is 2 cm dilated, 90% effaced, and –1 station with a cephalic presentation. Contractions are 5 to 6 minutes apart and palpate mild to moderate. What is indicated in her plan of care?
   1. Admit to the hospital's birthing unit.
   2. Begin GBS prophylaxis per Centers for Disease Control and Prevention guidelines.
   3. Discuss artificially rupturing her amniotic sac.
   4. Encourage continued labor at home.

30. A G1P0 woman presenting to the hospital verbalizes "it feels like my back is breaking" with contractions, which are 3 minutes apart and moderate to strong to palpation. Bag of water is intact, and she is dilated to 4 cm, is 100% effaced, and baby is at a –1 station with head slightly asynclitic. She has been trying to ambulate but finds it too difficult now. Which of the following should be considered?
   1. Consider placement of an intrauterine pressure catheter (IUPC).
   2. Discuss Pitocin (oxytocin) augmentation.
   3. Encourage hands and knees position in bed.
   4. Transition from intermittent to continuous fetal monitoring.

31. A woman who is a G3P2002 at 35 weeks is in town visiting family. She presents to labor and delivery noting "2 large gushes of bright red blood" in the last hour "heavier than my period." She denies loss of fluid otherwise, and has been having irregular, frequent contractions today. Which of the following is the most reasonable to include in the management plan at this point?
   1. Offer her the shower/tub for relief.
   2. Order an ultrasound.
   3. Perform a digital vaginal exam.
   4. Use nitrazine to check for ruptured membranes.

32. A woman just had a full-term uncomplicated vaginal birth following an uncomplicated pregnancy. The midwife notes a small gush of blood vaginally as the umbilical cord lengthens. Gentle cord traction is provided as the woman bears down. A modified Brandt-Andrews maneuver is performed, with no resulting change in cord length. Which of the following is the next most appropriate action?
   1. Administer Hemabate (carboprost tromethamine).
   2. Expectant management.
   3. Maintain continuous cord traction.
   4. Summon physician to room.

33. Which of the following is an expected outcome of immediate skin-to-skin placement of the neonate after birth?
   1. Length of the third stage of labor is decreased.
   2. Maternal postbirth nausea is decreased.
   3. Maternal cooperation with perineal inspection is enhanced.
   4. Transfer of heat to baby via conduction is facilitated.

34. A woman in active labor has been nauseated since the onset of labor 10 hours ago and has vomited multiple times. She is able to take in ice chips orally a few times an hour; drinking any clear fluids induces vomiting fairly quickly. She is afebrile, normotensive, with a pulse of 100 and respirations of 20. She last urinated 2 hours ago. What should be included in the management plan?
   1. Administer Bicitra (sodium citrate/citric acid).
   2. Continue to try to advance her from ice chips to clear liquids.
   3. Initiate an IV fluid drip.
   4. Recommend she get into the shower.

35. A G1P0 woman presented in labor 4 hours ago at 5 cm dilation, 90% effaced, and –1 station with a cephalic presentation, fetus left occiput anterior (LOA). She is now 8 cm, 100% effaced, and 0 station with a fetus in occiput anterior position. Her contractions occur every 2 to 3 minutes and palpate moderate. Fetal heart rate baseline is 145 bpm, with accelerations and occasional early decelerations noted. Which of the following should be included in the management plan?
   1. Amniotomy.
   2. Expectant management.
   3. IV hydration.
   4. Intrauterine pressure catheter placement (IUPC).

36. A G2P1001 woman at 39.4 weeks with an uncomplicated pregnancy is laboring sitting on her birth ball beside the bed. At last cervical exam she was 4 cm, 80% effaced, with the vertex at a –1 station and intact bag of waters. During a contraction she feels a large gush of fluid expelled. Of the following, which is most important to assess first?
   1. Cervical status.
   2. Fetal heart rate.
   3. Fluid odor.
   4. Presence of bloody show.

37. Inspection of the perineum after a vacuum-assisted vaginal birth reveals the following: a laceration that extends from inside the vagina through the perineum, involving the underlying vaginal muscles. The rectal sphincter and mucosa are intact. This laceration is classified as which of the following?
   1. First degree.
   2. Fourth degree.
   3. Second degree.
   4. Third degree.

38. As the fetal heads moves through the pelvis, there is a certain degree of pressure exerted on the head. What is the most common result of that noted in neonates?
    1. Caput succedaneum.
    2. Cephalohematoma.
    3. Molding.
    4. Subgaleal hematoma.

39. A nulliparous woman at 37.6 weeks is admitted in active labor. Her group B *Streptococcus* (GBS) culture result is not available because the test was just collected at her appointment yesterday. Bag of waters is intact. She is afebrile and normotensive. Which of the following is warranted based on current recommendations?
    1. Inform patient that baby will need a 48-hour stay.
    2. No treatment for GBS is indicated.
    3. Treat with IV penicillin G.
    4. Treat with IV Cefazolin.

40. Comparing both midline to mediolateral episiotomies, a midline episiotomy is associated with:
    1. Enhanced degree of difficulty to repair.
    2. Greater blood loss.
    3. Higher degree of pain.
    4. Higher incidence of rectal extension.

41. The relationship of the long axis of the fetus to the long axis of the mother is described as the fetal:
    1. Attitude.
    2. Lie.
    3. Position.
    4. Presentation.

42. Which of the following is a characteristic of the lithotomy position for birth as compared with nonlithotomy positions? Lithotomy position for birth:
    1. Enhances maternal cardiac output.
    2. Facilitates backward rotation of the sacrum.
    3. Facilitates intervention by the attendant.
    4. Results in a greater number of intact perineums.

43. Which of these fetal head diameters is the greatest?
    1. Occipitofrontal.
    2. Submentalbregmatic.
    3. Suboccipitobregmatic.
    4. Verticomental.

44. A patient presents for her initial prenatal intake. Clinical pelvimetry exam reveals inlet—oval; anteroposterior (AP) diameter is much greater than transverse diameter; forepelvis more narrow than posterior segment; sacrum posteriorly inclined; sagittal diameters long; wide sacrosciatic notch; side walls convergent; and ischial spines prominent. What is the patient's pelvis type?
    1. Android.
    2. Anthropoid.
    3. Gynecoid.
    4. Platypelloid.

45. Which pelvis type is associated with the fetus presenting in the posterior position?
    1. Android.
    2. Anthropoid.
    3. Gynecoid.
    4. Platypelloid.

46. What is considered a definitive diagnosis of ruptured membranes?
    1. Positive nitrazine test.
    2. Positive ferning of dried fluid on microscopy.
    3. Ultrasound showing low amniotic fluid levels.
    4. Visualization of fluid pooling in posterior fornix of the vagina.

47. A WHNP/midwife is discussing artificial rupture of membranes with a G2P1 at 38 weeks gestation being induced for gestational hypertension. The patient is currently 6 cm dilated with regular contractions and a cephalic vertex presentation with the head engaged. What information should the midwife include in her discussion?
    1. "There is a high risk of cord prolapse."
    2. "I will do the amniotomy between contractions to reduce the force of the rupture."
    3. "After rupturing your membranes, I will immediately remove my hands to reduce the risk of infection."

48. In making a differential diagnosis, the midwife knows that the following characteristic is more likely to occur when a laboring patient has chorioamnionitis rather than dehydration:
    1. Fetal tachycardia >160 bpm.
    2. Uterine tenderness.
    3. Maternal tachycardia >100 bpm.
    4. Maternal oral temperature of 38.0°C (100.4°F) for more than 1 hour.

49. On evaluation of the fetal heart tracing of a term fetus, you observe recurrent decelerations with the nadir of the deceleration occurring at the peak of the contraction with gradual return to baseline and moderate variability. What is the most appropriate next step for the midwife to take?
    1. Attempt fetal scalp stimulation to assess fetal well-being.
    2. Order an amnioinfusion.
    3. Assess the patient's dilation.
    4. Administer tocolytic therapy.

50. A G2P1 presents in labor with a protracted active phase. On exam, the WHNP/midwife feels the fetal sagittal suture directed toward the maternal sacral promontory. What does the midwife suspect is causing the protracted labor?
   1. Direct occiput posterior fetal lie.
   2. Anterior asynclitic fetus.
   3. Platypelloid pelvic type.
   4. Posterior asynclitic fetus.

51. A placenta is noted to be abnormally large and pale yellowish-gray. What should the midwife assess the fetus for?
   1. Erythroblastosis.
   2. Postmaturity.
   3. Syphilis.
   4. Fetal hydrops.

52. What factor increases a patient's risk for abruptio placentae?
   1. Polyhydramnios.
   2. Gestational diabetes.
   3. Obesity.
   4. History of heparin use in the pregnancy.

53. Exam of a vulvar hematoma characteristically reveals:
   1. Pink, indurated tissue.
   2. Painful swelling identified on high rectal exam.
   3. Blue-black discoloration of tissue.
   4. Mild pain on palpitation.

54. Recurrent decelerations are:
   1. Decelerations that are associated with uterine contractions.
   2. Decelerations that occur with at least every other contraction over the period of 1 hour.
   3. Decelerations in which the peak-to-trough is <6 bpm.
   4. Decelerations that occur with approximately half the contractions in a given 20-minute period.

Pharmacology

55. Targeted intrapartum antibiotic prophylaxis has demonstrated efficacy for prevention of group B *Streptococcus* (GBS) early-onset disease (EOD) in neonates born to women with positive antepartum GBS cultures, and women who have other risk factors for intrapartum GBS colonization. Which of the following is the appropriate treatment to help avoid GBS transmission?
   1. Oral antepartum antibiotics at time of positive GBS screening.
   2. Intramuscular antepartum antibiotics at time of positive GBS screening and repeat × 1 dose intrapartum.
   3. IV intrapartum antibiotic prophylaxis.
   4. Oral antepartum and intrapartum antibiotics at time of positive GBS screening.

56. Active management of the third stage guidelines include which of the following?
   1. Oxytocin (Pitocin) 10 mu IM.
   2. Oxytocin (Pitocin) 10 units IM.
   3. Oxytocin (Pitocin) 10 units IV push.
   4. Oxytocin (Pitocin) 20 mu to 1 L of IV fluid.

57. The midwife is reviewing the prenatal record of a patient who has been admitted in active labor with spontaneous rupture of membranes prior to admission. She is a G3P2 at 38.5 weeks gestation, and her previous deliveries were without complications. She has no medical problems and denies allergies to medications. The prenatal record indicates the patient is HIV-negative but a culture for group B *Streptococcus* (GBS) at 37 weeks was positive. Which therapy is the recommended intrapartum prophylaxis for this patient?
   1. Vancomycin (Vancocin).
   2. Clindamycin (Cleocin).
   3. Cefazolin (Ancef).
   4. Penicillin.

58. A patient who is 39^4 EGA is being admitted in active labor. Her history includes pulmonary embolism after her last pregnancy. She has been on prophylactic low-molecular-weight heparin injections during this pregnancy. The labor nurse is requesting orders for continued heparin therapy. What is the most appropriate order the midwife would write?
   1. Unfractionated heparin 1000 units subcut every 12 hours.
   2. Unfractionated heparin 3000 units subcut every 12 hours.
   3. Enoxaparin 40 mg subcut daily.
   4. Enoxaparin 1 mg/kg every 12 hours.

59. When would the midwife stop an oxytocin infusion?
   1. Contractions lasting longer than 2 minutes.
   2. Contractions occurring every 3 to 5 minutes.
   3. Resting intrauterine pressure is less than 15 mm Hg.
   4. Moderate pain with each contraction.

60. The midwife is considering prostaglandin administration for her patient to:
   1. Decrease amniotic fluid volume.
   2. Promote uteroplacental circulation.
   3. Cause the membranes to rupture.
   4. Ripen the cervix.

61. Obstetric interventions, when necessary, should not be delayed solely to provide 4 hours of antibiotic administration before birth for group B *Streptococcus* (GBS) prophylaxis. The midwife understands which is an appropriate intervention:
   1. Administration of oxytocin.
   2. Avoidance of fetal monitoring.
   3. Fundal pressure.
   4. Delay in epidural analgesia.

62. A patient who is a G2P0 at 39^2 EGA has been admitted in active labor. Her membranes ruptured spontaneously 1.5 hours before her admission and the patient reports the fluid was clear. The midwife examines the patient and finds the cervix is 5 cm dilated and 100% effaced with the fetal head at 0 station. Fetal heart tracing is reactive. After 2 hours, noting early decelerations on the fetal tracing, the midwife re-examines the patient to find the cervix is 5 cm dilated, and the fetal head is at +1 station. What is the midwife's next step in the management of this patient's labor?
   1. Order terbutaline (Brethine) to be given.
   2. Begin an amnioinfusion.
   3. Order oxytocin (Pitocin) augmentation.
   4. Notify the physician to discuss a cesarean section for arrest of descent.

63. The midwife is managing the induction of labor for a G3P2 who experienced an intrauterine fetal demise at 26 weeks of gestation. The patient's history includes blood type A+, and tests for group B *Streptococcus* (GBS), gonorrhea and chlamydia, HIV, and syphilis negative, and a diagnosis of cystic fibrosis. The labor nurse questions the order for misoprostol for induction rather than dinoprostone. The midwife's best explanation for this order is:
   1. Misoprostol is the drug of choice for intrauterine fetal demise labor induction prior to 28 weeks gestation.
   2. Misoprostol is contraindicated because of the patient's history of cystic fibrosis.
   3. Misoprostol is indicated to avoid the side effects of dinoprostone.
   4. Misoprostol is indicated because it is more effective than dinoprostone.

64. What antibiotic should be given for antimicrobial prophylaxis for perinatal group B *Streptococcus* (GBS) disease prevention to a penicillin-allergic woman at high-risk for anaphylaxis and unknown antibiotic susceptibility?
   1. Cefazolin.
   2. Clindamycin.
   3. Vancomycin.
   4. Erythromycin.

65. Which of the following applies to the use of nitrous oxide for labor and birth?
   1. A woman may not use nitrous oxide prior to receiving regional anesthesia.
   2. Decreased oxygen saturation is a complication of nitrous oxide use.
   3. Nitrous oxide causes neonatal depression.
   4. Nitrous oxide clears the woman's body quickly via the lungs.

66. QSEN The midwife is discussing intrapartum prophylaxis regimen for a patient without drug allergies and a positive group B *Streptococcus* (GBS) screening. According to the American College of Obstetricians and Gynecologists recommendation, what is the *preferred medication* and route of administration?
   1. IV penicillin (penicillin G).
   2. IM amoxicillin (Amoxil).
   3. IV first-generation cephalosporin, cefazolin (Ancef).
   4. IM clindamycin (Cleocin).

6 Answers and Rationales

Intrapartum Care

1. (3) Endogenous endorphin (beta-endorphin) released during labor will raise the woman's pain threshold and produce sedation. In addition, physiologic anesthesia of the perineal tissues, caused by the pressure of the presenting part, decreases the mother's perception of pain. During labor the blood pressure will increase during contractions and continue to remain somewhat elevated between them. Valsalva maneuver is discouraged during the second stage labor because it can cause fetal hypoxia.

2. (3) During the active pushing (descent) phase, the woman has strong urges to bear down as the presenting part of the fetus descends and presses on the stretch receptors of the pelvic floor. The vulva stretches and begins to bulge, encircling the fetal head. Birth of the head occurs when the station is +4. A 0 station indicates engagement. Bloody show occurs throughout the labor process and is not an indication of an imminent birth. Rupture of membranes can occur at any time during the labor process and does not indicate an imminent birth.

3. (3) Fetal position is denoted with a three-letter abbreviation. The first letter indicates the presenting part in either the right or the left side of the maternal pelvis. The second letter indicates the anatomic presenting part of the fetus. The third letter stands for the location of the presenting part in relationship to the anterior, posterior, or transverse portion of the maternal pelvis. Palpation of a round, firm fetal part in the fundal portion of the uterus would be the fetal head, which means that the fetus is in a breech position with the sacrum as the presenting part in the maternal pelvis. Palpation of the fetal spine along the mother's left side denotes the location of the presenting part in the mother's pelvis. Because the midwife can palpate the fetal spine, this is a fetus that is anteriorly positioned in the maternal pelvis. The description is of a fetus that is on the left side of the maternal pelvis with the sacrum as the presenting part and anteriorly positioned. LSA is the correct three-letter abbreviation to indicate this fetal position. LSP describes a fetus that is on the left side of the pelvis with the sacrum as the presenting part and posteriorly positioned. LOA describes a fetus that is on the left side of the pelvis with the occiput as the presenting part and anteriorly positioned.

4. (3) The normal attitude of the fetus is called general flexion. The fetal attitude is the relationship of the fetal body parts to each other. The horizontal lie is perpendicular to the mother; in the longitudinal (or vertical) lie, the long axes of the fetus and the mother are parallel. Vaginal birth cannot occur if the fetus stays in a transverse lie.

5. (2) The size of the maternal pelvis and the ability of the fetal head to mold affect the mechanism of labor process. Asynclitism is the deflection of the fetal head and refers to the position of a fetus in the uterus such that the head of the fetus is presenting first and is tilted to the shoulder, causing the fetal head to no longer be in line with the birth canal. The Leopold maneuver is a means of judging descent by palpating the mother's abdomen and determining position and presentation of the fetus. Restitution is the rotation of the infant's head after birth.

6. (1) With a nullipara's first pregnancy, the fetal descent down the birth canal is usually slow but steady. Multiparas have a more rapid descent, which results in a shorter duration of labor. The process of cervical effacement and dilation is the same for all labors. The experience of pain is unique for each woman and does not relate to the number of labors she has experienced.

7. (1) During each contraction, 400 mL of blood is emptied from the uterus into the maternal vascular system, which increases cardiac output by approximately 10% to 15% during the first stage of labor, and by approximately 30% to 50% in the second stage of labor. The heart rate increases slightly during labor. During the first stage of labor, uterine contractions cause systolic readings to increase by approximately 10 mm Hg. During the second stage, contractions may cause systolic pressures to increase by 30 mm Hg and diastolic readings to increase by 25 mm Hg.

8. (3) The Bishop score is used to evaluate for induction of labor. There are five parameters evaluated, which are dilation, effacement, station, cervical consistency, and cervical position. When the Bishop score totals 8 or more, induction of labor is usually successful.

9. (2) In cephalic presentations (headfirst), the presenting part is the occiput, which occurs in 96% of births. The sacrum emerges first with a breech presentation and occurs in approximately 3% of births. With a shoulder presentation, the scapula emerges first and this occurs in only 1% of births.

10. (3) Attitude is the relationship of the fetal body parts to one another. Lie is the relationship of the long axis (spine) of the fetus to the long axis (spine) of the mother. Position is the relationship of the presenting part of the

fetus to the four quadrants of the mother's pelvis identified by the letters L (left), R (right), A (anterior), and P (posterior).

11. (1) Induction of labor is contraindicated with prolapsed cord. Early induction of labor is indicated when there is mild placental abruption, gestational hypertension, preeclampsia, eclampsia, premature rupture of the membranes, fetal death, chorioamnionitis, postterm pregnancy, and fetal isoimmunization.

12. (3) With a breech presentation, the sacrum or lower limbs are the presenting fetal part. Fetal anus/sacrum/genitals/feet are palpable on vaginal exam. Leopold maneuver or ultrasound reveals head in fundal region. Terminal meconium is found during vaginal exam after rupture of membranes. The fetal heart rate is heard above the mother's umbilicus. Early gestational age is frequently found with a breech presentation and the risk decreases as gestational age advances.

13. (4) Group B *Streptococcus* (GBS) bacteriuria at any time during the pregnancy is considered positive GBS for current pregnancy. History of GBS-infected newborn requires GBS intrapartum prophylaxis for all pregnancies. Intrapartum antibiotic prophylaxis is based on current GBS screening. If a woman presents in labor at term with unknown GBS colonization status and does not have risk factors that are an indication for intrapartum antibiotic prophylaxis but reports a known history of GBS colonization in a previous pregnancy, the risk of GBS early-onset disease (EOD) in the neonate is likely to be increased. With this increased risk, it is reasonable to offer intrapartum antibiotic prophylaxis based on the woman's history of colonization. Health care providers also may consider discussing the option of empiric intrapartum antibiotic prophylaxis as a shared decision-making process in this clinical scenario.

14. (2) There are three types of breech presentations. Frank breech (hips flexed, knees extended; sacrum presents first in 40% to 60% of breech presentations at term), complete breech (hips and knees flexed; feet and sacrum present together), and footling breech (when one foot [single footling] or both feet [double footling] present before the buttocks).

15. (3) Electronic fetal monitoring is indicated in high-risk situations that include multiples, breech presentation, high body mass index, prior cesarean birth, postterm pregnancy, preterm labor, premature rupture of membranes, and the use of oxytocin (Pitocin). Evidence supports hands-on listening (intermittent auscultation)—a low-tech, high-touch approach—for women giving birth without known complications. Practice guidelines encourage the use of hands-on listening with low-risk pregnancies.

16. (1) Fetal hypoxia may cause decreased variability. Increasing IV fluids, lateral recumbent position, and maternal oxygen therapy all contribute to increased oxygenation to the fetus, which may resolve this finding. An amnioinfusion and fetal scalp stimulation will not correct fetal hypoxia. Although tocolytics may correct hypoxia, these are not nonpharmacologic therapies.

17. (4) Hydrotherapy allows the fluid to shift from the extravascular space to the intravascular space, which increases fluid excretion by the kidneys and may lead to dehydration. Hydrotherapy decreases the use of anesthesia and analgesia and has no effect on maternal breathing pattern.

18. (3) The midwife should assist the labor nurse to locate a more consistent fetal heart monitoring location. Fetal scalp electrode placement is contraindicated with infections, such as HIV and hepatitis B. Indications for surgical delivery and amnioinfusion do not include inability to perform continuous external fetal heart monitoring.

19. (2) In patients with no significant obstetric risk factors, the fetal heart rate should be auscultated, or the electronic monitor tracing evaluated at least every 30 minutes. The mother may ambulate, provided that intermittent monitoring ensures fetal well-being.

20. (4) Epidural analgesia is the most likely cause because it can be associated with maternal hypotension and decreased placental perfusion. Placental abruption would be accompanied by vaginal bleeding; a prolapsed cord would be felt on re-exam. The contraction pattern and uterine palpation does not indicate hyperstimulation due to oxytocin administration, a cause of fetal hypoxia.

21. (1) Application of counterpressure helps the woman cope with the sensations of internal pressure and pain in the lower back. Counterpressure lifts the occiput off the spinal nerves, thereby providing pain relief.

22. (3) Postmaturity is the most likely cause of late decelerations in this fetus. With uterine contractions every 2 minutes, tachysystole is not a cause. The fetal heart baseline in the 140s and maternal temperature at 37.4°C does not indicate an infection. The patient's BP is within normal range and her history indicates no medical problems (hypertension).

23. (1) The diagnosis of a placental abruption is entertained if a patient presents with painful vaginal bleeding in association with uterine tenderness, hyperactivity, and increased tone. Uterine rupture is characterized by the sudden onset of intense abdominal pain, and the most consistent clinical finding is an abnormal fetal heart rate pattern. The classic presentation of placenta previa is

painless vaginal bleeding in a previously normal pregnancy. Fetal bleeding does not present with maternal pain or changes in uterine tone.

24. (1) The physical exam should be focused on the assessment of blood pressure, edema, and reflexes, as well as on a qualitative assessment of urinary protein excretion with a dipstick. A positive screen for urine protein can be further investigated with a 24-hour urine collection for protein. Both the nonstress test and the biophysical profile evaluate the well-being of the fetus, not the mother.

25. (1) Cardiac patients should be delivered vaginally unless obstetric indications for cesarean delivery are present. They should be allowed to labor in the lateral decubitus position with frequent assessment of vital signs, urine output, and pulse oximetry. These women should avoid the lithotomy and supine positions. Reverse Trendelenburg position can increase the cardiac afterload.

26. (3) Obstetrics is the second highest litigated medical specialty in the United States. Midwives and WHNPs who provide obstetrical care must be acutely aware of the climate and what constitutes legal action. By not informing a patient of the available screening options, the provider has breached the duty to the patient.

27. (3) Particularly of late there has been a specific emphasis on correct diagnosis of labor and not admitting women to the hospital too early (i.e., prior to the onset of active labor). Therefore it is imperative that the midwife knows what constitutes "active" labor so that unnecessary intervention is not undertaken.

28. (1) Six centimeters marks the onset of active labor. From that point the patient should make steady progress to culminate in second stage. As a multiparous patient, for this woman to have progressed only 1 cm in 4 hours signifies that she has essentially "fallen off" the labor curve, which means that the provider does need to intervene at this point. Amniotomy will release prostaglandins and has been shown to be an appropriate method for augmentation of labor. Encouraging her to continue to ambulate, when she already has been doing it without any results, is incorrect for that reason. Encouraging her to nap ignores the fact that her progress is abnormal, and suggesting an epidural is incorrect for a number of reasons; she is comfortable, is not asking for medication, and it will likely slow her labor further with this contraction pattern.

29. (4) There has been recent evidence to note that women admitted too early in labor are more likely to experience a cascade of interventions. The movement has been toward not admitting women until in active labor. This woman is clearly in latent labor and should not yet be admitted, nor is any augmentation (like amniotomy) warranted in latent labor. Group B *Streptococcus* (GBS) prophylaxis is not initiated until active labor.

30. (3) The midwife should be able to recognize the signs of a fetus in occiput posterior position and further, what to do to facilitate repositioning of the fetus (which is hands/knees position). She is not yet in active labor, so augmentation is not warranted. She is actively contracting every 3 minutes so IUPC placement is unwarranted, particularly because she is not yet in active labor. Intermittent monitoring is still the most appropriate monitoring mode for her.

31. (2) The midwife should recognize when cervical exam is not only not warranted, but when it can be dangerous. Because this patient is from out of town there is likely no record of any ultrasounds that she may have had during pregnancy. Even if she were to be asked and respond that she knows of no issues with her placenta, the midwife should still want to prove that with an ultrasound. Performing a digital exam could lead to the midwife poking his/her finger through a placenta that may be a placenta previa. Nitrazine is inaccurate in the presence of blood making that an incorrect tool to use.

32. (3) The midwife should know what a Brandt-Andrew maneuver is done for (to check for separation of the placenta from the uterine wall). If the cord shortens on doing the maneuver, the placenta is not yet separated. If there is no change in cord length when the maneuver is done, the placenta has separated and can be delivered with gentle cord traction. Hemabate is given for hemorrhage (which this situation does not indicate). There is no need for physician consultation.

33. (4) Placing baby skin-to-skin immediately after birth has many benefits, including facilitating initiation of bonding and helping to maintain heat in the neonate. It does not affect length of the third stage of labor unless baby is put to breast, which would then potentially decrease the length of the third stage via oxytocin release with suckling. Skin-to-skin does not affect maternal nausea, nor does it enhance maternal cooperation for perineal inspection.

34. (3) Although laboring women should be encouraged to liberally take in oral fluids, some women experience nausea severe enough that they require IV hydration to replace fluid loss through vomiting. Labor requires a tremendous amount of energy both in terms of calories and fluids. If a woman is unable to take and keep in fluids orally, and particularly if she is vomiting, she is at risk to develop ketosis, which is counterproductive to her ability to progress in labor and maintain a reasonable state of homeostasis.

35. (2) Recognition of normal labor progression is paramount for midwives. This patient's pattern is indicative of normal labor progress, meaning that no augmentation is indicated. There is no indication that IV hydration is warranted (the stem does not indicate that she is dehydrated or unable to take in oral fluids; remember not to assume something if it is not in the stem). Because her progress has been normal, intrauterine pressure catheter placement (IUPC) is unwarranted.

36. (2) Because of the risk of prolapsed cord (although small) with rupture of membranes, the first thing to check after rupture is fetal heart rate.

37. (3) Identification of laceration by type is an imperative skill for the midwife. Laceration types have very specific parameters and are clearly defined in the literature. A laceration that involves the vaginal floor muscles but goes no deeper is classified as a second-degree laceration.

38. (3) Recognition of normal and abnormal signs that may appear on newborns is an expected skill of the midwife or nurse practitioner. The bones of the fetal skull "mold" to the passageway of the pelvis as the fetus descends through it to crowning. Molding is a very normal finding in a neonate.

39. (2) Recently, the American Society for Microbiology (ASM) commented about situations like this and superseded the American College of Obstetricians and Gynecologists (ACOG) recommendations, which state no prophylaxis in unknown status if there are no symptoms. ASM also added that a nucleic acid amplification test (NAAT) be done in labor and delivery and this must be negative to proceed with no treatment. Because the patient is afebrile, does not have prolonged ruptured membranes, and is term, she does not require GBS treatment at this point. Should she develop any risk factors during labor, the recommendation would then be to treat.

40. (4) Although mediolateral episiotomy is rarely warranted, in the event that the midwife must cut a mediolateral episiotomy, knowing the difference between the two in terms of side effects, outcomes, and others is imperative. Because the midline cuts in the direction of the rectum, it is more likely to extend into a rectal laceration than is a mediolateral episiotomy.

41. (2) The fetal attitude is the relationship of the fetal body parts to one another. Lie is the relationship of the long axis (spine) of the fetus to the long axis (spine) of the mother. Position is the relationship of the presenting part of the fetus to the four quadrants of the mother's pelvis identified by the letters L (left), R (right), A (anterior), and P (posterior). Presentation refers to the part of the fetus' body that leads the way out through the birth canal (called the presenting part).

42. (3) Lithotomy position was first instituted to allow the birth attendant easier access to the perineum. Beyond that it has very little to offer. Women lying on their back have decreased cardiac output, and greater chance for laceration because of the undue pressure on the perineum because of the legs spread wide.

43. (4) Verticomental is the greatest diameter, and least favorable, of the fetal head diameters.

44. (2) The inlet is oval in the anthropoid pelvis. In the gynecoid pelvis the inlet is rounded. In the android pelvis the inlet is heart-shaped, and in the platypelloid pelvis the inlet is flat. In the anthropoid pelvis the AP diameter is much greater than the transverse diameter. In the gynecoid pelvis the AP diameter is greater than or equal to the transverse diameter, and in the platypelloid pelvis the AP diameter is short, and the transverse diameter is wide. Side walls are convergent in the anthropoid pelvis, as well as the android and platypelloid pelves. In the gynecoid pelvis the side walls are straight.

45. (1) Because of the shape of the android pelvis, the fetus is more likely to assume a posterior position (occiput posterior). The gynecoid pelvis is most optimal for childbearing.

46. (4) Nitrazine can be easily contaminated by blood, urine, semen, and antiseptic agents, and cervicitis and vaginitis can also cause false-positive results. False-positive results of ferning can come from contamination with cervical mucus or semen, fingerprints, or technical area, such as contamination with blood or use of a dry swab to collect the sample. Ultrasound evidence of diminished amniotic fluid cannot confirm the diagnosis, but it may be suggestive of ruptured membranes. Other causes of oligohydramnios would need to be ruled out. Because visualization of pooling of clear fluid in the posterior fornix of the vagina or leakage of fluid from the cervical os are unlikely to have other causes, they are considered a definitive diagnosis of ruptured membranes.

47. (3) The fetal membranes should be ruptured between contractions to reduce the force of the rupture, which can increase risk of prolapse, and make sure membranes are not stretched tightly against the fetal head, which makes safely grasping them to tear them more difficult. Although amniotomy always presents some risk of cord prolapse, with an engaged head and term infant in a vertex, noncompound position, this patient is not at high risk for cord prolapse. There is a risk of uterine infection with prolonged rupture of membranes, but the fingers should always be left in the vagina through the

next contraction to evaluate the effect of the amniotomy on dilation and fetal position and station, as well as to ensure there is no prolapse of the cord.

48. (2) Both chorioamnionitis and dehydration can cause maternal and fetal tachycardia and maternal fever. However, fundal tenderness on palpation is unlikely to occur due to dehydration and is a relatively common finding with chorioamnionitis.

49. (3) The contraction pattern described is early decelerations, which are typically associated with head compression and often occur shortly before delivery when the perineal floor puts pressure on the head during contractions. Because early decelerations can indicate delivery is imminent and because there are not significant concerns about fetal well-being, checking a patient's dilation to determine proximity to delivery is the most appropriate next step. Amnioinfusion is the instillation of fluid into the amniotic cavity. The rationale is that augmenting amniotic fluid volume may decrease or eliminate problems associated with a severe reduction or absence of amniotic fluid, such as severe variable decelerations during labor. Fetal scalp stimulation is not an inappropriate measure to take here because of the decelerations. Given the early nature of decelerations, return to baseline and moderate variability, tocolytic therapy is not indicated.

50. (2) Asynclitism is suspected because the sagittal suture is not midway between the symphysis pubis and the sacral promontory but is instead directed to the maternal sacral promontory. Anterior versus posterior asynclitism is determined by which parietal bone is dominant. Because in this case the sagittal suture is closer to the sacral promontory, the anterior parietal bone has become dominant and anterior synclitism is suspected. In a direct occiput posterior position, the sagittal suture would be midline. Pelvic type is unlikely to be determined by assessment of fetal sutures.

51. (3) A syphilitic placenta is abnormally large and pale yellowish-gray, and a syphilitic fetus should be expected. Larger and heavier placentas than normal are also expected with erythroblastosis, although these placentas are typically lighter in color due to fetal anemia. Postmature placentas are similar in appearance to nonpostmature placentas, although they may have increased calcification. Fetal hydrops can cause a thick (>4 cm) placenta but is not associated with color change.

52. (1) A sudden decrease in uterine volume or size, such as with rupture of membranes when polyhydramnios is present, is a significant risk factor for abruptio placentae. Obesity, gestational diabetes, and history of C-section are not strongly associated with increased risk of placental abruption in the absence of other risk factors. There is some evidence that heparin can reduce risk of abruption, particularly in women with a history of preeclampsia.

53. (3) Vulvar hematomas typically present as a tense, fluctuant swelling and bluish or blue-black discoloration of tissue and with severe pain, out of proportion to the expected amount of pain. Painful swelling on high rectal exam is characteristic of broad ligament hematomas.

54. (4) Recurrent decelerations are typically defined as decelerations that occur with approximately 50% of contractions in any 20-minute segment. Decelerations that occur with uterine contractions are known as periodic patterns. The amplitude of decelerations is not related to contractions being recurrent.

Pharmacology

55. (3) Neither antepartum nor intrapartum oral or intramuscular regimens have been shown to be comparably effective in reducing group B *Streptococcus* (GBS) early-onset disease (EOD).

56. (2) Oxytocin is measured in units. Ten units is the correct dosage. Oxytocin is not given directly with IV push as it can cause circulatory collapse.

57. (4) IV penicillin remains the agent of choice for intrapartum prophylaxis of women who are positive group B *Streptococcus* (GBS). Vancomycin is recommended for women who report a high-risk penicillin allergy and whose GBS isolate is not susceptible to clindamycin. Clindamycin is the recommended alternative to penicillin in high-risk penicillin allergies only if the GBS isolate is known to be susceptible to clindamycin. Cefazolin is recommended for women whose reported penicillin allergy indicates a low risk of anaphylaxis or is of uncertain severity.

58. (3) Neither 1000 nor 3000 units of unfractionated heparin will achieve prophylactic anticoagulation. Enoxaparin 1 mg/kg every 12 hours is used for deep vein thrombosis dosing. Enoxaparin 40 mg subcut daily is used for prophylactic pulmonary embolus dosing.

59. (1) Oxytocin infusions should be stopped when contractions last longer than 1 minute. Mild to moderate pain is normal with contractions and so is the frequency of every 3 to 5 minutes. A resting intrauterine pressure greater than 15 to 20 mm Hg is a concern; normal should be less than 15 mm Hg.

60. (4) Prostaglandins are given to ripen the cervix (thin and soften) prior to elective labor induction. Uteroplacental perfusion or amniotic fluid volume are not altered by the

use of prostaglandins. The insertion of prostaglandin gel has no effect on rupturing the membranes.

61. (1) Appropriate obstetric interventions include, but are not limited to, administration of oxytocin, artificial rupture of membranes, or planned cesarean birth, with or without precesarean rupture of membranes. However, some variation in practice may be warranted based on the needs of individual patients to enhance intrapartum antibiotic exposure. Fundal pressure should always be avoided. Delays in intrapartum fetal assessment or maternal treatment for labor pain is not recommended.

62. (3) The patient is experiencing a protraction disorder of the active phase of labor (cervical dilation rate of less than 1.2 cm/hr in nulliparous women). The American College of Obstetricians and Gynecologists recommends the use of oxytocin for all protraction and arrest disorders. A cesarean section is not indicated at this time, terbutaline induces uterine relaxation, an amnioinfusion is not indicated for early decelerations.

63. (2) Prostaglandins are contraindicated in patients with a history of bronchial asthma or active pulmonary disease. Dinoprostone can be used from the 12th to the 28th week of gestation. After 28 weeks' gestation, if the condition of the cervix is favorable for induction and there are no contraindications, misoprostol, followed by oxytocin are the drugs of choice.

64. (3) If susceptibility testing has not been done and susceptibility is unknown, or if GBS is resistant to clindamycin or erythromycin, vancomycin should be given. Penicillin G or ampicillin are the preferred treatment for group B *Streptococcus* (GBS). In penicillin-allergic patients who are not at high risk of anaphylaxis, cefazolin can be given. However, penicillin-allergic patients who are at high risk of anaphylaxis should avoid cefazolin. These patients should ideally have clindamycin and erythromycin susceptibility testing performed on prenatal GBS isolates.

65. (4) Although nitrous oxide has been used for approximately 100 years in Europe during childbirth, it is relatively new in the US landscape. Providers need to be knowledgeable on it as a modality. Nitrous oxide has potent anxiolytic properties and may be used prior to any other analgesic or anesthetic. It has not been shown to decrease oxygen saturation. It is also eliminated very quickly via the lungs.

66. (1) First-line IV penicillin remains the agent of choice for intrapartum prophylaxis with IV ampicillin as an acceptable alternative. First-generation cephalosporins (i.e., cefazolin) are recommended for women whose reported penicillin allergy indicates a low risk of anaphylaxis or is of uncertain severity. For women with a high risk of anaphylaxis, clindamycin is the recommended alternative to penicillin only if the group B *Streptococcus* (GBS) isolate is known to be susceptible to clindamycin.

7

Postpartum

Postpartum Care

1. Which statement is accurate regarding physiologic changes in the immediate postpartum period for the mother?
   1. Within 12 hours the fundus is found approximately 1 cm below the umbilicus.
   2. Estrogen and progesterone levels rise quickly after expulsion of the placenta.
   3. Cardiac output is decreased immediately after birth, along with pulse rate.
   4. Leukocytosis occurs during the first week after birth.

2. During a postpartum assessment, the WHNP/midwife notes a cluster of external hemorrhoids. Which statement made by the patient indicates a need for additional teaching?
   1. "I can give myself an enema every other day to reduce constipation."
   2. "I can take sitz baths for pain."
   3. "I can decrease the swelling by using a topical hydrocortisone cream."
   4. "I can take a stool softener to decrease the pain of a bowel movement."

3. Ten days after delivery, a patient is diagnosed with mastitis. Which of the following would the WHNP/midwife expect to find on physical exam?
   1. Tender, hard, hot, and reddened area on breast.
   2. Dimpled skin on breasts and firm nodules around areola.
   3. Decreased milk production, inverted nipple, and firm, inflamed breast tissue.
   4. Soft, tender, palpable masses with cracked, bleeding nipples.

4. A patient with a history of bipolar disorder has just given birth. The WHNP/midwife should educate the patient and her spouse on the signs and symptoms of which postpartum complication?
   1. Postpartum blues.
   2. Postpartum psychosis.
   3. Taking-in phase.
   4. Taking-hold phase.

5. During a breast exam on a lactating woman, which finding is cause for concern?
   1. Leaking of "watery" fluid from left breast.
   2. Cracked nipples that are tender to touch.
   3. Warm breasts that are distended.
   4. Inverted left nipple and flat right nipple.

6. A new first-time mother is being evaluated for a complaint of breast pain. Her infant is 3 weeks old, and she is breastfeeding. The infant is gaining weight and seems satisfied after feeding. On exam, the WHNP/midwife finds red, irritated nipples on both breasts, but no masses or tenderness to the breasts themselves. What is an important part of the WHNP/midwife's evaluation?
   1. Mammogram of the breast.
   2. Exam of the infant's mouth.
   3. STAT complete blood count (CBC).
   4. Analysis of the milk.

7. The WHNP/midwife is completing the assessment of a patient the day after delivery. Where should the nurse be able to palpate the patient's fundus?
   1. 2 cm above the umbilicus.
   2. 1 to 2 cm below the umbilicus.
   3. Midline at the level of the umbilicus.
   4. Midway between the umbilicus and the symphysis pubis.

8. When do most nonnursing mothers resume menstruation after childbirth?
   1. 30 days.
   2. 7 to 9 weeks.
   3. 45 days.
   4. 2 to 4 weeks.

9. What risk factor is often associated with puerperal infection?
   1. Rupture of membranes 36 hours before delivery.
   2. Excessive weight gain during pregnancy.
   3. 10 hours in the labor process.
   4. Premature labor and delivery.

10. Which statement is correct regarding postpartum blues?
    1. Selective serotonin reuptake inhibitors (SSRIs) are generally effective and safe to use.
    2. Similar symptoms to nonpregnancy depression.
    3. Require outpatient psychotherapy along with antidepressant medication.
    4. Onset and resolution of symptoms are within the first 10 days postpartum.

11. To meet the goal of promoting feeding in a breastfed baby, which activity is the **least** effective?
    1. Alternate breastfeeding and formula for each feeding.
    2. Stop breastfeeding if her nipples get sore.
    3. Maintain on-demand breastfeeding for the first 4 weeks.
    4. Keep the newborn nearby to respond to feeding cues.

12. A new mother asks about changes to her skin that appeared during pregnancy. What change is most likely to completely disappear?
    1. Spider nevi.
    2. Chloasma.
    3. Darker pigmentation of the areolae.
    4. Acne.

13. What is the correct information to give to a postpartum patient on how to perform Kegel exercises?
    1. Have patient contract abdomen and buttocks daily.
    2. Encourage the patient to tighten thighs at intervals throughout the day.
    3. Tell the patient to try and stop the flow of urine midstream.
    4. Have patient raise lower legs slowly into the air four times a day.

14. The postpartum patient complains of severe perineal pain the first hour after delivery. The WHNP/midwife suspects:
    1. A soft, boggy uterus.
    2. Perineal hematoma.
    3. Presence of a cervical laceration.
    4. Increase in vaginal flow caused by retained placental fragments.

15. A woman (gravida 4, para 3) delivered a 10-lb 9-oz (4790 g) baby boy after 24 hours of labor. During the immediate postpartum period, what complication would this patient be at an increased risk to develop?
    1. Urinary retention.
    2. Puerperal infection.
    3. Thrombophlebitis.
    4. Postpartum hemorrhage.

16. A postpartum primipara asks, "What can I do if I experience breast engorgement when trying to breastfeed?" Which response is appropriate?
    1. "Feeding the baby every 2 hours often helps prevent the problem."
    2. "Apply chilled romaine lettuce leaves to the breasts inside a nursing bra."
    3. "Apply heat to the engorged breast area."
    4. "Take a warm shower after breastfeeding."

17. A primipara appears nervous and asks if she is holding her baby right. The new mother is in which phase of maternal postpartum adjustment?
    1. Taking-hold.
    2. Postpartum blues.
    3. Taking-in.
    4. Letting-go.

18. All of the following statements are accurate regarding postpartum fever *except*:
    1. Oral temperature 38°C (100.4°F) on two successive days of the first 10 days postpartum, exclusive of the first 24 hours.
    2. Involves colonization and infection of the tissues of the uterus, peritoneum, or surrounding organs.
    3. Vaginal deliveries have the highest prevalence of postpartum infection.
    4. Most common organism is group B *Streptococcus.*

19. At her 2-week postpartum visit, an exclusively breastfeeding patient reports sudden onset of very sore nipples and reports that the pain persists through feedings. On exam, you note a bright, pinkish-red color bilaterally that extends beyond nipple/areola. What is the most likely diagnosis?
    1. Candidiasis.
    2. Mastitis.
    3. Herpes simplex.
    4. Poor infant latch.

20. The WHNP/midwife has just diagnosed an exclusively breastfeeding patient with mastitis. The patient's infant is 3 weeks old. What information should the patient be given?
    1. Stress and fatigue increase the risk of mastitis.
    2. Discontinue breastfeeding the infant at the breast and switch to pumping to give the breasts time to heal and reduce infant exposure to bacteria.
    3. Antibiotics are necessary to resolve the mastitis.
    4. Avoid antipyretics as they are not safe for breastfeeding mothers.

21. The following findings are noted in a G1P1 patient at the 6-week postpartum exam: profuse reddish-brown lochia and a soft, nontender uterus larger than expected. What is the most likely diagnosis?
    1. Endometritis.
    2. Pelvic hematoma.
    3. Excessive physical activity.
    4. Subinvolution.

22. The WHNP/midwife is preparing to discharge home a healthy patient (G1P0) who is in postpartum day 2 and planning to exclusively breastfeed her infant. What nutrition information should the WHNP/midwife provide the patient?
    1. Increase your calories by 100 to 300 calories per day.
    2. Swordfish and king mackerel are good sources of protein and omega three fatty acids that aid in brain development.
    3. Avoid common allergens, such as peanuts, to help reduce your baby's risk of developing an allergy later in life.
    4. Keep caffeine consumption under 300 mg/day.

23. What group of breastfeeding patients would most benefit from B_{12} supplementation while breastfeeding?
    1. Those who do not consume red meat.
    2. History of gastric bypass.
    3. Consumption of fewer than 1800 kcals/day.
    4. Celiac disease on gluten-free diet.

24. What factor places a patient at highest risk for severe diastasis recti postpartum?
    1. Grand multiparity.
    2. Obesity.
    3. Long pregnancy intervals.
    4. Severe back pain.

25. The WHNP/midwife evaluates a patient who has just given birth vaginally. The exam reveals a laceration extending deep into the vagina involving the vaginal mucosa, posterior fourchette, perineal skin, and torn bulbocavernosus and transverse perineal muscles. How should the WHNP/midwife describe the tear?
    1. Second-degree laceration.
    2. Third-degree laceration.
    3. Fourth-degree laceration.
    4. Sulcus tear.

26. Which of the following statements regarding postpartum blood loss is accurate?
    1. Postpartum hemorrhage is defined as blood loss that exceeds 500 mL.
    2. The most common etiology is uterine atony.
    3. Hypotension is the first sign of hemorrhage and corresponds to visible blood loss.
    4. Blood work results will guide treatment.

27. Which of the following are recommendations for follow-up for a postnatal woman who has experienced gestational diabetes?
    1. Weekly fasting blood glucose levels for 1 year.
    2. 75 g oral glucose tolerance test at 6 to 12 weeks postpartum.
    3. Continue oral hypoglycemic agents for 4 months, then wean off of the oral agents.
    4. Monthly hemoglobin A1c levels for 1 year.

28. In a breastfeeding patient having difficulty with milk production, the WHNP/midwife understands that milk production will be increased by:
    1. More frequent suckling of infant.
    2. Longer duration of suckling.
    3. Cessation of suckling for 24 hours.
    4. Cold compresses to the breast.

29. The first postpartum day a woman's uterus would be expected to be located where?
    1. 1 fingerbreadth above the umbilicus.
    2. At the level of the umbilicus.
    3. Midway between the symphysis and the umbilicus.
    4. Not palpable at all in the abdomen.

30. A woman has had a third-degree laceration at birth that has been repaired. On postpartum day 2, which of the following would be most concerning? That she:
    1. Cannot sit comfortably in the bed/chair.
    2. Has not yet had a bowel movement.
    3. Is experiencing urinary incontinence.
    4. Is saturating a maxi pad every 1 to 2 hours.

31. A woman who gave birth several hours ago has summoned the nurse as she is noting "a lot of pain where my stitches are." The midwife is called by the nurse to come to the woman's room. On exam, the repaired second-degree vaginal laceration is noted to be intact. On the left side of the vulva there is marked edema, which is soft and painful to the touch. The nurse reports that the patient has voided twice since the birth, which was 5 hours ago, 300 and 250 cc each. What, if anything, is warranted at this time?
    1. Anesthetic spray to the perineum.
    2. Begin sitz baths.
    3. Catheterize the woman for residual.
    4. Renew the ice packs to the perineum.

Pharmacology

32. For the patient who wants to breastfeed and take oral contraceptives, the pill of choice is:
    1. 1/35 preparation.
    2. Triphasic preparation.
    3. Progestin-only preparation.
    4. 1/50 preparation.

33. The WHNP/midwife has diagnosed infectious mastitis in a 6-week postpartum patient. The patient has no known drug allergies. Which medication is appropriate for treatment?
    1. Doxycycline (Vibramycin) 100 mg PO bid for 10 days.
    2. Dicloxacillin (Dynapen) 250 mg PO qid for 10 days.
    3. Metronidazole (Flagyl) 500 mg PO bid for 10 days.
    4. Ciprofloxacin (Cipro) 500 mg PO bid for 7 days.

34. The WHNP/midwife would identify which situation as an indication for the administration of Rh immunoglobulin (RhIg)?
    1. A woman who has been Rh-sensitized in the past two pregnancies.
    2. An infant with increased hemolysis of red blood cells because of ABO incompatibility.
    3. An infant with an increase in serum bilirubin levels as a result of the presence of Rh factor antibodies.
    4. A primigravida who is Rh-negative and is pregnant with an infant who is Rh-positive.

35. Rho(D) immunoglobulin (RhIg) would be administered in all of the following situations *except*:
    1. After chorionic villus sampling.
    2. History of Rh exchange transfusion in a previous pregnancy.
    3. Following a spontaneous abortion.
    4. Positive indirect Coombs test at 28 weeks.

36. All of these medications can be used to stop postpartum bleeding *except*:
    1. Tranexamic acid (Lysteda).
    2. Oxytocin (Pitocin).
    3. Misoprostol (Cytotec).
    4. Carboprost tromethamine (Hemabate).

37. Acute medical management of postpartum hemorrhage is critical in improving outcomes in maternal mortality. The patient's estimated blood loss is 800 mL from vaginal delivery with repaired second-degree laceration. Oxytocin 10 units has already been given intramuscularly. The WHNP/midwife orders misoprostol (Cytotec) 800 mcg rectally for treatment of continued uterine atony. Which is an expected side effect of this treatment?
    1. Urticaria.
    2. Diarrhea.
    3. Wheezing.
    4. Angioedema.

38. Indications for routine administration of postpartum antibiotic prophylaxis include:
    1. Prolonged labor with rupture of membranes.
    2. Manual removal of placenta.
    3. Episiotomy.
    4. History of mitral valve prolapse.

7 Answers and Rationales

Postpartum Care

1. (4) During the first 4 to 7 days after birth, a leukocytosis occurs and along with an elevated sedimentation rate can obscure a diagnosis of an acute infection. Within 12 hours after birth, the fundus rises approximately 1 cm above the umbilicus. The fundus descends 1 to 2 cm every 24 hours. By the sixth postpartum day the fundus is normally located halfway between the umbilicus and the symphysis pubis. Estrogen and progesterone levels drop markedly after expulsion of the placenta and reach their lowest levels 1 week after birth. Cardiac output is increased immediately after birth over prelabor values; it returns to prelabor values within 1 hour. By 2 weeks postpartum, cardiac output continues to decrease and gradually returns to prepregnant levels by 6 to 8 weeks following birth.

2. (1) An enema every other day to reduce constipation would negatively affect the normal bowel movement pattern and deplete the patient's natural intestinal flora. Sitz baths, antiinflammatory and analgesic topical ointments and sprays, stool softeners, and increased bulk in the diet would be indicated in the management of the external hemorrhoids.

3. (1) A tender, hard, hot, and reddened area on breast over the affected area is typically found with mastitis. The patient with mastitis will also typically be febrile. Dimpled skin (peau d'orange or orange-peel appearance) is a potential sign of breast cancer. Decreased milk production, inverted nipple, and firm breast tissue may be complications of engorgement. Cracked nipples may result from improper positioning or oversuckling. Soft, tender breast masses may be engorged milk ducts.

4. (2) Postpartum psychosis is rare and begins 2 weeks after childbirth. The patient's history of bipolar disorder increases this risk. Postpartum blues occurs within a few days of giving birth. The blues are brief and a normal response, and no medicine is required. During the taking-in phase, the mother is primarily concerned with her own needs and is reacting to the intense, physical effort expended during delivery. The taking-hold phase is when the mother is transitioning into her role of mothering.

5. (2) Cracked nipples are a sign of irritation and may eventually cause skin breakdown with severe pain and possible infection.

6. (2) Breast irritation in nursing mothers is often caused by *Candida albicans*. The source of infection is most likely the infant's mouth (thrush).

7. (2) Within 12 hours after delivery, the fundus may be approximately 1 cm above the umbilicus. The fundus descends approximately 1 to 2 cm every 24 hours. By the sixth postpartum week, the fundus is normally halfway between the symphysis pubis and the umbilicus.

8. (2) Most nonnursing mothers will resume menstruation 7 to 9 weeks after birth. Approximately one-half of them will ovulate during the first cycle. Most lactating women will resume menstruation in 12 weeks, although some do not menstruate during the entire lactation period.

9. (1) Prolonged rupture of the membranes is defined as membrane rupture more than 24 hours before delivery. The rupture provides an increased opportunity for bacterial growth. Excessive weight gain and premature delivery are not associated with postpartum infection. Ten hours in labor is well within the normal time for labor.

10. (4) Postpartum blues or baby blues after pregnancy are feelings of sadness during the first few days postpartum. They feelings usually go away on their own, and do not require any treatment. Unlike the baby blues, postpartum depression is a more serious problem. Postpartum depression is similar to nonpregnancy depression (sleep disorders, anhedonia, psychomotor changes, etc.); it most often has its onset within the first 12 weeks postpartum yet can occur within 1 year after delivery. Psychotherapy and antidepressant medication is often prescribed.

11. (1) The mother should be taught to feed the baby on cue for at least the first 4 weeks, until lactation is well established. This encourages the mother to look for cues the infant is hungry rather than waiting so long that the baby is demanding to be fed, for example, crying, turning red, and others. Feeding should start when subtle cues first start to increase likelihood of a good latch, especially early on. Feeding only breast milk frequently stimulates milk production. Nipple soreness is one of the most common problems; however, the use of a cream to soften the nipples is often helpful, as well as offering a pacifier to meet the sucking needs of the newborn after lactation has been established. The newborn needs to learn how to suckle effectively and not how to suck on a pacifier until later. Adequate rest and good fluid intake help promote

milk production. Keeping the newborn nearby will assist the mother in recognizing and responding to the infant's feeding cues.

12. (4) Many women have acne during pregnancy and some notice that it gets worse during pregnancy, if they had it before. Other women who may always have had clear skin will develop acne while they are pregnant. Acne typically goes away shortly after delivery. Chloasma (mask of pregnancy) usually disappears at the end of pregnancy; however, in some women it may fade, but still persist. For some women, spider nevi persist indefinitely, as does permanent darker pigmentation of the areolae and linea nigra.

13. (3) Kegel exercises help to strengthen the perineal muscles and encourage healing. To have the patient understand which muscles should be contracted 24 to 100 times per day, tell her to try and stop or pretend to stop the passing of urine midstream, which will replicate the sensation of tightening in an upward and inward movement the pelvic floor muscles. The patient should not try and contract the buttocks, abdomen, or thighs but concentrate on the pelvic floor muscles. Raising and lowering the legs describes leg raises that strengthen the abdominal wall muscles.

14. (2) A mother's complaint of excruciating perineal pain after delivery is frequently related to the development of a perineal hematoma. A soft, boggy uterus will cause an increase in the bloody flow but is usually not associated with pain. A cervical laceration may be painful at the time it occurs, but not after delivery.

15. (4) Hemorrhage is always a consideration with a large baby and numerous past pregnancies because the uterine wall muscles may contract poorly. Urinary retention may occur in any patient during the immediate postpartum period. Thrombophlebitis and puerperal infection may develop several days after delivery, but not in the immediate postpartum period.

16. (1) Frequent feeding of the infant and completely emptying the breast of milk helps to prevent and/or relieve engorgement. If engorgement occurs, the patient can take ibuprofen as needed. Chilled cabbage leaves around the breasts help relieve engorgement, not lettuce leaves, and ice rather than heat (which causes increased blood flow to the area) is helpful. A warm shower before breastfeeding stimulates the let-down response and facilitates emptying of the breast as the infant feeds, not a shower after breastfeeding.

17. (3) The taking-in phase is characterized by passiveness and dependency with the focus on herself and meeting basic needs. The mother may feel overwhelmed and seeks support from the WHNP/midwife to meet needs for comfort, rest, closeness, and nourishment. The new mother is excited and talkative during taking-in and desires to review the birth experience with family and friends. In the taking-hold phase the mother is more confident, although she may still need reassurance. The letting-go phase is characterized by the mother accepting the infant into her family unit. Postpartum blues is a transient period of depression following childbirth and appears during the taking-hold phase.

18. (3) Postpartum infection occurs after approximately 2% of vaginal births and 10% to 15% of cesarean births. The most common infecting organisms are the numerous streptococcal and anaerobic organisms that colonize and infect the tissues of the uterus, peritoneum, and surrounding organs.

19. (1) Candidiasis should be suspected if sore nipples develop rapidly after breastfeeding without discomfort, persistent pain through breastfeeding, and a striking deep pink color, possibly with tiny blisters. Mastitis is typically unilateral, appears as a hot, reddened, and tender area on the breast, and is accompanied by systemic signs of infection, such as fatigue, fever, and headache. Herpes simplex may present as chickenpox-like ulcerations, a combination of scabbed healing lesions, active oozing ulcerations, and new lesions that are tiny and bright-red flat. Poor infant latch can present in numerous ways, such as crescent-shaped abrasions above or below nipple, but do not typically extend beyond the nipple/areola, and discomfort and pain are not typically sudden onset.

20. (1) Stress and fatigue are considered risk factors for mastitis. Patients with mastitis should be provided with guidance on this and information about how to reduce stress and fatigue to prevent recurrence of mastitis. Breastfeeding should not be discontinued; frequent feedings should continue. Although antibiotics should be used judiciously for treatment of mastitis, untreated cases heal almost as quickly as untreated ones and may not be necessary, especially if fever is already subsiding. Early in the course, 12 to 24 hours after symptoms start, symptomatic treatment is appropriate for infectious mastitis. The patient would be seen in the clinic within that early period to establish the diagnosis. Antipyretics, such as Tylenol, are safe for breastfeeding patients and can be safely used in women to reduce fever.

21. (4) Persistent lochia and a stationary fundal height are classic signs of subinvolution. Endometritis is not typically a concern at 4 to 6 weeks unless tenderness or pain of the adnexa or on movement of the uterus is noted, which is not here. Although excessive physical activity can cause persistent lochia, it is unlikely to prevent the

uterus from decreasing in size. Pelvic hematomas are typically accompanied by significant pain, a well-contracted uterus, and no excessive vaginal bleeding.

22. (4) Because caffeine is transmitted through breastmilk, keeping caffeine consumption moderate (under 300 mg) is recommended to prevent interference with infant sleep. General guidelines suggest increasing calories by 500 extra calories per day for breastfeeding; an increase of 100 to 300 calories per day is recommended during pregnancy. The US Dietary Association and Food and Drug Administration recommend breastfeeding women avoid swordfish and king mackerel due to their high mercury levels. Although it is recommended that breastfeeding women include a large variety of food to expose babies to diverse flavors, there is no research to suggest that limiting exposure to allergens reduces the risk of an infant developing allergies.

23. (2) Women with a history of gastric bypass require vitamin B_{12} supplementation to reduce the risk of vitamin B_{12} deficiency in themselves and their nursing infant. Good sources of vitamin B_{12} include fortified cereal, meat, fish, shellfish, poultry, and dairy, so avoidance of red meat alone would not necessitate supplementation. Breastfeeding patients who are consuming less than 1800 kcals/day may not be meeting overall nutritional needs and should be advised to consume nutrient-rich foods and consider a general multivitamin supplement but would not be at risk of B_{12} deficiency specifically. Patients with treated or controlled celiac disease typically have normal B_{12} concentrations, but patients with untreated celiac disease may be at risk for B_{12} deficiency.

24. (1) Regaining good abdominal muscle tone becomes more difficult with increasing parity. Obesity alone is not a risk factor, although general condition and muscle tone do affect severity of diastasis recti. Short rather than long pregnancy intervals are a risk, as short intervals limit the time a patient has to regain muscle tone prior to another pregnancy. Severe back pain is a symptom rather than cause of diastasis recti.

25. (1) A second-degree laceration extends into the perineal muscles. Third- and fourth-degree lacerations also involve the external anal sphincter, and fourth-degree lacerations involve the anal sphincter and anterior rectal wall. Sulcus tears are second-degree lacerations, but instead of tearing in the middle, sulcus tears occur in the vaginal tissue unilaterally or bilaterally along the sides of the vagina. This patient's laceration includes the bulbocavernosus and transverse perineal muscles but not the anal sphincter or rectal wall and it is in the midline, so it should be described as second degree.

26. (2) Uterine atony is the most common cause of postpartum hemorrhage. Normal postpartum blood loss is up to 1000 mL, which is a newer definition. Typical signs of hypovolemia (hypotension, tachycardia, hematocrit, hemoglobin) are delayed in the postpartum patient. Hematocrit and hemoglobin changes are slow to reflect the degree of blood loss in the postpartum patient.

27. (2) A patient who has experienced gestational diabetes is at risk for continued insulin resistance, glucose intolerance, and development of type II diabetes during the next 10 years. A 75 g oral glucose tolerance test performed at 6 to 12 weeks postpartum is recommended by the American College of Obstetricians and Gynecologists (ACOG). Weekly fasting blood glucose levels would be costly and not recommended. The increased insulin resistance caused by pregnancy hormones ends with the delivery of the placenta, thus medications are not usually needed after delivery. Monthly hemoglobin A1c levels would be inappropriate and costly.

28. (1) More frequent suckling will increase production of milk more effectively than increasing the duration of suckling. Stopping or decreasing breastfeeding or applying cold compresses to the breasts will decrease milk production.

29. (2) The uterus rises above the umbilicus immediately postpartum and then recedes by approximately 1 fingerbreadth per day after that.

30. (4) A woman having recently given birth vaginally may experience urinary incontinence briefly during the postpartum period. Not yet having had a bowel movement is normal on the second postpartum day. With a third-degree laceration it would be expected that she would have a certain degree of discomfort when sitting. Having that heavy of a flow on the second postpartum day would be abnormal regardless of the type of laceration.

31. (4) There is no evidence of a hematoma, which would be indicated by induration, as well as pain to the touch. Vulvar edema can be noted postpartum, particularly after long pushing sessions. Anesthetic spray will not help specifically with the discomfort from the edema. Sitz baths are not warranted until 24 hours postpartum. She is voiding normally so there is no need for catheterization. Maintaining ice to the perineum will do the most for keeping the edema under control.

Pharmacology

32. (3) Estrogen inhibits milk production. Progestin-only preparations are ideal for the breastfeeding patient because they do not contain estrogen, and therefore do

not inhibit milk production. The other oral contraceptives listed contain estrogen in varying amounts.

33. (2) Dicloxacillin will treat *Staphylococcus aureus*, which is the most common organism associated with mastitis. None of the other medications are appropriate for treatment of mastitis, and both doxycycline and ciprofloxacin are contraindicated when breastfeeding.

34. (4) The medication RhIg is given to prevent maternal sensitization to the Rh antibodies to women who are Rh-negative. RhIg will not prevent or treat the problem if it has already occurred. RhIg is not given to the infant.

35. (4) Rho(D) immunoglobulin (RhIg) is administered to Rh-negative women whose indirect Coombs tests are negative. Women who are sensitized are not given RhIg, which would include a woman with a history of Rh exchange transfusion in a previous pregnancy and a positive indirect Coombs test at 28 weeks (a negative indirect Coombs test means sensitization has not occurred). Also, it is not necessary to give RhIg if the infant is Rh-negative. It is given within 72 hours of an Rh-negative mother's delivery of an Rh-positive infant following amniocentesis, chorionic villus sampling, ectopic pregnancy, miscarriage, elective abortion, abruptio placentae, placenta previa, or trauma at 28 weeks' gestation (with a negative indirect Coombs test result).

36. (1) Tranexamic acid is used for the treatment of menorrhagia, heavy menstrual bleeding. Oxytocin and misoprostol are powerful uterotonic agents and are effective in stopping postpartum hemorrhage due to uterine atony. Carboprost tromethamine suppresses bleeding primarily by causing intense uterine contractions and partly by causing direct vasoconstriction.

37. (2) Uterotonic agents should be the first-line treatment for postpartum hemorrhage caused by uterine atony. The specific agent selected, outside of recognized contraindications, is at the health care provider's discretion because none have been shown to have greater efficacy than others for the treatment of uterine atony. The following are common medical agents, for example, oxytocin, methylergonovine, 15-methyl prostaglandin F2α, and misoprostol. It is common for multiple uterotonic agents to be used, assuming there are no contraindications, and without adequate uterine response and ongoing hemorrhage, they should be used in rapid succession. Diarrhea is a common side effect with use of prostaglandins. The remaining options are a possible allergic reaction.

38. (2) Current recommendations are for administration of prophylactic antibiotics after manual removal of placenta due to high risk of puerperal infection from the intrauterine manipulation. Although episiotomy and prolonged labor with rupture of membranes do increase the risk of postpartum puerperal infection, current evidence does not support the use of routine administration of prophylactic antibiotics for these conditions in the absence of fever or other signs/symptoms of infection. Antibiotic prophylaxis for infective endocarditis prophylaxis in patients with mitral valve prolapse is not recommended at any time based on current evidence.

8

Neonatal Care (Midwifery Only)

Newborn

1. The midwife is measuring a newborn's frontal-occipital circumference. The correct technique involves:
   1. Placing the paper tape measure at the maximal occipital prominence and just above the eyebrows.
   2. Placing the cloth tape measure at a level 2 inches above the ears.
   3. Using a cloth tape to prevent inaccuracy due to stretchable materials.
   4. Having another person hold the tape in the center of the forehead and repeating the measurement.

2. Which newborn screening tests are mandatory state requirements?
   1. Complete blood count (CBC) and urinalysis.
   2. Thyroid function test and phenylketonuria (PKU).
   3. PKU and alpha-fetoprotein.
   4. Glucose and thyroid function tests.

3. The midwife notes an undescended testicle on a newborn. She understands that testicular function and the ability to produce healthy sperm as an adult may be impaired if the repair is not made by age:
   1. 6 years.
   2. 2 years.
   3. 1 year.
   4. 6 months.

4. The midwife correctly identifies the bluish discoloration on the neonate's hands and feet that may occur during the first 24 hours following birth as:
   1. Circumoral cyanosis.
   2. Central cyanosis.
   3. Pseudocyanosis.
   4. Acrocyanosis.

5. The midwife is examining a full-term infant who developed physiologic jaundice and is being treated with phototherapy. What is the mechanism of action of phototherapy in the treatment of this infant?
   1. The light is absorbed by bilirubin and promotes the conversion of a toxic bilirubin to an unconjugated product that can be excreted in the bile.
   2. It increases hemolysis of the excessive red blood cells that are received by the full-term infant during labor and delivery.
   3. The ultraviolet light decreases sensitivity to the destruction of red blood cells secondary to the Rh incompatibility.
   4. It increases enzymatic activity in breaking down the unconjugated bilirubin to a nontoxic form to be eliminated by the kidneys.

6. A 4-day-old infant who is being breastfed begins to develop jaundice. What is a common theory regarding the precipitating cause of this jaundice?
   1. Decreased intake in the first few days and the subsequent weight loss.
   2. Decreased tolerance and digestion of the breast milk.
   3. Increased destruction of red blood cells with release of bilirubin.
   4. Antigen–antibody reaction that increases destruction of fetal red blood cells.

7. Which infant is at an increased risk for development of "bronze baby syndrome"?
   1. Premature infant with ABO incompatibility.
   2. Asian infant who is bottle fed.
   3. White infant who is breastfed.
   4. Presence of obstructive liver disease.

8. A mother brings her 6-week-old infant to the office with concern over the child's "constant crying." She states she did not have this problem with her other two children. She is bottle feeding the infant, and there is no problem with feeding. The infant has a bowel movement every day, and the stools are soft. The infant is afebrile with no evidence of ear, throat, lung, or abdominal problems. What is the best diagnosis for this infant?
   1. Infantile colic.
   2. Spastic colon.
   3. Infant stress syndrome.
   4. Lactose intolerance.

9. The midwife suspects infantile colic in a 4-week-old infant. A complete physical exam reveals no abnormalities. What further study might the midwife order?
   1. Chest radiograph.
   2. Complete blood count and differential.
   3. Blood culture.
   4. None of the above.

10. The midwife is discussing with the parents the care of their 1-month-old infant, who has been diagnosed with infantile colic. What is important to explain to the parents?
    1. The problem may be decreased by not feeding the infant more often than every 3 hours.
    2. No specific medication is indicated to treat the problem.
    3. The problem is often related to increased stress in the home; family therapy may be indicated.
    4. The formula should be changed from a milk-based to a soy-based formula.

11. The midwife is assessing an infant who was delivered by cesarean section. What is a complication frequently associated with cesarean delivery?
    1. Increased levels of serum bilirubin.
    2. Respiratory distress.
    3. Meconium aspiration.
    4. Hypoglycemia.

12. A newborn's Apgar score at 1 minute is determined to be 3. Which of the following findings support this score?
    1. Heart rate and respiratory effort absent, flaccid, no reflex response, body cyanotic.
    2. Heart rate 120 beats/min, good cry effort, well flexed extremities, grimace, body pink with acrocyanosis.
    3. Heart rate 100 beats/min, good cry, some flexion of extremities, pink color.
    4. Heart rate 90 beats/min, slow respiratory effort with weak cry, flaccid muscle tone, no reflex response, body slightly pink with blue extremities.

13. The midwife is assessing an infant's respiratory status immediately after birth. Breath sounds are normal, no retractions present, acrocyanosis present, respirations of 70 breaths per minute and irregular with 5-second periods of apnea, pulse regular at 160 beats per minute, and first and second heart sounds normal with no murmurs. What is the initial interpretation of these findings?
    1. Normal newborn findings for immediately after birth.
    2. Symptoms suggestive of respiratory distress syndrome.
    3. Increased probability of neonatal asphyxia.
    4. Presence of choanal atresia.

14. The midwife is performing a newborn assessment on a full-term infant approximately 6 hours after birth. When evaluating the infant's head, the midwife identifies an edematous area that crosses the cranial suture lines, is soft, and varies with size. The cranial suture lines have minimal space between them. What is the midwife's interpretation of these findings?
    1. A cephalohematoma is present.
    2. The cranial suture lines indicate premature closing.
    3. Molding of the infant's head is present.
    4. A caput succedaneum is present.

15. The nurse is evaluating an infant 8 hours after delivery. The infant was full term, weighed 10 lbs. at birth, and is being breastfed. The mother has a history of gestational diabetes during the pregnancy. What findings indicate the need for further evaluation?
    1. Blood glucose of 50 mg/dL with glucose screening strips.
    2. Respirations of 70 breaths per minute, tremors, and jitteriness.
    3. Bilirubin level 3 mg/dL.
    4. No passage of meconium stool.

16. A 10-day-old breastfed infant is brought to the clinic because the mother is concerned about the infant's "yellow-orange" color. History and findings are as follows: mother's blood type is AB-positive; infant's blood type is B-negative, and total bilirubin 15 mg/dL. The midwife understands that this is most likely caused by:
    1. Hemolytic jaundice.
    2. Breastfed jaundice.
    3. Obstructive jaundice.
    4. Physiologic jaundice.

17. The midwife understands that the test ordered for all newborns to screen for cystic fibrosis (CF) is:
    1. Serum amylase.
    2. Immunoreactive trypsinogen (IRT).
    3. Sweat chloride test.
    4. DNA analysis.

18. Why does an infant have increased loss of scalp hair 2 to 4 months after delivery?
    1. Increased number of hairs in telogen.
    2. Hyperthyroidism.
    3. Fatigue.
    4. Sudden postpartum cardiovascular changes.

19. When does the anterior fontanel close?
    1. 2 months.
    2. 12 months.
    3. 18 months.

20. An infant of a diabetic mother is a risk for all of the following *except*:
    1. Respiratory distress syndrome.
    2. Stillbirth.
    3. Anemia.
    4. Hyperbilirubinemia.

21. A patient delivers a healthy newborn with a cleft lip and cleft palate. Which action by the midwife would promote maternal-infant bonding?
    1. Explain how effective orofacial surgery will completely correct the defect.
    2. Have the mother begin taking care of the newborn immediately after delivery.
    3. Explain to the mother how the problem is not significant.
    4. Show the mother the newborn's normal characteristics.

22. Which of the following statements regarding neonatal apnea is accurate?
    1. It is characterized by periodic breathing.
    2. Prematurity is the most common cause of apnea.
    3. Postterm infants have a high frequency of apnea associated with chronic intermittent hypoxia.

23. A mother presents to the clinic with her 1-week-old infant who has developed a copper-colored maculopapular rash on the palms and soles. There were no associated infections at the time of delivery. The midwife suspects:
    1. Herpes simplex virus infection.
    2. HIV infection.
    3. Congenital syphilis.
    4. Cytomegalovirus (CMV) inclusion disease.

24. The midwife notes tremors in a newborn who was born 2 hours ago at 37 weeks gestation, weighing 5.2 kg. The midwife suspects the tremors are due to which of the following conditions?
    1. Hypocalcemia.
    2. Seizures.
    3. Hypoglycemia.
    4. Hypercalcemia.

25. A woman had ruptured membranes and has been in labor for 25 hours. She had a cesarean delivery due to a stalled labor and delivers a newborn with Apgar scores of 5 and 6 at 1 and 5 minutes, respectively. Physical exam by the midwife notes that the newborn is pale, lethargic, has tachypnea and tachycardia, dry mucous membranes, and sunken fontanelle. Considering the findings and labor history, what is the most likely cause of the newborn's distress?
    1. Sepsis.
    2. Hyperglycemia.
    3. Respiratory distress syndrome.

26. A pregnant woman who is HIV-positive asks the midwife about transmission of HIV. Which statement regarding the method of transmission is most accurate?
    1. HIV is spread only during the postpartum period.
    2. HIV is transmitted in utero only by the fetus ingesting of amniotic fluid.
    3. HIV can be spread via the ingestion of breast milk.

27. All of the following are metabolic disorders that are obtained in a routine screening of newborns *except*:
    1. Galactosemia.
    2. Phenylketonuria (PKU).
    3. Thalassemia.
    4. Cytomegalovirus (CMV).

28. When completing a physical exam on a male infant, the midwife notes drainage of urine from the umbilical cord. The midwife suspects which condition?
    1. Hypospadias.
    2. Umbilical cord infection.
    3. Exstrophy of the bladder.
    4. Patent urachus.

29. When completing a newborn assessment, the midwife notes the following as normal newborn respiratory findings:
    1. Grunting after first respiratory efforts.
    2. Obligate nose breathing.
    3. Respiratory rate 60 to 80 breaths per minute.
    4. No diaphragmatic or abdominal breathing.

30. Which condition is prenatally acquired and associated with microcephaly in the newborn?
    1. Hepatitis B.
    2. Zika infection.
    3. Group B streptococcal infection.

31. Which of the following correctly states the voiding and stool pattern in the breastfed normal newborn?
    1. At day 7, 6 to 7 wet diapers and 3 stools (bright yellow, seedy texture).
    2. At day 3, 3 wet diapers and 3 stools (transitional).
    3. At day 2, 2 wet diapers and 1 stool (green, pasty texture).
    4. At day 1, 1 wet diaper and 2 to 3 meconium stools (sticky texture).

32. The midwife notes that a newborn has a plexus injury. A diagnosis of Erb palsy is made. Which of the following would be noted on the physical exam?
    1. Hyperactive bicep deep tendon reflex (DTR).
    2. Symmetric Moro reflex.
    3. Limp shoulder, adducted, and internally rotated.
    4. Arm flaccid and no reflexes present.

33. Which tool can the midwife use to assess gestational age in a newborn?
    1. New Ballard score.
    2. Naegele rule.
    3. Piaget stage.
    4. Denver Developmental Screening Test II (DDST-II).

34. A newborn has contracted a TORCH (toxoplasmosis, other [syphilis, varicella-zoster, parvovirus B19], rubella, CMV, and herpes) infection. The new mother reports having a cat for a pet. What is the most likely cause of the infection?
    1. Rubella.
    2. Toxoplasmosis.
    3. Rubeola.
    4. Tularemia.

35. All of the following are intrapartum risk factors for neonatal sepsis *except*:
    1. Chorioamnionitis.
    2. Meconium aspiration.
    3. Presence of a cervical cerclage.
    4. Group B *Streptococcus* (GBS) colonization.

36. The midwife is providing discharge teaching to a 20-year-old mother who has had her first male child. Which statement by the mother demonstrates that she understands the discharge teaching regarding his circumcision?
    1. "I will observe the whitish-yellow drainage on his penis, but I will not remove it."
    2. "I will bring him back to the clinic in 3 days to have the drainage removed."
    3. "I will use antibiotic ointment on his penis with every diaper change."
    4. "I will rub the area briskly with a washcloth to remove the discharge."

37. A neonate is being discharged home with a fiberoptic blanket for treatment of physiologic jaundice. What is important to include in the discharge instructions?
    1. Cover the infant's eyes during the treatment.
    2. Reduce the daily number of formula feedings.
    3. Encourage frequent feeding to increase intake.
    4. Expect a constipated stool until jaundice clears.

38. A newborn is suspected of having esophageal atresia with a tracheal esophageal fistula. What clinical findings would assist in validating the presence of a fistula?
    1. Clammy skin and a croupy cough.
    2. Crying and chest retractions.
    3. Choking and coughing.
    4. Chin tug and circumoral pallor.

39. In performing the initial newborn assessment, which finding is associated with Down syndrome?
    1. Asymmetry of the gluteal folds.
    2. Hypertonicity of the skeletal muscles.
    3. A rounded occiput and high-set ears.
    4. Simian creases on the palms and soles.

40. The midwife is assessing a 4-hour-old neonate. Which of the following would be a cause for concern?
    1. Anterior fontanel is ¾-inch (1.9-cm) wide, head is molded, and sutures are overriding.
    2. Color is dusky, axillary temperature is 97°F (36.1°C), and the baby is spitting up excessive mucus.
    3. Hands and feet are cyanotic, abdomen is rounded, and the infant has not voided or passed meconium.
    4. Irregular abdominal respirations and intermittent tremors in the extremities are noted.

41. All of the following instructions are appropriate for the new mother in regard to actions that may prevent sudden infant death syndrome (SIDS) *except*:
    1. Place the infant on the back to sleep.
    2. No smoking should be allowed in the home with an infant.
    3. Use a soft sleeping surface, such as a pillow, placed in the bassinet.
    4. Offer a pacifier at naptime and at bedtime.

42. The midwife is performing a blood glucose test every 4 hours on a large-for-gestational-age newborn of a mother with diabetes. Which laboratory value for the infant's blood glucose would be of concern?
    1. 35 mg/dL (1.94 mmol/L).
    2. 45 mg/dL (2.50 mmol/L).
    3. 50 mg/dL (2.78 mmol/L).
    4. 120 mg/dL (6.67 mmol/L).

43. At a 2-week clinic visit, a mother explains to the midwife that her infant has been having a distended abdomen that "seems to move after feeding." What disorder does the midwife suspect?
    1. Intussusception.
    2. Pyloric stenosis.
    3. Gastritis with colic.
    4. Congenital esophageal stricture.

44. Which statement is accurate regarding thermoregulation in the transitional period?
    1. Newborn shivering produces heat and is similar to adult shivering activity.
    2. Brown fat is located in the abdominal area in the newborn.
    3. Evaporation, conduction, radiation, and convection are four mechanisms used for heat production.
    4. Metabolism of brown fat (brown adipose tissue) functions to produce heat under the stress of cooling.

45. What are characteristic signs and symptoms of an overstimulated newborn?
    1. Yawning, tremors, disinterested in sucking or nursing.
    2. Generalized hypotonia, hyporeflexic DTRs, falling asleep when feeding.
    3. Poor or flaccid muscle tone, lethargy, slow regular breathing.
    4. Cranky, excessive crying, turning head away from mother, moving in a jerky way.

46. Which condition may be characterized by a birthmark or hairy patch above the defect?
    1. Myelomeningocele.
    2. Meningocele.
    3. Spina bifida occulta.
    4. Spina bifida manifesta.

47. The midwife correctly identifies a large for gestational age newborn with the following:
    1. Birth weight less than the 10th percentile.
    2. Birth weight less than the 90th percentile.
    3. Weight 4000 g.
    4. Absent lanugo and minimal vernix caseosa.

48. Retinopathy of prematurity is a potential hazard for preterm newborns. What causes this problem?
    1. Sustained oxygen levels of 40% or higher.
    2. Short exposures to 50% oxygen levels.
    3. Rigidity of the retinal vessels.
    4. PaO2 levels of 50 to 70 mm Hg in the full-term infant.

49. Using the new Ballard scale, the midwife correctly identifies the gestational age of the following newborn: complete Moro reflex with arm extension and open-fingers, frog-like posture, excellent arm recoil, skin wrinkled and dry, overgrown nails, thinning of lanugo, creases over entire sole, breast tissue 5 mm bud, pendulous testes, and deep rugae.
    1. 34 weeks.
    2. 36 weeks.
    3. 40 weeks.
    4. 42 weeks.

50. The midwife understands that an Apgar score of 10 at 1 minute after birth indicates:
    1. An infant in respiratory distress who needs immediate attention.
    2. A positive prediction of cardiorespiratory adaptation after birth.
    3. An infant having no difficulty adjusting to extrauterine life but who should be assessed again at 5 minutes after birth.
    4. An infant having no difficulty adjusting to extrauterine life and ready to be transferred to the nursery.

51. The midwife understands that the following are signs and symptoms of opioid withdrawal in the newborn:
    1. Seizures, a high-pitched cry, skin mottling, tremor, hypertonicity, and excoriation.
    2. Jitteriness, agitation, crying, shivering, increased muscle tone, breathing, and sucking problems.
    3. Hypertension, tachycardia, hyperthermia, agitation, hallucinations, and seizure.
    4. Low birth weight, microcephaly, facial abnormalities, cardiac defects, and fussy behavior.

52. What condition is the infant of a mother with gestational diabetes at risk of developing?
    1. Microsomia.
    2. Shoulder dystocia.
    3. Hyperglycemia.
    4. Diabetes type 1.

53. The midwife determines the 5-minute Apgar score on a newborn who has a heart rate of 100 beats/min, good lusty cry, some flexion of extremities, body pink with acrocyanosis.
    1. 4.
    2. 6.
    3. 8.
    4. 10.

54. The classic triad of congenital rubella syndrome includes:
    1. Deafness, cataracts, cardiac defects.
    2. Deafness, kidney defects, cataracts.
    3. Deafness, cardiac defects, kidney defects.
    4. Deafness, cataracts, cleft palate.

55. On exam of an apparently healthy newborn after a spontaneous vaginal delivery, the midwife notes swelling across the suture lines on the top of the infant's head. What is the most likely diagnosis?
    1. Molding.
    2. Caput succedaneum.
    3. Cephalohematoma.
    4. Subgaleal hemorrhage.

Pharmacology

56. The midwife is aware that fetal exposure to tetracycline causes:
    1. Blindness.
    2. Hearing loss.
    3. Tooth discoloration.
    4. Limb deformities.

57. A primigravida has just delivered a healthy newborn. The midwife is about to administer erythromycin ointment in the newborn's eyes when the mother asks, "What is that medicine for?" How should the midwife respond?
    1. "It protects the newborn's eyes from contracting herpes simplex."
    2. "It provides a lubricant to prevent the newborn's eyes from dryness."
    3. "It is given prophylactically to protect the infant's eyes from bacteria he may have been exposed to during birth."
    4. "It is important to keep the infant's eyes as clean as possible, and the ointment will help flush out any bacteria."

58. A mother has been diagnosed with a TORCH infection. Which medication and corresponding condition is correct for the treatment of the newborn?
    1. Syphilis: pyrimethamine and sulfadiazine.
    2. Herpes: penicillin G.
    3. CMV: ganciclovir.
    4. Rubella: no specific antiviral agent indicated.

59. A newborn is diagnosed with a group B *streptococcal* (GBS) infection. Which medication would be prescribed for this condition?
    1. Ciprofloxacin.
    2. Penicillin.
    3. Chloramphenicol.
    4. Tetracycline.

60. The midwife understands that the following substance when used during pregnancy can lead to cognitive impairment, facial abnormalities, and microcephaly in the infant:
    1. Heroin.
    2. Cocaine.
    3. Marijuana.
    4. Alcohol.

61. The midwife prepares to give phytonadione (AquaMephyton) for the prophylaxis and treatment of vitamin K deficiency in a neonate. What is the correct dosage?
    1. 0.5 to 1 mg IM within 1 hour of birth.
    2. 10 mcg IM within the first 24 hours after delivery.
    3. 0.1 to 0.2 mg subq within 1 hour of birth.
    4. 10 mg subq within the first 24 hours after delivery.

62. Which selective serotonin reuptake inhibitor (SSRI) taken during pregnancy is associated with cardiac defects in the newborn?
    1. Duloxetine (Cymbalta).
    2. Sertraline (Zoloft).
    3. Paroxetine (Paxil).
    4. Imipramine (Tofranil).

8 Answers and Rationales

Newborn

1. (1) Using a paper or a plastic tape, rather than cloth, prevents error because of the stretching of the fabric. Measurements should be repeated to confirm accuracy. The tape should not lie over the ears.

2. (2) Neonatal screening for PKU and congenital hypothyroidism is done in all states. Other tests are generally mandated by the state or obtained by the provider due to family history. Alpha-fetoprotein is usually a maternal blood test done during the prenatal period to screen for genetic defects, primarily neural tube anomalies.

3. (3) Normal morphology and testes tissue development will be impaired if the testes are not descended by age 1 year. These children are at higher risk for development of testicular cancer in the male young adult (20–30 years old).

4. (4) Acrocyanosis is characterized by a bluish discoloration of the newborn's hands and feet and is considered a normal finding in the first 24 hours after birth. Acrocyanosis may appear intermittently over the first 7 to 10 days following birth when the newborn is exposed to cold temperature. In the newborn, transient periods of duskiness while crying are common immediately after birth. Central cyanosis is abnormal and is an indicator of hypoxemia. Central cyanosis findings include a bluish-purple hue to the lips and mucous membranes, head, and torso. Pseudocyanosis is an uncommon condition that can mimic peripheral cyanosis; however, there is no response to attempted "blanching" of the skin by applying pressure. Pseudocyanosis is generally due to drug exposure (e.g., amiodarone) or exposure to gold or silver salts.

5. (1) Phototherapy is effective secondary to the absorption of the light by bilirubin across the infant's skin. The light energy is absorbed by bilirubin and promotes the conversion of bilirubin to a nontoxic form that can be excreted in the bile and eliminated in the urine and stool. The increase in hemolysis will increase the bilirubin level, and this is physiologic jaundice, which is not associated with an Rh-incompatibility problem.

6. (1) Neonatal jaundice is more common in breastfed infants and is thought to result from the decreased intake in the first few days. It usually begins between 4 and 7 days after birth, and the bilirubin levels range from 10 to 30 mg/dL. Increasing the infant's intake of water does not improve the condition. Breastfeeding may be temporarily interrupted, but phototherapy is usually unnecessary.

7. (4) Bronze baby syndrome describes a grayish-brown pigmentation that occurs in neonates. It may occur in infants undergoing phototherapy but is usually associated with infants who have obstructive liver problems. The pigmentation is not permanent but may last for several months.

8. (1) Infantile colic is unexplained crying and restlessness that lasts longer than 3 hours/day, 3 days a week. Most often it stops spontaneously at approximately 3 months. Other causes, particularly infections, should be ruled out. Spastic colon and lactose intolerance are unlikely and would include problems with diarrhea and constipation. Infant stress syndrome is not a valid problem.

9. (4) With a normal physical exam, in the absence of fever or sepsis, the listed lab tests are not necessary to diagnose colic. If there were positive findings or fever, the complete laboratory workup should be obtained, with the addition of urinalysis and lumbar puncture.

10. (2) After the infant has been carefully evaluated and there is no evidence of other problems, it is important to explain to the parents that no medication is available to treat the condition. The condition is not resolved by changing the feeding schedule of the infant nor is it related to stress within the home, and a change to soy formula will not solve the problem. The parents must be informed that the colic most often resolves with no residual problems by age 3 months.

11. (2) The physiology of normal vaginal delivery causes pressure against the infant's thorax and helps remove amniotic fluid. If the cesarean section was done as an emergency before term, the infant may have inadequate surfactant for good pulmonary function. A cesarean delivery does not increase the risk of elevated bilirubin, meconium aspiration, or hypoglycemia.

12. (4) The Apgar score permits a rapid assessment of the newborn's transition to extrauterine life based on five signs that indicate the physiologic state of the neonate. In this instance, the newborn's score is based on: (1) heart rate under 100 (score 1); (2) respiratory effort, slow with weak cry (score 1); (3) muscle tone, flaccid (score 0); (4) reflex irritability, no response (score 0); and (5) body pink with acrocyanosis (score 1).

13. (1) These are normal newborn findings. The respiratory rate is increased but is usually increased immediately after birth (transient tachypnea) and during the second period of reactivity. Continued tachypnea is abnormal. The respiratory rate should be counted for a full minute because of the irregularity of the infant's breathing. Periodic pauses may occur for up to 10 seconds, but apnea lasting longer than 20 seconds is abnormal. Acrocyanosis is normal immediately after birth. Choanal atresia occurs when one or both of the nasal passages are blocked by an abnormality of the septum. In respiratory distress syndrome, the infant exhibits other symptoms that are consistent with hypoxia.

14. (4) Caput succedaneum results from pressure against the mother's cervix during labor. The edematous area crosses the suture lines and will resolve within hours to days after birth. There is normally a space between the cranial suture lines; if there is no space or an overriding suture line, it may be caused by molding. Widening of the suture line may indicate increased intracranial pressure. Cephalohematoma is characterized by bleeding between the bone and the periosteum, and it does not cross the suture line.

15. (2) Early signs of hypoglycemia are jitteriness, poor muscle tone, tremors, and symptoms of respiratory difficulty. The blood sugar of 50 mg/dL is within normal limits at this time (40–60 mg/dL the first 24 hours). If blood sugar levels are less than 45 mg/dL on the screening strip, a follow-up serum glucose should be done. The meconium stool should be passed within the first 24 hours, and the bilirubin level is normal.

16. (2) This is a type of exaggerated physiologic jaundice that occurs frequently in breastfed babies because of the infant's inadequate caloric intake before the mother's milk comes in. It typically occurs between 7 and 15 days of life, whereas physiologic jaundice occurs most often between the second and fourth day of life. Hemolytic jaundice occurs in an Rh-negative mother who has an Rh-positive infant who becomes isoimmunized.

17. (2) In all states cystic fibrosis (CF) newborn screening starts with evaluating infants for an elevated serum IRT, which is a biomarker for trypsinogen. When there is blockage in the pancreatic exocrine ducts that occurs in CF, this prevents the release of trypsinogen in the small intestine. The increased circulating trypsinogen is because of blockage cause by decreased CF transmembrane conductance regulator activity, which is a protein that acts on the chloride channel. If the infant's serum Immunoreactive trypsinogen (IRT) is elevated, a second step is required, which is DNA analysis looking for common mutations. If one or more mutations are found, the infant is referred to a Cystic Fibrosis Foundation accredited care center for sweat chloride confirmative testing. The sweat chloride test has been the primary way to confirm a diagnosis of CF. A sweat chloride test measures the amount of chloride in the infant's sweat. A chloride value of 60 mmol/L or greater has been considered positive for a diagnosis of CF.

18. (1) Normally, 15% to 20% of hairs are in telogen (resting phase of hair cycle). In late pregnancy, this is reduced to less than 10%. After delivery the percentage increases and by 2 months postpartum, 20% of hairs are in telogen; therefore, a marked increase occurs in hair loss at 2 to 4 months after delivery.

19. (3) The anterior fontanel is the larger of the two fontanels and closes by 18 months after birth. The posterior fontanel closes at 6 to 8 weeks after birth. The remaining option is too early for the anterior fontanel to close.

20. (3) Infants of diabetic mothers are at risk for hypoglycemia, hyperbilirubinemia, macrosomia, stillbirth, respiratory distress syndrome, and congenital heart defects. They are not at risk for anemia.

21. (4) When a newborn has visible facial defects, it is important to allow the mother the opportunity to accept that her newborn has a congenital defect before encouraging her and assisting her to take care of the newborn. It is helpful to point out and show her the normal characteristics of the newborn, which allows her to put the cleft lip and cleft palate problem in perspective. The congenital defect is significant, and the mother will focus on the defect, so it is not helpful to explain that the problem is insignificant. Orofacial surgery will provide closure of the defect but will not completely correct due to scarring that occurs.

22. (2) Prematurity is the most common cause of apnea. Periodic breathing is a normal neonatal breathing pattern, defined by 3 or more pauses, each 3 or more seconds, with less than 20 seconds of regular respiration between pauses. Preterm infants (not postterm) with a high frequency of apnea associated with chronic intermittent hypoxia need prolonged respiratory support.

23. (3) The rash of congenital syphilis is bullous, peeling and/or maculopapular (copper-red) with or without desquamation, "blueberry muffin" spots, with symmetric distribution on palms and soles (but can be generalized), and petechiae. The lesions may extend over the trunk and extremities. This rash is not an indication that the neonate has contracted CMV because the rash associated with CMV is petechial or purpuric in appearance and often the neonate is asymptomatic. The HIV-infected neonate is asymptomatic at birth for the first 2 to 3 months. The "classic" herpes simplex virus rash consists

of vesicles on an erythematous base, which subsequently ulcerate, become friable, and bleed easily.

24. (3) The newborn weighs 5.2 kg (11.5 lbs.). A newborn diagnosed with fetal macrosomia has a birth weight of more than 8 lbs., 13 oz (4000 g), regardless of his or her gestational age. A newborn diagnosed with macrosomia is more likely to be born with a blood sugar level that is lower than normal. Symptoms of hypoglycemia in a newborn are cyanosis, tremors, shakiness, irritability or listlessness, hypothermia, poor feeding, and hypotonia. Symptoms of hypocalcemia include hypotonia, tachycardia, tachypnea, apnea, poor feeding, jitteriness, tetany, and seizures. Symptoms and signs of neonatal hypercalcemia include anorexia, gastroesophageal reflux, nausea, vomiting, lethargy or seizures or generalized irritability, and hypertension.

25. (1) Early onset sepsis occurs due to prolonged rupture of membranes and the increased risk for infection that a neonate has due to their immature immune system. The physical exam findings of paleness, lethargy, tachypnea, tachycardia, dry mucous membranes, and sunken fontanelle suggest sepsis, along with hypothermia, irritability, poor sucking reflex, hypotension, and abdominal distention. Hypoglycemia and meconium aspiration syndrome would be included in a differential diagnosis. With respiratory distress syndrome, the physical exam would reveal tachypnea, grunting, nasal flaring, subcostal and intercostal retractions, decreased breath sounds, and cyanosis.

26. (3) HIV can be transmitted in breast milk. Women with HIV should not breastfeed their babies. Infant formula is a safe and healthy alternative to breast milk, especially for women in the United States who have access to clean water. Women who take HIV medicines during pregnancy and childbirth and whose babies receive HIV medicines for 4 to 6 weeks after birth have a low risk of vertical (mother to child) transmission of HIV.

27. (4) Galactosemia, phenylketonuria (PKU), and thalassemia are just three of the many tests that are part of a newborn screening tests. Cytomegalovirus (CMV) screening is not part of the battery of tests.

28. (4) The male infant has a patent urachus, which is the persistence of a fetal opening between the bladder and the umbilical cord. The condition can be treated surgically. Exstrophy of the bladder is a rare birth defect in which the bladder develops outside the fetus and can be repaired surgically. The condition is more common in male infants than in female infants. Hypospadias is a congenital birth defect in which the opening of the urethra is on the underside of the penis instead of at the tip or end of the penis. Signs of infection would not be urine, but purulent drainage.

29. (2) Newborns are obligate nose breathers (breathe through nose not mouth). Respiratory rate is 40 to 60 breaths per minute. Respiratory distress is characterized by increased rate, nasal flaring, grunting, and intercostal retractions. Diaphragmatic and abdominal breathing is normal.

30. (2) Findings in the congenital Zika syndrome include microcephaly (skull may be partially collapsed), congenital contractures (clubfoot), and hypertonia. Hepatitis B (may cause prematurity and low birth weight), and group B *streptococcal* infection do not cause microcephaly.

31. (1) By days 5 to 7, the breastfed normal newborn should have 6 to 7 wet diapers and 3 stools (bright mustard yellow, seedy texture). At day 3, there should be 5 to 6 wet diapers and 3 stools (transition stools to looser dark green to yellow). At day 2, there should be 2 wet diapers and 3 stools (thick, tarry, black). At day 1, within the first 24 hours of life, the newborn should have 1 wet diaper and 1 meconium stool (thick, tarry, black).

32. (3) Erb palsy is the most commonly encountered plexus injury and is associated with downward force on the head and neck during delivery, leading to upper plexus injuries. Characteristic signs include limp shoulder, adducted, and internally rotated. Biceps and brachioradialis DTRs are absent with an asymmetric Moro reflex. A complete plexus injury ("flail" arm or pan-plexus) is characterized by flaccidity of the entire extremity and shoulder girdle with areflexia.

33. (1) The new Ballard score is commonly used to determine gestational age. Scores are given for six physical and six nerve and muscle development (neuromuscular) signs of maturity. The scores for each may range from –1 to 5. The scores are added together to determine the neonate's gestational age. The total score may range from –10 to 50. Premature newborns have a low score, and post-term newborns have a high score. The Denver Developmental Screening Test II was devised to provide an easy method to screen for evidences of slow development in children from birth to age 6. Naegele rule is a method for calculating gestational age and estimated date of delivery and used in the antepartum period. The estimated date of delivery is calculated by counting back 3 months from the last menstrual period and adding 7 days. Piaget's four stages are marked by important characteristics of thought processes (theory of intellectual and cognitive development).

34. (2) Toxoplasmosis is a disease resulting from infection by the *Toxoplasma gondii* protozoan parasite. Infection usually occurs by eating undercooked contaminated meat, exposure from infected cat feces, or mother-to-child transmission during pregnancy. A person can become infected if they fail to wash their hands after

cleaning a cat's litter box. Pregnant women should avoid handling cat litter and raw meat, consuming raw/undercooked meat, and unpasteurized goat milk. They should wear rubber gloves for meat preparation and gardening. Rubella is the R in TORCH infections, not rubeola. Rubella is also called German or 3-day measles. Congenital rubella infection has been reduced significantly by vaccination. Rubella in the first trimester can cause serious birth defects and is the most common cause of congenital deafness. Rubeola infections during pregnancy for mothers who are not immunized may cause miscarriage, stillbirth, low birth weight, and an increased risk of preterm delivery. Tularemia is not part of the TORCH group of infections and is often called rabbit fever or deer fly fever.

35. (2) Meconium aspiration is an infant risk factor for sepsis, along with low Apgar scores, prematurity, galactosemia, and compromised skin integrity. Chorioamnionitis, presence of a cervical cerclage, and Group B *Streptococcus* (GBS) colonization are considered to be intrapartum risk factors.

36. (1) The whitish-yellowish exudate around the glans penis is granulation tissue and is normal. It will usually disappear within 2 to 3 days. It is not an infection; therefore antibiotic ointment is not appropriate. Soap and water cleansing after each diaper change is appropriate. A small sterile petrolatum gauze dressing may be applied to the area during the first 2 to 3 days (if circumcision was performed with a Gomco or Mogen clamp). If a PlastiBell was used, keep the area clean; application of petrolatum jelly is not necessary; the plastic ring will dislodge when the area has healed (5 to 7 days).

37. (3) Feedings and fluids should be encouraged to promote excretion of the bilirubin. It is not necessary to cover the neonate's eyes when a fiberoptic blanket is used; however, there should be a covering pad between the infant's skin and the fiberoptic blanket. The stool would be loose, rather than constipated, while the jaundice is resolving.

38. (3) The classic three Cs—choking, coughing, and cyanosis—plus frothy saliva and constant drooling are the characteristic signs of esophageal atresia with a tracheoesophageal fistula. The other options are incomplete descriptions of the signs and symptoms.

39. (4) Simian creases, low-set ears, a small depressed nasal bridge, and inner epicanthal folds in the eyes are characteristic of infants with Down syndrome. Asymmetry of the gluteal folds is indicative of developmental dysplasia of the hip. Hypertonicity of the skeletal muscles may be associated with drug-addicted newborns. A rounded occiput and high-set ears would not be classified as abnormal findings.

40. (2) Skin color is expected to be pink-tinged or ruddy, saliva should be scant, and the normal axillary temperature ranges from 97.5°F to 99°F (36.4°C to 37.2°C). Overriding sutures and molding, when present, may persist for a few days. Acrocyanosis may be present for 2 to 6 hours. Passage of meconium and voiding are expected within the first 24 hours after birth. Neonatal tremors are common in a term neonate; however, they must be evaluated to differentiate them from seizures.

41. (3) Parents should use only a firm sleeping surface and avoid very soft surfaces, such as pillows or multiple blankets, which may occlude the infant's airway. Infants should be placed only on their backs to sleep. A correlation has been found between pacifier use at bedtime and a decreased risk of sudden infant death syndrome (SIDS), so offering a pacifier at naptime and at bedtime would be appropriate. In addition, avoid overheating the infant by keeping the room temperature between 68°F and 72°F (20°C and 22.2°C). Secondhand smoke is an irritant to the respiratory tract and increases the risk of SIDS.

42. (1) Hypoglycemia during the early period after delivery is a concern for the infant of a mother with diabetes, not hyperglycemia. Hypoglycemia is defined as a blood glucose concentration of less than 35 mg/dL (1.94 mmol/L) or a plasma concentration of less than 40 mg/dL (2.22 mmol/L) in the newborn. Blood glucose levels should be checked initially between 30 minutes and 2 hours of life and repeated every 30 minutes to 1 hour until the levels are within normal limits. Glucose levels may be monitored every 4 hours until the risk period of hypoglycemia has passed, and the newborn has stabilized.

43. (2) Typical clinical findings for pyloric stenosis are epigastric distention, visible gastric peristalsis after feeding, and a firm ("olive-like") mass palpable in the right upper quadrant (historically 70%–90% of the time). In addition, mothers often report projectile vomiting after feeding, increasing in frequency and severity, emesis may become blood-tinged from vomiting-induced gastric irritation, hunger due to inadequate nutrition, decrease in bowel movements, and weight loss. The primary symptom of esophageal stricture is dysphagia. Intussusception generally occurs in an older infant (>3 months) and is characterized by paroxysms of colicky pain with episodes of calmness interspersed with fussiness, persistent vomiting, and blood stool (currant jelly stools), which represent mucosal sloughing. The history of an infant experiencing gastritis with colic includes nausea, vomiting after feedings (may be bloody), diarrhea (dark or black stools), poor feeding, and weight loss.

44. (4) The metabolism of brown fat (brown adipose tissue) functions to produce heat under the stress of cooling. Brown fat is metabolized and utilized within several

weeks after birth. Heat is generated immediately by shivering; newborn shivering is characterized by increased muscular activity, restlessness, and crying during the transitional period. Newborn shivering activity is not as apparent or similar to adult shivering activity. Brown fat is located in the intrascapular region, in the posterior triangle of the neck, in the axillae, behind the sternum, and around the kidneys. Newborns readily lose heat and body temperature through all four mechanisms of heat loss, including evaporation, conduction, radiation, and convection.

45. (4) When newborns are stressed or overstimulated, they show changes in their body and behavior. The signs and symptoms are changes in color (becoming more red or pale), changes in breathing (becoming more irregular or choppy), changes in movement (becoming jerky or having more tremors), crying and becoming unsettled, grizzle (crying continuously, but not loudly), behave as if they are hungry and want to suck, "spacing out" (going from an alert state to a drowsy state), "switching off" (gaze aversion, or looking away from parent), and "shutting down" (going from drowsy to a sleep state).

46. (3) There are two types of spina bifida: spina bifida occulta and spina bifida manifesta (meningocele and myelomeningocele). Spina bifida occulta is the mild malformation in which the spinal cord fails to close, where the spinal cord or meninges do not herniate or protrude through the defect, and there is no abnormality of the spinal cord, nerve roots, or meninges. Skin typically covers the opening in the spinal cord. There can also be a bulge under the skin where the ends of the spinal cord terminate in fatty tissue. Often a birthmark or a hairy patch is present above the defect. Spina bifida manifesta occurs predominantly in the lumbar or lumbosacral. A meningocele is a herniation of the meninges at the site of the defect in the vertebral column and is typically covered by skin. The newborn's neurologic function tends to be normal unless other abnormalities are present. A myelomeningocele is a herniation of the meninges and spinal cord at the site of the defect, with or without skin or vertebral covering. Because the nerves are involved, there are motor and sensory deficits below the lesion in myelomeningocele.

47. (3) The large for gestational age newborn is above the 90th percentile for weight: 4000 g or greater. Absent lanugo and minimal vernix caseosa are noted in the postterm newborn. A birth weight less than the 10th percentile is the small for gestational age newborn.

48. (1) The basis for the damage that occurs from retinopathy of prematurity comes from the degree of immaturity, the concentration of oxygen, and the length of exposure to oxygen. This occurs with sustained exposure to oxygen above a level of 40%.

49. (4) The findings indicate a postterm newborn of 42 weeks: dry, loose, peeling skin, overgrown nails, absent or bald places of lanugo, large amount of hair on the head, full areola (5–10 mm bud), thick cartilage around ears, visible creases on palms and soles of feet, small amount of fat on the body, tests pendulous with deep rugae and in females labia majora cover clitoris and labia minor, and neuromuscular maturity (frog-like posture, complete Moro reflex), alert and "wide-eyed."

50. (3) The 1-minute Apgar score is a rapid evaluation of the status of the neonate's intrauterine oxygenation. A score of 10 is a good sign of healthy adaptation; however, it is unlikely for a newborn to have an Apgar of 10 at 1 minute. Most newborns do not have an Apgar of 10 at 5 minutes, either. The Apgar must be repeated at 5 minutes of age to evaluate the neonate's response to cardiorespiratory adaptation after birth.

51. (1) Neonates with opioid withdrawal can have seizures, a high-pitched cry, skin mottling, frequent yawning or sneezing, poor feeding and sucking, tachypnea, vomiting, diarrhea, hypothermia or hyperthermia, sweating, and abnormal sleep cycle. Neonatal withdrawal from selective serotonin reuptake inhibitors (SSRIs) may result in jitteriness, agitation, crying, shivering, increased muscle tone, breathing and sucking problems, as well as seizures. Hypertension, tachycardia, hyperthermia, agitation, hallucinations, and seizures are noted in sedative-hypnotic withdrawal. Alcohol withdrawal and fetal alcohol syndrome effects include microcephaly, facial abnormalities, cardiac defects, fussy behavior, jitteriness, increased tone and reflex responses, irritability, and seizures.

52. (2) Infants of mothers who have gestational diabetes are at risk for the following: shoulder dystocia, fetal anomalies, intrauterine fetal demise, macrosomia, birth trauma, perinatal asphyxia, hypoglycemia, and hyperbilirubinemia.

53. (3) The Apgar score permits a rapid assessment of the newborn's transition to extrauterine life based on five signs that indicate the physiologic state of the neonate. In this instance, the newborn's score is based on: (1) heart rate over 100 (score 2); (2) respiratory effort based on good cry (score 2); (3) muscle tone, based on degree of flexion and movement of the extremities (score 1); (4) reflex irritability, based on a good, lusty cry (score 2); and (5) generalized skin color (score 1).

54. (1) Rubella spreads through the circulatory system of the fetus thereby affecting all organs. Deafness, cataracts, and cardiac defects are the hallmarks of congenital rubella syndrome, although other organs may be affected.

55. (2) Molding is caused by the overriding of skull bones and although it often accompanies caput succedaneum it would not be felt as a swelling. Cephalohematoma

is felt as swelling but it is limited to individual bones, typically parietal bones, and does not cross any suture lines, whereas caput succedaneum crosses sutures lines as a generalized swelling. Subgaleal hemorrhage occurs beneath the epicranial aponeurosis and may extend to orbits and nape of neck; it is very rare, is strongly associated with vacuum delivery, and is typically accompanied by other symptoms.

Pharmacology

56. (3) Tetracycline binds with developing enamel and discolors the deciduous teeth between 26 weeks of gestation and 6 months of infancy.

57. (3) Prophylactic ophthalmic ointment is mandatory in the United States regardless of method of maternal delivery. Protecting the infant's eyes from an infection is the best answer. It will increase the mother's anxiety considerably if she is told her infant could have been exposed to gonorrhea or chlamydia. Instillation of 0.5% erythromycin ophthalmic ointment in both eyes is administered after birth to prevent ophthalmia neonatorum. Erythromycin is used to prevent an eye infection caused by gonorrhea, not the herpes simplex virus, and is given to prevent infection, not for lubrication to prevent eye dryness or to flush out any bacteria.

58. (3) CMV can be treated with ganciclovir in newborns with central nervous system symptoms. Syphilis is treated by administration of aqueous crystalline penicillin G. Toxoplasmosis is treated with pyrimethamine, sulfadiazine, and folinic acid. The recommended treatment for herpes is acyclovir.

59. (2) Penicillin and ampicillin are two antibiotics commonly used to treat group B *streptococcal* (GBS) infection, along with gentamicin and a third-generation cephalosporin (cefotaxime or ceftriaxone). In patients allergic to penicillin, vancomycin and clindamycin can be administered.

60. (4) Infants of mothers who drink alcohol during pregnancy can have fetal alcohol spectrum disorders. Because alcohol is a teratogen, this condition causes brain damage and growth problems. When compared with normal infants, infants with fetal alcohol spectrum disorders tend to weigh less, have microcephaly, facial abnormalities, cardiac defects, and fussy behavior. When they grow up, they have lifelong problems in how they think and act—intellectual disability. Marijuana crosses the placenta, and there is little or no evidence of teratogenic effects. The effects seen in the newborn are a shortened gestation, a higher incidence of intrauterine growth restriction, and fine tremor, prolonged startle response, irritability, and poor habituation to visual stimuli. Heroin crosses the placenta and can lead to "opioid withdrawal syndrome" in the newborn, along with intrauterine growth restriction, stillbirth, infection from mother's intravenous drug use, and congenital anomalies. Compared with cocaine and alcohol, there are minimal long-term effects.

61. (1) Neonates are born vitamin K deficient. To prevent hemorrhagic disease in neonates, it is recommended that all newborns be given an injection of phytonadione (0.5 to 1 mg IM) after delivery.

62. (3) Two selective serotonin reuptake inhibitors (SSRIs), paroxetine and fluoxetine, may cause septal heart defects and the medications should be avoided both during pregnancy and in women considering pregnancy. In addition, the use of fluoxetine and other SSRIs late in pregnancy poses a small risk of two adverse effects in the newborn: (1) neonatal abstinence syndrome, and (2) persistent pulmonary hypertension of the newborn. Duloxetine is a serotonin/norepinephrine reuptake inhibitor and interferes with fetal and postnatal development leading to reduced fetal weight, decreased postnatal survival, and neurologic disturbances. Imipramine is a tricyclic antidepressant.

PART 4 Primary Care

9

Health Promotion and Maintenance

Health Screening and Promotion

1. What is an example of a secondary level of prevention measure for an older adult patient?
   1. Dietary counseling.
   2. Focus on preventing complications related to disease processes.
   3. Assessment of bone mineral density.
   4. Identification of smoking based on self-report of patient.

2. What are the current American Cancer Society (ACS) dietary recommendations for cancer prevention?
   1. Maintaining a desirable body weight and eating a variety of foods, including fruits and vegetables, as well as foods that are high in fiber.
   2. Increasing the amount of protein in the diet.
   3. Alcohol use in small to moderate amounts.
   4. Increase in consumption of fresh fruits, refined grain products, and white rice.

3. Which of the following is recommended by the US Preventive Services Task Force (USPSTF) as an annual screening test for colorectal cancer in a patient who is 51 years old?
   1. Guaiac-based fecal occult blood test (gFOBT) at-home test.
   2. Digital rectal exam.
   3. Sigmoidoscopy.
   4. Stool sample (gFOBT) collected at the office.

4. The American Diabetes Association recommends screening adults starting by at least age 45 years with a fasting plasma glucose test every:
   1. 1 year.
   2. 3 years.
   3. 5 years.
   4. 10 years.

5. Which of these health promotion screenings should be completed annually for the patient who is over age 50 years?
   1. Chest x-ray.
   2. Pneumococcal vaccination.
   3. Colonoscopy.
   4. Guaiac-based fecal occult blood test (gFOBT).

6. QSEN The WHNP/midwife is performing an annual Medicare exam on a 77-year-old patient. Which of the following recommendations would be of greatest benefit in maintaining optimal health?
   1. "Exercise your arms and legs as much as you can each day."
   2. "Sleeping at least 9 hours will improve your energy level."
   3. "Urinate every 2 hours while awake to prevent accidents."
   4. "You should avoid soda and other types of junk food."

7. The WHNP/midwife is discussing making lifestyle changes that will decrease the older adult's risks for cardiovascular disease. Which of the following is most important to include in this discussion?
   1. Decrease smoking, increase vitamin supplements, and increase protein intake.
   2. Control hypertension, stop smoking, maintain normal weight, and exercise regularly.
   3. Maintain normal levels of serum blood sugar and decrease cholesterol intake.
   4. Have a yearly physical examination, increase fiber in the diet, and exercise regularly.

8. Which of the following is an example of a community health promotion activity?
   1. High school–based family planning clinic.
   2. Work-site urgent care clinic.
   3. Asthma follow-up clinic in an elementary school.
   4. Employer-sponsored multiphasic health screening.

9. In a follow-up visit, a new mother asks about fevers, the WHNP/midwife knows that:
   1. Fevers over 104°F (40°C) can cause brain damage.
   2. Most fevers over 104°F (40°C) are usually of bacterial origin.
   3. Children under 6 months of age are especially susceptible to brain damage from a fever.
   4. Fevers may precipitate convulsions in children between 6 months and 5 years of age.

10. A new mother asks about the differences between human milk and cow's milk. The WHNP/midwife explains that:
    1. Human milk has more lipase and linoleic acid.
    2. Human milk has more calcium, phosphorus, sodium, and potassium.
    3. Cow's milk has low protein and casein content.
    4. Cow's milk has high linoleic acid and low saturated fatty acids.

11. When screening for intimate partner violence (IPV), it is important for the WHNP/midwife to understand that the following statement is true:
    1. Only men with psychological problems abuse women.
    2. IPV occurs in a small percentage of the population.
    3. Only people who come from abusive families end up in abusive relationships.
    4. One-fourth of all women experience IPV.

12. A client of Latino heritage is refusing treatment at the clinic and wants a curandero called. What should the WHNP/midwife understand about the practices of a curandero?
    1. Curanderos are folk healers who use holistic healing practices.
    2. Clients who believe in magic and witchcraft want the assistance of a curandero.
    3. Curanderos are religious leaders in Hispanic and Latino communities.
    4. Clients cannot receive medical treatment unless it is approved by the curandero.

13. QSEN The number one cause of accidental death in patients older than 65 years of age is:
    1. Motor vehicle accidents.
    2. Poisoning.
    3. Falls.
    4. Drowning.

14. According to US Preventive Services Task Force (USPSTF) guidelines, which test is considered an important screening test to be done every 2 years for women between the ages of 50 and 74 years?
    1. HIV test.
    2. Colonoscopy.
    3. Mammogram.
    4. Chlamydia test.

15. At what age should a routine screening mammography begin for women who have average risk of breast cancer, according to the US Preventive Services Task Force (USPSTF) 2016 recommendations?
    1. 30 years.
    2. 35 years.
    3. Begin at age 25 years.
    4. Begin at age 50 years.

Immunizations

16. What would be an appropriate postexposure immunization for hepatitis A for an adult over age 40 years who has not been previously immunized?
    1. Immunoglobulin M (IgM).
    2. Twinrix.
    3. Shingrix.
    4. GamaSTAN S/D

17. According to the Centers for Disease Control and Prevention, which two immunizations are recommended as primary prevention for adults ages 60 years and older?
    1. Flu and shingles.
    2. Yearly tetanus prophylaxis.
    3. Flu and human papilloma virus (HPV).
    4. Adult who has had previous allergic reaction to an immunization.

18. The WHNP/midwife understands that the only contraindication to hepatitis B vaccination is:
    1. Pregnancy and lactation.
    2. History of poliomyelitis.
    3. Prior anaphylaxis or severe hypersensitivity.
    4. Mild viral illness.

19. Immunizations and chemoprophylaxis offered routinely to patients age 65 years or older are:
    1. Tdap/Td, influenza, shingles, and PPSV23 vaccine.
    2. Td, varicella, or shingles vaccine.
    3. Td and influenza; for those with a weakened immune system, offer the shingles vaccine.
    4. Offer influenza and Td vaccines to those who have not had these vaccines in the last 10 years.

20. At what patient age should the WHNP/midwife recommend routine use of the single-dose PPSV23 vaccination?
    1. 65 years or older.
    2. 60 years or older.
    3. 55 years or older.
    4. 50 years or older.

21. The Advisory Committee on Immunization Practices (ACIP) recommends that healthy older adults receive the Td or tetanus booster vaccination:
    1. Every 5 years.
    2. Every 10 years.
    3. At age 65 years.
    4. At age 50 years.

22. A 66-year-old woman inquires about her vaccination requirements regarding the pneumococcal vaccine. She received a single PCV13 vaccination at age 65 years because of the presence of risk factors. She has never received any other pneumococcal vaccinations. Which of the following should the WHNP/midwife recommend?
    1. Administer PPSV23 vaccine now.
    2. No further vaccination is necessary.
    3. Administer PCV13 vaccine now.
    4. Administer PPSV23 vaccine at age 67 years.

23. Immunizations recommended for healthy young adults include:
    1. Measles, rubella, varicella, and hepatitis B.
    2. PPSV23, influenza, and rubella.
    3. Tetanus, influenza, varicella, Pneumovax, and hepatitis B.
    4. Influenza, hepatitis B, rubella, measles, and tetanus.

24. Primary prevention of Neonatal Abstinence Syndrome (NAS) includes:
    1. Prescribing a reliable form of birth control for a patient being treated for chronic pain with opioids.
    2. Universally screen pregnant women for substance abuse and make referrals to treatment when appropriate.
    3. Never prescribe opioids to a woman of childbearing age.
    4. Obtain a patient's records from the state prescription drug monitoring program if you suspect she is getting opioids from another provider.

25. The human papilloma virus (HPV) vaccine should be recommended to:
    1. A 40-year-old woman who did not finish the vaccine series as a teen.
    2. Girls ages 11 or 12.
    3. At birth.
    4. Women with compromised immune systems (including HIV infection) through age 50 years, if they did not get the HPV vaccine when they were young.

26. The following person should **not** receive the Shingrix vaccine:
    1. A 62-year-old patient who previously had chickenpox.
    2. A 45-year-old patient who was exposed to chickenpox.
    3. A 50-year-old patient who has a history of having shingles.
    4. A 39-year-old patient who is pregnant.

27. Immunizations recommended for a healthy 40-year-old adult who has had her childhood series include:
    1. Measles, rubella, varicella, and hepatitis B.
    2. PPSV23, influenza, and rubella.
    3. Tetanus, influenza, varicella, Pneumovax, oral polio vaccine (OPV), and hepatitis B.
    4. Influenza, hepatitis A, hepatitis B, varicella, measles/mumps/rubella (MMR), and tetanus.

28. A 30-year-old pregnant woman presents to your office for a routine visit. Her last full-term pregnancy was 2 years ago. She indicates that she wants to make sure that she is up-to-date on all her vaccinations. Which vaccinations are safe for her to have and are also indicated?
    1. Tdap, flu vaccine.
    2. PPSV23, hepatitis A, Tdap.
    3. Tdap, Gardasil, Shingrex.
    4. Flu vaccine, Tdap, MMR.

9 Answers and Rationales

Health Screening and Promotion

1. (3) Secondary prevention measures focus on detection and management of potential disease states through diagnostic testing and scheduled examinations; thus assessment of bone mineral density helps to establish a baseline. Dietary counseling and identifying smoking are examples of primary level of prevention measures because they focus on preventing the occurrence of disease and identifying relevant risk behaviors. Focusing on preventing complications related to disease is an example of a tertiary level of prevention because the disease process is already established.

2. (1) The ACS recommends maintenance of a desirable body weight; research has shown an association between increased mortality resulting from various cancers and varying degrees of being overweight. Another recommendation is to eat a wide variety of foods, consistent with the ChooseMyPlate guide of the US Department of Agriculture and the US Department of Health and Human Services. A variety of fruits and vegetables should be included in the daily diet (make half your plate fruits and vegetables) because research has shown an association between lower cancer rates and high fruit and vegetable consumption. Whole grain foods should be chosen instead of refined grain products and brown rice instead of white rice. High-fiber foods are also recommended; a lower risk of colon cancer is seen in those who consume a high-fiber diet. Currently, there are no recommendations to increase the amount of protein in the diet. Because of the high consumption of red meat in the American diet, many people are already receiving large quantities in their current diets. It is recommended that red meat and processed foods should be limited. The ACS recommends limiting the daily consumption of alcohol to two drinks for men, one drink for women, and no drinks for pregnant women. They also state that ideally, no alcohol should be consumed; regular alcohol consumption has been shown to increase the risk of various cancers.

3. (1) The US Preventive Services Task Force (USPSTF) recommends screening for colorectal cancer using high sensitivity gFOBT, sigmoidoscopy, or colonoscopy beginning at age 50 years and continuing until age 75 years. Of course, a colonoscopy is the best test and it is okay to have a standalone screening of gFOBT, as long as colonoscopy is recommended first. The multiple gFOBT stool take-home test should be used. One gFOBT test obtained by the WHNP/midwife in the office is not adequate for testing. A colonoscopy should be scheduled if the gFOBT test result is positive.

4. (2) The American Diabetes Association recommends screening adults starting at least by age 45 years and repeating the fasting plasma glucose every 3 years. The US Preventive Services Task Force (USPSTF) recommends screening for abnormal blood glucose as part of cardiovascular risk assessment in adults aged 40 to 70 years who are overweight or obese.

5. (4) The guaiac-based fecal occult blood test (gFOBT) will assist in identifying any problems with intestinal bleeding, polyps, and cancer and is recommended to be started at age 50 years. Pneumococcal vaccination is not a screening test. A colonoscopy is recommended at age 50 years and then every 10 years thereafter, not annually. Annual chest x-rays are recommended for adults ages 55 to 80 years who have a 30 pack per year smoking history and currently smoke or have quit within the past 15 years.

6. (1) Maintaining muscle strength reduces the risk of immobility. Immobility is a predictor of loss of independence, depression, reduced quality of life, falling, institutionalization, and death. Sleeping long hours is not associated with improved energy. Optimal nutrition and urinary incontinence are not as great a threat to loss of independence as immobility is. Preventing falls is a Healthy People 2020 goal.

7. (2) Hypertension, smoking, and hyperlipidemia are the major risk factors in the development of cardiovascular disease. Controlling hyperglycemia, increasing high dietary fiber intake, and taking vitamin supplements assist in maintaining a healthy lifestyle, but they are not as important in preventing cardiovascular disease.

8. (4) Multiphasic health screening is a form of periodic health surveillance in which participants undergo a battery of laboratory or diagnostic tests to determine risk factors and disease detection. The other three settings described are not examples of community health promotion activities; they are secondary care settings. The locations of the two clinics are in community settings.

9. (4) Febrile seizures are benign and do not lead to brain damage. Most febrile illnesses in children result from a virus rather than bacteria and are associated with a high fever.

10. (1) Human milk has more lipase and linoleic acid. Cow's milk is not as good a nutritional source as human milk because cow's milk has more mineral content (calcium, phosphorus, sodium, potassium), which causes a larger

renal solute load. In addition, cow's milk is high in protein, casein, and saturated fat, and is lower in carbohydrates than human milk.

11. (4) One-fourth of all women experience IPV. IPV can occur in any primary care setting. Most abused women report that their partner was the first person to abuse them. Many batterers are successful professionals, including politicians, ministers, physicians, and lawyers, as well as men with psychological problems.

12. (1) Latino clients may use home remedies and consult folk healers known as curanderos or curanderas rather than traditional Western health care providers. Curanderos provide a holistic form of healing, which combines prayer, herbal remedies, rituals, psychic healing, spiritualism, and massage. Curanderos believe in the hot and cold theory of disease.

13. (3) Falls are the major cause of morbidity and mortality in the older adult. A fall is often the precipitating event for a cascade of problems leading to death. Complications from falls include fractures, pneumonia, pressure ulcers, pain, and immobility.

14. (3) Starting at age 50 years, a screening mammogram should be performed every 2 years through age 74 years. At ages 75 years and older, the patient needs to check with a health care provider to see if screening is required because of previous findings and current risk factors. Patients should be tested for chlamydia or HIV if they are sexually active and at increased risk. Starting at age 50 years, a patient should be screened for colorectal cancer with colonoscopy every 10 years unless there are increased risk factors or polyps are present.

15. (4) According to the 2016 US Preventive Services Task Force (USPSTF) recommendations, screening mammography in women prior to age 50 years should be an individual decision. Women may choose to begin biennial screening between the ages of 40 and 49 years. Biennial screening mammography is recommended for women aged 50 to 74 years with average risk. The American Cancer Society (ACS) current recommendations are that women aged 40 to 44 years should have the choice to start annual breast cancer screening with mammograms if they wish to do so, and women aged 45 to 54 years should get mammograms every year and switch to every 2 years at the age of 55.

Immunizations

16. (4) GamaSTAN S/D is the only intramuscular preparation for immune globulin (IG). IG is also preferred over hepatitis A vaccine for persons aged older than 40 years; however, vaccine may be used if IG cannot be obtained. Poscctexposure prophylaxis with IG or hepatitis A vaccine prevents infection with hepatitis A virus when administered within 2 weeks of exposure. Twinrix provides immunization for both hepatitis A and B. Shingrix is an immunization for herpes zoster. Immunoglobulin M (IgM), which is found mainly in the blood and lymph fluid, is the first antibody to be made by the body to fight a new infection.

17. (1) The Centers for Disease Control and Prevention recommends that adults age 60 years and older should receive immunizations for seasonal flu and herpes zoster. Yearly tetanus prophylaxis is not indicated because the required time interval for a booster is every 10 years and/or in response to an injury. An adult who has had a previous allergic reaction to an immunization should be further evaluated to determine potential adverse reactions to specific components before any immunization schedule is started.

18. (3) Prior anaphylaxis and severe hypersensitivity would be considered a contraindication; a mild viral illness would not. The patient who is pregnant or lactating may be immunized. A history of poliomyelitis is not a contraindication.

19. (1) The Advisory Committee on Immunization Practices (ACIP) continues to recommend that all adults aged 65 years and older receive 1 dose of pneumococcal polysaccharide vaccine (PPSV23). A single dose of PPSV23 is recommended for routine use among all adults aged 65 years and older. Annual influenza immunizations are recommended for those who are age 65 years and older. Shingles vaccination is recommended as a 2-dose series (2–6 months apart). Tdap for all adults aged 65 years and older is recommended for those who never received a Tdap as an adult because then they would just get Td booster every 10 years because this is recommended at all ages older than 19 years. Boostrix should be used for adults aged 65 years and older; however, the ACIP concluded that either vaccine (Adacel or Boostrix) administered to a person 65 years and older is immunogenic and provides protection. Shingles vaccine is contraindicated in women who are pregnant and in individuals who have a weakened immune system.

20. (1) The pneumococcal polysaccharide vaccine (PPSV23) is recommended in patients without risk factors starting at age 65 years. PPSV23 vaccination is indicated only for those ages 2 to 64 years if additional risk factors or comorbidities are present, including smoking, immunosuppression, or serious disease.

21. (2) Td is usually given as a booster dose every 10 years, but it can also be given earlier after a severe and dirty wound or burn. For adults aged 19 through 64 years who previously have not received a dose of Tdap, a single

dose of Tdap should replace a single decennial (occurring every 10 years) Td booster dose. Persons aged 65 years and older (e.g., grandparents, child care providers, and health care practitioners) who have or who anticipate having close contact with an infant aged less than 12 months and who previously have not received Tdap should receive a single dose of Tdap to protect against pertussis and reduce the likelihood of transmission. For other adults aged 65 years and older, a single dose of Tdap vaccine may be administered instead of Td vaccine in persons who previously have not received Tdap. Boostrix should be used for adults aged 65 years and older; however, the Advisory Committee on Immunization Practices (ACIP) concluded that either vaccine (Boostrix or Adacel) administered to a person aged 65 years and older is immunogenic and would provide protection.

22. (1) The Advisory Committee on Immunization Practices (ACIP) continues to recommend that all adults aged 65 years and older receive 1 dose of PPSV23. If a patient wants to receive both PCV13 and PPSV23, then administer 1 dose of PCV13 first then give 1 dose of PPSV23 at least 1 year later. If the patient already received PPSV23, give the dose of PCV13 at least 1 year after they received the most recent dose of PPSV23. Anyone who received any doses of PPSV23 before age 65 should receive 1 final dose of the vaccine at age 65 or older. Administer this last dose at least 5 years after the prior PPSV23 dose. There is no need to wait to administer the PPSV23 for this patient.

23. (4) A percentage of young adults (5%–20%) are susceptible to measles and/or rubella. Influenza and hepatitis B vaccinations are recommended for young adults who have exposure to a large number of people. Tetanus is recommended every 10 years, especially in high-risk situations (young adults who participate in outdoor sports). PPSV23 is indicated in a young adult who has a chronic disease (e.g., diabetes, chronic pulmonary disease, chronic cardiovascular disease) and is also indicated for young adults who are immunocompromised.

24. (1) Pregnancy prevention is the primary prevention for NAS. Universal screening and referrals to treatment are recommended, but they do not prevent NAS. There will be times when childbearing-age women must be prescribed opioids. Although consulting the drug monitoring program does help decrease health care provider shopping, it does not prevent NAS.

25. (2) All boys and girls ages 11 or 12 years should get vaccinated. Catchup vaccines are recommended for males through age 21 years and for females through age 26 years. It is recommended for men and women with compromised immune systems (including people living with HIV infection) through age 26 years if they did not get fully vaccinated when they were younger. The vaccine is also recommended for gay and bisexual men (or for any man who has sex with a man) through age 26 years. The Advisory Committee on Immunization Practices (ACIP) does not recommend the vaccine over age 26 years but rather promotes shared decision-making.

26. (4) A person should not receive Shingrix if they have ever had a severe allergic reaction to any component of the vaccine or after a dose of Shingrix, tested negative for immunity to varicella zoster virus, currently have shingles, or currently are pregnant or breastfeeding. Women who are pregnant or breastfeeding should wait to get Shingrix. Healthy adults 50 years and older should get two doses of Shingrix, separated by 2 to 6 months. The patient should get Shingrix even if in the past if they have had shingles, received Zostavax, or are not sure if they had chickenpox. There is no maximum age for getting Shingrix. If a patient had Zostavax (the other shingles vaccine) in the recent past, the patient should wait at least 8 weeks before getting Shingrix.

27. (4) It would be important to start the hepatitis B series, considering her age, because this was not included as part of her childhood vaccination series. Hepatitis A is also recommended, especially if the person travels to foreign countries, along with varicella because these immunizations were not available during her childhood. A MMR immunization is required for adults born in 1957 or later who have no laboratory proof of immunity or documentation of either previous vaccination or a health care provider–documented case of measles. Tetanus vaccination is recommended every 10 years, especially in high-risk situations (adults who participate in outdoor sports). PPSV23 is indicated for an adult who has a chronic disease, such as diabetes, chronic pulmonary disease, or chronic cardiovascular disease, and it is also indicated for adults who are immunocompromised. If the adult did not receive the oral polio vaccine (OPV) series as a child, it is recommended to vaccinate the adult with injectable enhanced-potency inactivated polio virus vaccine because the risk of vaccine-associated poliomyelitis is lower.

28. (1) Pregnant women should have a Tdap with each pregnancy (usually in the third trimester, preferably at 27–36 weeks) due to risk of exposure to infant once they are born. Flu shot is indicated every flu season. Hepatitis is only needed if there is a risk of exposure. PPSV23 is indicated for 65 years of age and older patients, unless a younger patient is at an increased risk of serious pneumococcal infection. Gardasil is indicated for ages 9 to 26 years. HPV vaccination is not recommended until after pregnancy. Shingrex is for shingles and is indicated for patients over 50 years of age. MMR is for children ages 6 months to 10 years of age—if there is any question of immunity, a titer followed by a booster for MMR is appropriate. An MMR is given to a woman planning to get pregnant, who has not been vaccinated, and should be administered at least 1 month before becoming pregnant.

10

Cardiovascular

Disorders

1. The diagnosis of hypertension (HTN) should be established on the basis of:
   1. An average of two or more readings taken during at least two separate clinic visits.
   2. At least five readings 1 month apart.
   3. One reading of 140 mm Hg systolic blood pressure (BP) and 90 mm Hg diastolic BP or higher.
   4. One reading taken in three different positions.

2. A 60-year-old woman presents to the clinic for ongoing management of HTN. Which physical finding, if noted by the WHNP/midwife, would warrant further inquiry?
   1. 20/20 vision screening.
   2. Presence of nosebleeds.
   3. Brisk capillary refill bilaterally.
   4. Occasional nonproductive cough in response to self-identified seasonal allergies.

3. What are the cardiovascular risk factors predisposing a woman to cardiovascular disease (CVD)?
   1. Absence of estrogen adversely affects lipoprotein metabolism.
   2. Fat deposited on the hips mobilizes, raising serum cholesterol.
   3. Coronary arteries are longer and wider in diameter.
   4. Resting ejection fraction is lower.

4. The WHNP/midwife is planning the treatment of an older adult patient newly diagnosed with hypertension (HTN). What parameters are most important in determining the appropriate pharmacologic therapy?
   1. Determine medications and dosage on the basis of the patient's weight, age, and drug availability.
   2. Begin treatment using diuretics.
   3. Initiate lifestyle changes before beginning medications.
   4. Determine other medical conditions for which the patient is being treated.

5. Which of the following would be appropriate dietary therapy recommendations for a patient with hyperlipidemia?
   1. Limiting intake of salt, sweets, and sugar-sweetened beverages.
   2. Increasing the average daily protein intake to 70 g/day.
   3. Decreasing total fat to less than 37% of the daily total calories per day.
   4. Limiting carbohydrate intake.

6. In an overweight older adult female patient with an elevated cholesterol level and abnormal lipoprotein profile, the first step in treatment includes:
   1. Prescribing a bile acid sequestrant agent.
   2. Initiation of a diet and exercise program.
   3. Prescribe statin therapy.
   4. Referral to a cardiologist.

7. Which of the following would **not** be considered as contributing to the development of thrombophlebitis?
   1. Excessive use of oral anticoagulants.
   2. Trauma to the leg or arm.
   3. Recent intravenous therapy.
   4. Secondary to pregnancy.

8. A patient describes to the WHNP/midwife that she experiences "white coat syndrome." What does this signify?
   1. BP reading in the clinic is higher than BP at home.
   2. BP at home that is higher than BP in the office.
   3. BP that only increases early in the morning on awakening.
   4. BP that is higher in the right arm when taking a home measurement.

Pharmacology

9. An adult patient who is being treated for hyperlipidemia prefers to take a "natural" medication approach. On the basis of this patient's request, the WHNP/midwife would order which medication?
   1. Ezetimibe (Zetia).
   2. Gemfibrozil (Lopid).
   3. Colesevelam (Welchol).
   4. Niacin (Niaspan).

10. A WHNP/midwife is reviewing a female patient's medication profile during her annual wellness examination. The patient's past medical history includes recent treatment for hypertension (HTN) that began 8 months ago with a prescribed lisinopril (Prinivil) dosage of 10 mg daily. The patient now states that she may be considering having a child. Which action should be taken by the WHNP/midwife at this time?
    1. A referral of the patient to an obstetrician/gynecologist.
    2. Maintain dosage of prescribed beta blocker.
    3. Discontinue lisinopril (Prinivil).
    4. Decrease the dosage of prescribed angiotensin-converting enzyme (ACE) inhibitor.

11. A patient is recovering from an acute episode of thrombophlebitis and is being treated with warfarin (Coumadin) 5 mg by mouth daily. In reviewing the patient's medication information, the WHNP/midwife would include what information in her teaching?
    1. Do not take a multivitamin supplement.
    2. Limit dairy products.
    3. Aerobic exercises are the most effective.
    4. Maintain a daily record of intake and output.

12. The WHNP/midwife has prescribed losartan (Cozaar) 50 mg by mouth daily. This medication promotes vasodilation by:
    1. Blocking the action of angiotensin II.
    2. Promoting release of aldosterone.
    3. Promoting synthesis of prostaglandin.
    4. Inhibiting calcium influx into smooth muscle cells.

13. The WHNP/midwife, in using best practice, should discuss which methods of prevention for patients who are over age 40 years with a history of CVD risk factors?
    1. ACE inhibitor medication and potassium chloride.
    2. A beta blocker.
    3. Aspirin 81 mg daily in conjunction with a statin.
    4. Lifestyle modification with diet, exercise, and smoking cessation.

14. A patient with a history of hypertension (HTN) is started on spironolactone (Aldactone) 50 mg by mouth daily. The WHNP/midwife instructs the patient to call the clinic if which symptoms are experienced?
    1. Increased irritability, abdominal cramping, and lower extremity weakness.
    2. Decreased reflex response, nausea, and vomiting.
    3. Muscle twitching, numbness, tingling, burning sensations of the limbs, and diarrhea.
    4. Weight gain, excessive thirst, and fever.

15. A patient with a serum cholesterol level of 256 mg/dL, high-density lipoprotein (HDL) of 38 mg/dL, and low-density lipoprotein (LDL) of 172 mg/dL is instructed on dietary modifications and taking niacin (nicotinic acid) 1 g by mouth three times daily. Specific instructions include:
    1. Limiting daily fluid intake.
    2. Taking measures to minimize flushing.
    3. Administering the drug 1 hour after eating.
    4. Avoid exposure to direct sunlight.

16. When monitoring for the therapeutic effects of verapamil (Calan SR), the WHNP/midwife would assess for:
    1. Increase in heart rate.
    2. Decrease in systemic vascular resistance.
    3. Increase in BP.
    4. Decrease in ventricular premature beats.

17. A 45-year-old African American patient with essential hypertension (HTN) is treated by the WHNP/midwife with sodium restriction and chlorothiazide (Diuril) 25 mg by mouth daily. There is no history of diabetes or chronic kidney disease. After 3 months of therapy, the patient's BP is measured at 160/110 mm Hg. Which of the following is the next best step in the plan of care?
    1. Begin enalapril (Vasotec) 5 mg daily.
    2. Begin 50 mg of metoprolol (Toprol XL) daily.
    3. Add 5 mg of amlodipine (Norvasc) daily.
    4. Discontinue Diuril and change to captopril (Capoten) 50 mg three times daily.

18. The WHNP/midwife initiates antihypertensive therapy for a middle-aged nonsmoking woman. One week later, the patient returns for a follow-up visit and complains of a recurrent dry cough since initiating the medications. This is most likely a side effect of:
    1. Beta blocker.
    2. Thiazide diuretic.
    3. ACE inhibitor.
    4. Calcium channel blocker.

19. A patient who is mildly hypertensive and takes hydrochlorothiazide presents with red, painful swelling of the great toe. In addition to treating the gout, the WHNP/midwife also knows to:
    1. Order laboratory studies for diabetes.
    2. Explore for possible alcohol abuse.
    3. Advise patient to lose weight.
    4. Change the patient's thiazide antihypertensive medication.

20. The patient is instructed to take the lovastatin daily:
    1. In the morning with breakfast.
    2. 30 minutes before eating breakfast.
    3. In the evening.
    4. Around noon.

10 Answers and Rationales

Disorders

1. (1) A diagnosis of HTN based on a single measurement of BP elevation should not be done. A minimum of two readings on two or more separate occasions with an average greater than or equal to systolic BP of 140 mm Hg and diastolic BP of 90 mm Hg establishes the diagnosis. The 2017 American College of Cardiology guidelines recommend out of office BP measurements, as well as ambulatory BP monitoring to assist diagnosis. An average of two or more readings taken at each of two or more visits should follow an initial screening. The patient should be seated with the arm at heart level. No caffeine or nicotine ingestion should be allowed for 30 minutes before the reading. The room should be quiet for at least 5 minutes, and an appropriate cuff should be used.

2. (2) Clinical confirmation of nosebleeds in a patient who already has a diagnosis of HTN may be significant. As such, the WHNP/midwife should follow this physical symptom for its potential impact on the patient's vascular status. A 20/20 vision screening and brisk capillary refill bilaterally are normal findings. An occasional nonproductive cough in response to the patient's self-identified seasonal allergies is considered a normal finding.

3. (1) Cardiovascular risk factors predisposing women to cardiovascular disease (CVD) include smaller body size, declining estrogen level, heart, and thoracic cavity smaller and lighter, coronary arteries smaller in diameter, shorter PR interval, and a higher resting ejection fraction. Increased body fat percentage and fat distributed in the abdomen may be mobilized more easily in response to stress. This may raise serum cholesterol and blood glucose levels. Females after menopause are more likely to develop microvascular disorders as well from the reduction of estrogen. Estrogen levels can also fall in younger women suffering from persistent stress. This may lead to increased risk of CVD.

4. (4) The WHNP/midwife must consider the geriatric patient's other medical problems and treatment along with race before prescribing medications for hypertension (HTN). Frequently, geriatric patients cannot take beta blockers because of chronic pulmonary conditions; they may already be taking diuretics for problems of fluid retention. Therapy is individualized and should include consideration of existing comorbidities. Lifestyle changes should be initiated, and medications adjusted as changes are made.

5. (1) The adult treatment panel (i.e., ATP IV), the American College of Cardiology, and American Heart Association cholesterol guidelines recommend lifestyle modifications for patients with hyperlipidemia, including increasing vegetables, fruits, and whole grains, and limiting sodium, sweets and sugar-sweetened drinks, red meats, and saturated fats, and should include less than 10% of unsaturated fat. The amount of fat in the average diet should be between 20% and 35% of the total calories. Daily protein intake should be between 10% and 35%. Carbohydrate intake should be monitored in the maintenance of a healthy weight.

6. (2) Diet and exercise are the mainstays of any treatment program and would be used initially in all cases. First-line pharmacologic treatment is statin therapy, and the choice of a high- or moderate-intensity statin is based on calculated cardiovascular risk. A bile acid sequestrant agent, ezetimibe, or PCSK9 inhibitors may be added if no improvement is seen with diet and exercise therapy plus statin therapy. Referral to a cardiologist is not necessary unless the patient develops symptoms or shows resistance to treatment.

7. (1) Superficial inflammation of a vein may be caused by trauma (e.g., blow to the arm or leg) or recent intravenous therapy with irritating fluids, or it may occur secondary to pregnancy, especially during the postpartum period because of the increase in clotting factors (thromboplastin). Excessive use of oral anticoagulants can lead to bleeding but not to thrombophlebitis. Deep vein thrombosis associated with thrombophlebitis results from prolonged bed rest, major surgical procedures, injury to the blood vessel wall, and hypercoagulable states, such as the use of oral contraceptives (especially in women who smoke or have cancer), cancer, and polycythemia vera.

8. (1) White coat syndrome or white coat hypertension (HTN) is when the patient's BP reading in the clinic is higher than BP readings taken at other settings outside of the clinic, that is, at home. Masked HTN is defined as normal BP in the clinic but elevated at home, which is the opposite or reverse of white coat HTN.

Pharmacology

9. (4) Niacin (Niaspan) is also known as vitamin B_3 and as such would be considered to be a "natural" medication approach. Niacin boosts high-density lipoprotein (HDL) levels and modestly reduces low-density lipoprotein (LDL). It is generally only effective at higher doses. The

other medications represent medication classes: a cholesterol absorption inhibitor (Zetia), a fibric acid derivative (Lopid), and a bile acid sequestrant (Welchol).

10. (1) A female patient who is being treated with lisinopril (Prinivil) is being treated with an ACE inhibitor, which is contraindicated in pregnant women in the second and third trimesters. If a woman becomes pregnant on an ACE inhibitor, research has not shown adverse effects to the fetus in the first trimester, but the medication should be discontinued. A referral is indicated at this time because the patient is considering pregnancy and is discussing potential concerns at this time. The obstetrician/gynecologist will more than likely order an antihypertensive drug considered safe during pregnancy, such as methyldopa or labetalol. A change in BP medication is warranted at this time on the basis of the patient's voiced concerns. The medication should not be discontinued or dosage decreased until the patient has met with the obstetrician/gynecologist.

11. (1) Vitamin K is an antidote for warfarin. Also, multivitamin supplements may contain additional vitamin K. Increased intake of green leafy vegetables could cause an increase in vitamin K levels and decrease the effectiveness of the medication. Patients should be instructed that if they desire eating green leafy vegetables, they may but should eat the same amount each day. The warfarin dose may need to be higher than those who do not need greens, but this is acceptable. Eating varying amounts of greens will lead to inconsistent international normalized ratio (INR) results.

12. (1) Angiotensin II receptor blockers (ARBs), such as losartan (Cozaar), block access of angiotensin II to its receptors in blood vessels, the adrenals, and all other tissues. By blocking the action of angiotensin II, losartan relaxes muscle cells and dilates blood vessels (arterioles and veins), thereby reducing BP. By blocking angiotensin II receptors in the adrenals, ARBs decrease the release of aldosterone, which increases renal excretion of sodium and water. Sodium and water excretion are further increased through dilation of renal blood vessels.

13. (4) Previously, best practice for patients with a history of CVD risk factors was to start low-dose aspirin therapy in conjunction with a statin to help reduce the risk of potential cardiac events. In 2019, the American College of Cardiology released new guidelines on primary prevention of cardiovascular disease (CVD). Aspirin therapy is no longer recommended for the prevention of disease unless the patient is at high risk. In older adults, aspirin risk may outweigh the benefit because of bleeding risk. Statin therapy is also determined by level of risk. Lifestyle modifications are recommended. Initiating an ACE inhibitor medication and potassium chloride would be contraindicated because the mechanism of action of an ACE inhibitor would lead to hyperkalemia. Initiation of a loop diuretic and beta blocker or a beta blocker and a thiazide diuretic would not be warranted unless there is specific clinical evidence to support this therapy.

14. (3) Aldactone is a potassium-sparing diuretic. Patients should be instructed on the early signs of hyperkalemia, which include muscle twitching, numbness, tingling, and burning sensations of the limbs; diarrhea; palpitations; and skipped heartbeats. Hypokalemia symptoms are characterized by irritability; confusion followed by lethargy, abdominal cramping, distention, and constipation; and lower extremity weakness.

15. (2) Niacin can cause vasodilation, leading to intense flushing of the face, neck, and ears. The flushing can be mitigated by gradually increasing the dose, taking the medication with food, or by taking 325 mg of aspirin 30 minutes prior to each dose. Aspirin reduces flushing by preventing synthesis of prostaglandins, which mediate the flushing response. Antihyperlipidemic drugs may cause constipation. Antihyperlipidemic effectiveness is enhanced when the drug is taken before or with meals.

16. (2) Calcium channel blockers (1) depress the rate of discharge from the sinoatrial node and conduction velocity through the atrioventricular node, causing a decrease in heart rate; (2) relax the coronary and systemic arteries, producing vasodilation (decrease in afterload and BP); and (3) decrease myocardial contractility (negative inotropic effect).

17. (3) According to the Eighth Joint National Committee, initial antihypertensive treatment should include a thiazide diuretic, calcium channel blocker, ACE inhibitor, or ARB in the general nonblack population or a thiazide diuretic or calcium channel blocker in the general black population. African American patients without diabetes or chronic kidney disease (CKD) should be prescribed calcium channel blockers alone or in combination with a thiazide-type diuretic in the treatment of HTN. Amlodipine (Norvasc) is a calcium channel blocker. A combination drug is valsartan, which has amlodipine and hydrochlorothiazide, a thiazide diuretic. Enalapril and captopril are ACE inhibitors, which should be used with caution in African Americans as they may be at increased risk for the development of angioedema. Metoprolol is a beta blocker and not recommended in the Eighth Joint National Committee guidelines for the treatment of hypertension (HTN) unless comorbidities, such as atrial fibrillation, exist.

18. (3) Adverse side effects of ACE inhibitors include cough (1%–30% of patients), headache, dizziness, and hyperkalemia. Patients who experience a cough side effect should be switched to a different medication. The cough will resolve within 10 to 14 days of discontinuation. Adverse

effects of calcium channel blockers include peripheral edema, dizziness, headache, nausea, and tachycardia. Adverse effects of thiazide diuretics include nausea, vomiting, diarrhea, dizziness, and headache. Side effects of beta blockers include fatigue, bradycardia, impotence, depression, and shortness of breath.

19. (4) The most likely precipitating cause of this patient's gout is the thiazide diuretic used to control hypertension, because it blocks the excretion of uric acid, leading to hyperuricemia. Although gout may be more common in obese, alcoholic, and diabetic patients, these conditions are not indicated here.

20. (3) Because most cholesterol is synthesized when the body is in a state of fasting (between midnight and 3:00 am), hydroxymethylglutaryl-CoA reductase inhibitors (HMG-CoA) (lovastatin) are best taken in the evening.

11

Respiratory

Disorders

1. The WHNP/midwife understands that the following characteristic is more likely to occur when the adult patient has pneumonia (due to *Streptococcus pneumoniae*) rather than bronchitis:
   1. Purulent sputum production.
   2. Nonproductive cough.
   3. Dyspnea.
   4. Wheezing.

2. What would be a priority intervention for a patient experiencing respiratory arrest who has a pulse?
   1. Starting chest compressions at 30 compressions followed by two breaths.
   2. Starting rescue breathing, which is 1 breath every 5 to 6 seconds or approximately 10 to 12 breaths per minute.
   3. Giving oxygen using a rebreathing mask at 10 L/min.
   4. Pinching the nose and giving two breaths.

3. A young adult presents at the college clinic with complaints of tingling in the face and hands, sudden shortness of breath, vague chest discomfort, and concern about a missed menstrual period. The patient appears very anxious and denies any history of respiratory problems. On exam, hands are cool to the touch; vital signs include respirations of 34 breaths per minute, pulse regular at 100 beats per minute, BP 110/76 mm Hg, and normal temperature. Respiratory examination reveals bilateral breath sounds with tachypnea, no adventitious sounds, and normal percussion and visual examination of the chest. What is the best immediate treatment?
   1. Relaxation techniques and encouraging controlled diaphragmatic breathing.
   2. Two puffs of short-acting bronchodilator (albuterol) with metered-dose inhaler (MDI).
   3. Oxygen at 4 L and arterial blood gases after 30 minutes.
   4. Rebreathing into paper bag to increase $Paco_2$ levels.

4. An adult patient arrives at the family practice clinic complaining of difficulty breathing, a cough, and chest pain. History indicates that she was discharged from the hospital 2 days ago after a cesarean section and has a 15-pack per year smoking history. What would be an appropriate action?
   1. Obtain a sputum specimen for culture and sensitivity.
   2. Order a chest x-ray, pulmonary CT scan, and angiogram.
   3. Perform spirometry testing.
   4. Immediately transfer to the emergency department.

5. The WHNP/midwife is aware that the flu or influenza:
   1. Can be caused by receiving a live attenuated influenza vaccine when one's resistance is low.
   2. Is characterized by a slow, insidious onset of chills, fever, and muscle aches.
   3. In older adults, may persist for weeks and increase the prevalence of bacterial pneumonia.
   4. Is primarily contagious in the early autumn and spring.

6. An adult patient with a history of asthma calls to tell the WHNP/midwife that she is achieving 65% of her personal best on the peak flowmeter. She is talking in phrases and sounds calm. What advice would the WHNP/midwife give this patient?
   1. Call an ambulance immediately.
   2. Use a bronchodilator now and come in for evaluation in the office today.
   3. Use a corticosteroid inhaler now and every 4 hours as needed.
   4. Refer to a pulmonologist.

7. An older adult patient presents with signs and symptoms that suggest community-acquired pneumonia (CAP). What might the WHNP/midwife assess specific to an older adult patient with this condition?
   1. Chest pain with inspiration.
   2. Confusion/disorientation with or without a low-grade fever.
   3. Productive cough.
   4. Fever with leukocytosis.

8. In developing a plan for a healthy older patient with typical pneumonia, the WHNP/midwife understands that 60% to 65% of community-acquired pneumonia (CAP) is caused by which organism?
   1. *Hemophilus influenzae.*
   2. *Klebsiella pneumoniae.*
   3. *Mycobacterium tuberculosis.*
   4. *Streptococcus pneumoniae.*

9. What would be most appropriate to include in the health promotion plan for an older adult patient who is at risk for developing pneumonia?
   1. Administer the pneumococcal vaccine annually.
   2. Administer the influenza vaccine annually.
   3. Sputum culture annually along with a chest x-ray.
   4. Purified protein derivative (PPD) skin test every 3 to 5 years.

10. The WHNP/midwife evaluates an adult patient with a current history of alcoholism. The patient presents with an elevated temperature, congested cough with rusty sputum, and occasional chills. The suspected diagnosis is bacterial pneumonia. The Gram-stained sputum smear would most likely reveal which organism?
    1. *Haemophilus influenzae.*
    2. *Klebsiella pneumoniae.*
    3. *Staphylococcus aureus.*
    4. *Pseudomonas aeruginosa.*

11. The WHNP/midwife knows the following regarding asthma in older adult patients:
    1. Subcutaneous epinephrine is standard therapy.
    2. Spirometry is not needed to diagnose or manage this condition in the older adult.
    3. It can be confused with ischemic heart disease.
    4. Clinical presentation is usually dyspnea, costal retraction, and fever.

12. Clinical signs and symptoms of late-phase antigen exposure in asthma include:
    1. Bronchoconstriction refractory to bronchodilator therapy.
    2. Sneezing, watery eyes, and cough.
    3. Wheezing and increased sputum production.
    4. Bronchodilation secondary to the release of histamine.

13. The WHNP/midwife is assessing a patient for asthma. What is a common clinical manifestation of asthma?
    1. Pruritus.
    2. Diffuse crackles.
    3. Nocturnal exacerbation.
    4. Chronic hypoxemia.

14. During a routine follow-up visit for a patient with asthma, the patient states that she has been doing fine except that when she goes out for dinner, she has increased bronchospasm and wheezing. Which of the following would be an appropriate response by the WHNP/midwife?
    1. "Have you been taking your medication?"
    2. "Do you usually have wine with dinner?"
    3. "I recommend you do not go out for dinner."
    4. "Does going out to dinner make you feel stressed?"

15. A patient reports being exposed to secondhand smoke frequently at their place of employment. The WHNP/midwife knows that secondhand smoke exposure:
    1. Does not increase the patient's risk of cancer.
    2. Decreases with risk of stroke by approximately 10%.
    3. Could cause lung cancer even though the patient does not smoke.
    4. Does not increase the risk of heart disease.

Pharmacology

16. An adult patient with asthma has had uncontrolled symptoms after starting treatment 3 months ago. Before considering any step-up in treatment, the WHNP/midwife should consider that the current treatment may be ineffective because:
    1. The patient continues to use albuterol for shortness of breath.
    2. The patient is only using inhaled corticosteroids (ICSs) twice daily.
    3. The patient is using the inhaler incorrectly.
    4. The patient is taking montelukast concurrently for seasonal allergies.

17. When selecting a pharmacologic agent to assist in smoking cessation the WHNP/midwife recognizes a medication that binds potently with nicotine receptors is:
    1. Nortriptyline (Pamelor).
    2. Nicotine transdermal patch (NicoDerm).
    3. Bupropion (Zyban).
    4. Varenicline (Chantix).

18. QSEN The WHNP/midwife is following up on a patient who is experiencing acute asthma problems. Albuterol (Proventil) by metered-dose inhaler (MDI) (2 puffs) has been ordered as treatment. Which patient response would indicate to the WHNP/midwife that the patient understands how to take the medication?
    1. "I will take 1 puff of the medication, and then wait 1 minute before taking the second puff."
    2. "I will take 2 puffs of the medication every 4 hours, even if I am not short of breath."
    3. "It is important for me to take this medication on a regular cycle to prevent future attacks."
    4. "I will take 2 puffs, one right after the other, whenever I begin to get short of breath."

19. A patient with a history of bronchial asthma is seen in the clinic for increased episodes of difficulty breathing. She has been taking theophylline 100 mg orally three times a day. She is 40 years old and obese with an 18 pack per year history of cigarette smoking and excessive intake of coffee daily. She eats a low-carbohydrate, high-protein diet. Which identified factors decrease the therapeutic effects of the theophylline?
    1. Age and gender.
    2. Coffee intake and weight.
    3. Age and weight.
    4. Smoking history and diet.

20. In adults with asthma, the most common reason outpatient treatment fails resulting in hospitalization is:
    1. Exposure to allergens.
    2. Increased use of steroids.
    3. Improper inhaler technique.
    4. Use of cromolyn inhalers.

21. Which medication is most effective in promoting a decrease in airway inflammation, as well as providing long-term medication coverage in a patient with asthma?
    1. Montelukast (Singulair).
    2. Beclomethasone (Vanceril; Beclovent).
    3. Albuterol (Proventil; Ventolin).
    4. Salmeterol (Serevent).

22. The WHNP/midwife is planning regular daily treatment for a patient with asthma. Which is the preferred medication for the asthmatic patient who is not currently experiencing an exacerbation?
    1. Antibiotic.
    2. Inhaled corticosteroid (ICS).
    3. β_2 Agonist.
    4. Leukotriene receptor antagonist.

23. Patients with asthma need to be instructed to:
    1. Begin inhaled corticosteroids (ICSs) as soon as symptoms appear.
    2. Take 1 to 2 puffs of β_2 agonist as needed using a metered-dose inhaler (MDI).
    3. Use ICSs when they experience bronchospasm.
    4. Start antibiotic regimen when they experience bronchospasm.

24. The WHNP/midwife understands that one of the following over-the-counter preparations in high doses can cause euphoria, disorientation, paranoia, and hallucinations and has been known to be abused by adolescents.
    1. Pseudoephedrine.
    2. Diphenhydramine.
    3. Guaifenesin.
    4. Dextromethorphan.

25. An adult patient is started on ciprofloxacin (Cipro) for an infection. Five days later, on return to the clinic, the patient notes increased pain in her posterior ankle. Understanding the potential complications with fluoroquinolone therapy, the WHNP/midwife knows:
    1. The posterior ankle pain is an unrelated condition.
    2. This is a known side effect and the ciprofloxacin (Cipro) should be continued as prescribed.
    3. This is a known adverse reaction and the ciprofloxacin (Cipro) should be discontinued.
    4. Ciprofloxacin (Cipro) should not be used for treatment of an infection.

26. Which three statements relate to pregnancy considerations with asthma?
    1. Pregnant patients with poorly controlled asthma have low-birth-weight infants, increased prematurity, and perinatal mortality.
    2. Albuterol is the preferred short-acting β_2 agonist (SABA) for pregnant patients.
    3. The inhaled corticosteroid (ICS), budesonide, is the preferred ICS due to its excellent safety profile.
    4. All ICSs should be avoided as they can cause fetal defects.
    5. Long-acting β_2 agonists (LABA) should be only used as monotherapy in pregnancy.
    6. Montelukast and zafirlukast pose a high risk for teratogenicity and should not be used in pregnancy.

27. The WHNP/midwife is teaching a patient about the role of medications in the treatment of asthma. Which statement by the patient would require further teaching?
    1. "My albuterol is my quick-relief medication."
    2. "The salmeterol that I take provides me with long-term control."
    3. "I do not need to use a spacer with my MDI."
    4. "I need to use my peak flow meter to self-monitor how I am doing."

28. A pregnant woman comes in for a follow-up visit for her asthma treatment. The WHNP/midwife knows that a worse outcome of pregnancy-related complications would most likely be caused by:
    1. Regular daily inhaled corticosteroid (ICS) usage.
    2. Increased short-acting β_2 agonist (SABA) due to increased symptoms.
    3. Taking zafirlukast as prescribed.
    4. Poor symptom control.

29. The WHNP/midwife is treating a patient with community acquired pneumonia (CAP). There has been a high rate of macrolide resistant *Streptococcus pneumoniae* in the area. The patient should be started on:
    1. Clarithromycin 500 mg twice daily for 5 days.
    2. Doxycycline 100 mg twice daily for 5 days.
    3. Amoxicillin 1 mg three times daily for 10 days.
    4. Levofloxacin 750 mg daily for 5 days.

30. Which two medications are prescribed and used in smoking cessation?
    1. Cetirizine (Zyrtec).
    2. Valacyclovir (Valtrex).
    3. Varenicline (Chantix).
    4. Bupropion (Zyban).
    5. Lisinopril (Zestril).

11 Answers and Rationales

Disorders

1. (1) Community-acquired pneumonia (CAP) due to *S. pneumoniae* often presents abruptly with high fever, shaking chills (rigor), cough productive of purulent sputum, and pleuritic chest pain. In acute bronchitis, cough is the primary symptom and initially is dry and nonproductive. Fever, dyspnea, wheezing, and possible mucoid sputum production are also characteristic of acute bronchitis.

2. (2) According to the American Heart Association, the protocol for respiratory arrest (has a pulse) is rescue breathing, which is to give 1 breath every 5 to 6 seconds or approximately 10 to 12 breaths per minute. Pulse should be checked every 2 minutes, if no pulse, then begin CPR with 30 chest compressions followed by 2 breaths.

3. (1) The situation described is hyperventilation syndrome; treatment should be concentrated on patient education through reassurance and suggested breathing and relaxation techniques. Albuterol, oxygen, and arterial blood gases are not appropriate initial treatments. Breathing into a paper bag is not recommended because significant hypoxemia and death has occurred in the past from this treatment. This immediate treatment would be followed up with a pregnancy test.

4. (4) The patient is at risk for a pulmonary embolism as a result of hypercoagulation related to giving birth, smoking, and vascular injury (recent surgery). Immediate testing and treatment is critical to survival of someone with a pulmonary embolism, so they should be referred or transferred to the highest level of care available. Assessment reveals common symptoms of a pulmonary embolism: dyspnea, cough, and pleuritic pain. Diagnostic tests include D-dimer test, chest x-ray, ventilation/perfusion scan, CT scan, and/or pulmonary angiogram, which would be ordered at the emergency department.

5. (3) The flu or influenza is a highly contagious respiratory infection that occurs epidemically during the winter months and may increase the prevalence of bacterial pneumonia. It is characterized by a sudden onset of chills, elevated temperature (101°F–104°F [38.3°C–40°C]), headache, fatigue, muscle pain, dry cough, laryngitis, rhinorrhea, and red eyes occurring 24 to 48 hours after exposure directly through respiratory droplets from an infected person or indirectly by drinking from a contaminated glass. Flu vaccines do not cause the flu regardless of being manufactured with a live attenuated (nasal vaccine) or killed virus (injection).

6. (2) According to the Global Initiative for Asthma (2019) guidelines, this patient does not need immediate transfer to an acute care facility because she is not achieving less than 60% of her personal best on her peak flow meter, remains calm, and is speaking in phrases. The patient should use her bronchodilator immediately and be evaluated urgently. If she does not improve or becomes worse, she will need emergency intervention. Inhaled corticosteroids (ICSs) are used for maintenance therapy and are not for "rescue" symptoms. A referral to a pulmonologist may be necessary at some point, but not immediately.

7. (2) Confusion/disorientation with or without a low-grade temperature may be the first sign that the older adult patient has an infection. The older adult patient may not have a fever or leukocytosis; however, leukopenia may suggest severe community-acquired pneumonia (CAP) and require hospitalization. The older adult patient may not experience any discomfort or a cough with the onset of infection.

8. (4) *Streptococcus pneumoniae* is the most common cause of community-acquired and nursing home–acquired bacterial pneumonia. *Haemophilus influenzae* is common in older adult patients with underlying chronic diseases (e.g., chronic obstructive pulmonary disease (COPD), diabetes). *Klebsiella pneumoniae* and other gram-negative bacteria are pathogens in patients with alcoholism, immunocompromised hosts, and hospitalized patients. *Mycobacterium tuberculosis* is an infrequent cause of pneumonia.

9. (2) The pneumococcal vaccination should be given to all adults 65 years or older but is not administered annually. The influenza immunization given annually will decrease complications and hospitalizations for the older adult patient. There is no evidence to support the use of an annual sputum culture or chest x-ray for pneumonia prevention. The purified protein derivative skin test should be done annually for high-risk patients and only detects exposure to tuberculosis.

10. (2) *Klebsiella pneumoniae* is an important pathogen in patients with alcoholism. *Staphylococcus aureus* generally affects older adult patients recovering from influenza and is also common in hospitalized patients with diabetes and in intravenous drug users. *Pseudomonas aeruginosa* is most likely found in someone with structural lung disease (e.g., bronchiectasis).

11. (3) In older individuals, asthma can be confused with ischemic heart disease or left ventricular failure. Asthma symptoms can be discounted as old age or a lack of fitness. Dyspnea, costal retraction, and fever are more likely to be infection. Subcutaneous epinephrine is not standard treatment for asthma at any age but may be indicated in emergency situations. Spirometry is an important part of diagnosis and management in the older adult.

12. (1) Late-phase asthma occurs at 8 to 12 hours after the initial or acute bronchoconstrictive phase. The inflammatory response is the result of mast cell degranulation and the release of inflammatory mediators, including histamines and leukotrienes. The mediators act on the lung by causing bronchoconstriction, vascular permeability, and vasodilation. In late-phase asthma, bronchoconstriction is refractory to most bronchodilator therapy.

13. (3) Nocturnal exacerbation of asthma is a clinical sign. It is linked to variations in circulating cortisol, epinephrine, inflammatory mediators, and vagal tone. Chronic hypoxemia and diffuse crackles are seen in the patient with chronic bronchitis. Pruritus is often seen in contact allergic reactions.

14. (2) Asking the patient about the consumption of wine with dinner is the most appropriate response. Many wines, especially white wines, contain sulfites, which can trigger a mild allergic response.

15. (3) Secondhand smoke is a known carcinogen and increases the patient's risk of lung cancer. In addition, there is a 20% to 30% increase in stroke and heart disease when there is significant exposure to secondhand smoke.

Pharmacology

16. (3) When initiating pharmacologic therapy for asthma, patients should use a short-acting β_2 agonist (SABA) as needed for shortness of breath. Most inhaled corticosteroids (ICSs) should only be taken once or twice daily. Montelukast is indicated for the treatment of seasonal allergies and for the treatment of asthma. Up to 80% of patients use inhalers incorrectly.

17. (4) Varenicline (Chantix) prevents nicotine stimulation of the mesolimbic dopamine system associated with nicotine addiction. Varenicline stimulates dopamine activity but to a much smaller degree than nicotine, resulting in decreased craving and withdrawal symptoms.

18. (1) A 1-minute lapse between the two puffs is necessary for the medication to be most effective. The first puff opens the upper airways, allowing more effective penetration of the lower tract with the second puff. Albuterol (Proventil) should not be used as maintenance therapy. Only inhaled corticosteroids (ICSs) should be taken on a regular schedule.

19. (4) Because tobacco increases the metabolism of theophylline, a higher dose is required in smokers than in nonsmokers. A high-protein, low-carbohydrate diet increases the metabolism of theophylline and decreases serum concentrations. Coffee (and other xanthine-containing beverages) may increase the central nervous system effects of xanthine derivatives.

20. (3) One of the most common causes of outpatient treatment failure is improper inhaler technique. Exposure to allergens may trigger an asthma attack, but proper use of inhalers will control the attacks in many cases. Use of both steroids and cromolyn inhalers have decreased the severity of asthma attacks.

21. (2) Beclomethasone is a long-acting corticosteroid that stabilizes mast cells and greatly reduces mast-cell degranulation when exposed to allergens. Albuterol is a short-acting bronchodilator used as a rescue medication. Salmeterol is a long-acting bronchodilator most useful in controlling nocturnal asthma symptoms. Montelukast, a leukotriene receptor antagonist, inhibits bronchoconstriction and is used as an adjunct to bronchodilators and corticosteroids.

22. (2) Preferred, regular daily treatment (long-term treatment) of the patient with asthma includes inhaled corticosteroids (ICSs) for their antiinflammatory effects. Antibiotics are indicated if there is a concurrent infection, such as acute bronchitis. β_2 agonists are used for their bronchodilator effects and rapid onset of action when a patient may need "rescue" or acute treatment of symptoms with quick-relief medications. Leukotriene receptor antagonist is another option, but not preferred to ICSs for regular daily treatment.

23. (2) Patients with asthma should be instructed to keep their inhaled β_2 agonists with them at all times in case of bronchospasm and use them as necessary (prn). The β_2 agonists are effective in reversing bronchospasm and should only be used for rescue symptoms. Inhaled corticosteroids (ICSs) are long acting and will not give immediate relief, so the patient should be instructed to use them as prescribed. Antibiotics are not indicated for acute bronchospasm.

24. (4) Dextromethorphan is a widely used cough suppressant and is found in many cough and cold remedies. At low doses used for cough suppression, dextromethorphan lacks psychologic effects. However, at doses 5 to 10 times higher, dextromethorphan can cause euphoria, disorientation, paranoia, and altered sense of time, as well as visual, auditory, and tactile hallucinations. Guaifenesin is an expectorant; pseudoephedrine is a decongestant; and diphenhydramine is an antihistamine.

25. (3) Posterior ankle pain is suggestive of Achilles tendonitis. Tendon ruptures are a known adverse reaction to fluoroquinolone therapy, and there have been a significant number of cases in the United States. If tendon inflammation or pain occurs, the fluoroquinolone should be discontinued immediately. Ciprofloxacin (Cipro) is recommended for 60 days as part of empiric treatment of anthrax, as postexposure prophylaxis.

26. (1, 2, 3) Pregnant women with poorly controlled asthma have low-birth-weight, infants, increased risk of prematurity, and perinatal mortality. Albuterol is the preferred short-acting β2 agonist (SABA), and budesonide is the preferred inhaled corticosteroid (ICS) due to an excellent safety profile. SABA is the most effective rescue therapy for acute asthma symptoms. ICSs are the preferred long-term control therapy for patients of all ages. Other ICS agents and leukotriene inhibitors have not been associated with increased incidence of fetal abnormalities. Long-acting β_2 agonists (LABA), such as salmeterol or formoterol, should not be used as monotherapy, as doing so leads to an increased risk of severe outcomes, including death.

27. (3) It is important to emphasize how to take medications correctly. The metered dose inhaler (MDI) usually has three parts: mouthpiece, cap that goes over the mouthpiece, and a canister of medicine. A spacer device will help to avoid getting less medication in the mouth. The spacer connects to the mouthpiece. The inhaled medicine goes into the spacer tube first. The patient takes two deep breaths to get the medicine into the lungs: waiting a full minute between the two breaths. Using a spacer wastes a lot less medicine than spraying the medicine into the mouth. MDI technique is important, as well as understanding the use of the devices, such as the prescribed valved holding chamber, spacer, and nebulizer.

28. (4) Poor symptoms control and exacerbations are associated with worse outcomes for both the baby and the mother. Well-controlled asthma throughout a pregnancy has shown no increase in risk of adverse maternal or fetal complications. Regular daily inhaled corticosteroid usage (ICS), taking zafirlukast as prescribed, and increasing the short-acting β2 agonist (SABA) to treat increased asthma symptoms are all good strategies for asthma control.

29. (2) In the presence of macrolide resistance, clarithromycin (a macrolide) would not be a safe choice. Doxycycline is the best alternative. In cases in which the patient is unable to take doxycycline, a combination β-lactam and macrolide or a respiratory fluroquinolone should be considered.

30. (3, 4) Bupropion, originally marketed as an antidepressant and later for smoking cessation under the trade name of Zyban, is thought to reduce cravings for nicotine and symptoms of withdrawal because of its capacity to block neural reuptake of the neurotransmitters: dopamine, and norepinephrine. Varenicline (Chantix) interferes with nicotine receptors in the brain, which decreases the pleasurable effects of the nicotine and reduces symptoms of nicotine withdrawal. Valacyclovir (Valtrex) is used in the treatment of herpes virus infections, including shingles, cold sores, and genital herpes. Lisinopril (Zestril) is an ACE inhibitor used to treat high three high blood pressure and heart failure. Cetirizine (Zyrtec) is an antihistamine used to relieve allergy symptoms.

12

Head, Eyes, Ears, Nose, and Throat (HEENT)

Disorders

1. An adult patient presents to the WHNP/midwife for evaluation of a "red" right eye for 24 hours. The patient states that when she awoke, the eye was matted shut. The patient denies trauma to the eye, eye pain, and any changes in vision. During the exam, it is noted that the pupils are equal and reactive, and there is mild conjunctival hyperemia bilaterally and a significant amount of yellowish discharge. The WHNP/midwife treats this patient for:
   1. Allergic conjunctivitis.
   2. Corneal abrasion.
   3. Viral conjunctivitis.
   4. Bacterial conjunctivitis.

2. Which of the following organisms is *least likely* to cause otitis media?
   1. *Moraxella catarrhalis.*
   2. *Streptococcus pneumoniae.*
   3. *Staphylococcus aureus.*
   4. *Haemophilus influenzae.*

3. An adult patient presents to the WHNP/midwife's office with the following complaints for the past 10 days: fever and complaints of right facial pain, copious yellow nasal discharge, and acute pain and headache, primarily when bending over. The physical exam is significant for right maxillary sinus tenderness on palpation. The most likely diagnosis is:
   1. Chronic sinusitis.
   2. Acute sinusitis.
   3. Dental abscess.
   4. Giant cell (temporal) arteritis.

4. The WHNP/midwife notes a nasal septal perforation on a young adult. What does the WHNP/midwife suspect as the cause?
   1. Deviated nasal septum.
   2. Chronic epistaxis.
   3. Nose picking.
   4. Cocaine use.

5. An adult patient presents to the clinic complaining of sinus infection and states that symptoms started 3 days ago. The patient is complaining of rhinorrhea/congestion with green/yellow discharge from the nose. The patient reports a slight cough and postnasal drip. The patient denies fever, facial pain, or tooth pain. The patient requests an antibiotic to help him clear up this sinus infection. An appropriate response to this patient's request would be:
   1. "I agree, this is a sinus infection requiring an antibiotic. Here is a prescription for amoxicillin/clavulanate (Augmentin)."
   2. "Before we proceed with any treatment options, we should do some tests first. I will order a CT scan of your sinuses before prescribing any medication."
   3. "A viral infection associated with a common cold cause 98% of sinus infections that clear up on their own. An antibiotic will not be helpful in clearing a viral infection and can actually do harm if taken for nonbacterial sinusitis. Let us talk about other treatment options that will help you feel better."
   4. "I am going to order some blood work. A white blood cell count lab test can help us distinguish between viral and bacterial infections. I will call you with results and treat you accordingly. In the meantime, use a saline nose spray twice a day."

6. A rare complication of streptococcal pharyngitis that leads to contralateral uvular deviation, asymmetric tonsillar hypertrophy, muffled voice on exam but no stridor, drooling, or difficulty breathing or swallowing is recognized by the WHNP/midwife as:
   1. Peritonsillar abscess.
   2. Peritonsillar cellulitis.
   3. Retropharyngeal abscess.
   4. Epiglottitis.

7. A 20-year-old patient presents to the WHNP/midwife's office with a chief complaint of "severe sore throat" for 3 days. The patient states that he also "ran a fever, but does not know how high it got," and has been very fatigued. Physical exam reveals enlarged tonsils with large, patchy exudate; erythematous pharynx; and nontender posterior cervical lymphadenopathy. The remainder of the exam is unremarkable. The WHNP/midwife would most likely make a diagnosis of:
   1. Infectious mononucleosis.
   2. Leukemia.
   3. Scarlet fever.
   4. Oral candidiasis.

8. Which of the following clinical findings is most likely associated with bacterial streptococcal pharyngitis?
   1. Rhinorrhea.
   2. Cough.
   3. Enlarged erythematous tonsils with exudate.
   4. Small oral vesicles.

Pharmacology

9. An adult patient returns to the office of a WHNP/midwife 1 week after he was diagnosed with acute otitis externa and was started on otic ciprofloxacin/dexamethasone (Ciprodex). He explains that his symptoms of pain and itching of his left ear have worsened with the use of the medication. In addition, he now notes a white discharge from his left ear. Exam reveals a mildly edematous erythematous ear canal with white discharge and a normal tympanic membrane. An appropriate treatment for this patient would include:
   1. Continue the current medication and prescribe antipyrine/benzocaine (Auralgan).
   2. Discontinue Ciprodex and prescribe carbamide peroxide (Debrox).
   3. Discontinue Ciprodex, irrigate the ear canal, and prescribe clotrimazole 1% (Canesten) solution.
   4. Continue the current medication and prescribe oral amoxicillin twice daily.

10. When the WHNP/midwife decides to prescribe an antibiotic for the treatment of acute sinusitis, which antibiotic is recommended as first-line empiric therapy for nonpenicillin-allergic adults:
    1. Amoxicillin (Amoxil).
    2. Doxycycline (Vibramycin).
    3. Azithromycin (Zithromax).
    4. Amoxicillin-clavulanate (Augmentin).

11. The treatment plan for a patient diagnosed with infectious mononucleosis includes which of the following?
    1. Resting during the acute phase.
    2. Avoiding exercise during the acute phase.
    3. Corticosteroids during the acute phase.
    4. Ampicillin orally for 10 days.

12. A woman in the second trimester of pregnancy has a positive throat culture for *Streptococcus pyogenes* (strep throat). She denies allergies but becomes nauseated and has diarrhea when she has been prescribed erythromycin. Which of the following is the best choice for this pregnant patient?
    1. Penicillin (Pen VK).
    2. Ofloxacin (Floxin).
    3. Clarithromycin (Biaxin).
    4. Trimethoprim-sulfamethoxazole (Bactrim DS).

12 Answers and Rationales

Disorders

1. (4) Bacterial conjunctivitis presents with infection of the conjunctiva, no pain, and with a history of purulent discharge. Bacterial conjunctivitis is usually in one eye, and viral conjunctivitis is more common in both eyes. Viral conjunctivitis will usually present with acute onset of a red eye with itching, photophobia, and excessive watery discharge. Unlike conjunctivitis with infectious causes, allergic conjunctivitis typically presents simultaneously in both eyes with the predominant feature of itching. The chief complaint of a corneal abrasion is pain.

2. (3) The key factor that contributes to acute otitis media is a dysfunctional eustachian tube. The actual cause is unknown, but it may be sequelae of upper respiratory tract infections or allergies that result in edema of the eustachian tube, or it may result from reflux of nasopharynx bacteria into the eustachian tube. The most frequent bacterial organisms that infect the middle ear, especially in children, are similar to those of the nasopharynx: *Streptococcus pneumoniae*, *Haemophilus influenzae*, and *Moraxella catarrhalis*. *Staphylococcus aureus* is one of the most common causative organisms in otitis externa.

3. (2) The patient is experiencing the classic characteristics of acute sinusitis. Viral causes of sinusitis have improved or resolved by day 10, and bacterial sinus infections persist longer. A dental abscess can cause pain that radiates to the sinuses but more often causes constant, severe, tooth-associated pain and jaw tenderness. Giant cell (temporal) arteritis causes pain in the jaw and face but no nasal discharge.

4. (4) Nasal snorting of cocaine results in nasal congestion and discharge. Because cocaine is a potent sympathomimetic, the nasal passages appear similar to what is found on physical exam of patients who abuse nasal decongestants (e.g., oxymetazoline [Afrin]). Chronic use of cocaine causes the nasal septal mucosa to become ischemic, which leads to tissue atrophy and eventual septal perforation, which is noted on physical exam and should be followed up with questions about snorting cocaine.

5. (3) Most sinus infections are viral. It is recommended to avoid antibiotics during the first 7 to 10 days unless there is strong supporting evidence of bacterial infection, which this patient does not have. A CT scan is not typically taken at the initial visit unless there is treatment failure. All patients with chronic sinusitis should have a CT scan. A white blood cell count is also not helpful initially in most mild to moderate cases. Initial treatment is focused on pain relief, nasal irrigation, and nasal decongestants.

6. (1) Asymmetrical tonsillar hypertrophy with contralateral uvular deviation are hallmark signs of peritonsillar abscess, whereas peritonsillar cellulitis is associated with deep erythema that extends beyond the tonsils and pharynx without structural changes. Retropharyngeal abscess is a deep soft tissue infection that is difficult to diagnose on exam but is frequently accompanied by stridor. Drooling, tripoding, and dysphagia are a classic clinical triad indicating epiglottitis.

7. (1) Mononucleosis is often seen in adolescents and young adults. It often presents with sore throat, fever, tonsillar exudate, lymphadenopathy, and malaise. Leukemia presents with symptoms of fever, fatigue, and weight loss, as well as lymphadenopathy and bone pain. Scarlet fever, a complication of streptococcal pharyngitis, presents with sore throat, fever, abdominal pain, headache, erythematous fine rash, and strawberry tongue. Oral candidiasis presents with white, curd-like plaques on erythematous mucosa. The tongue is red with a white coat.

8. (3) The clinical presentation of pharyngitis varies and depends on the causative agent. Characteristics of bacterial pharyngitis include sore throat, headache, erythema of the tonsils with white or yellow exudate, dysphagia, tender anterior cervical adenopathy, and fever. Small oral vesicles are seen with herpangina, an infection caused by the coxsackievirus. Cough is typically the primary symptom of acute bronchitis; the presence of cough decreases likelihood of streptococcal pharyngitis. Rhinorrhea is associated with allergic rhinitis.

Pharmacology

9. (3) The WHNP/midwife recognizes that the patient's condition is a result of otomycosis, a fungal infection of the external auditory canal that occurs either as a solitary infection or as a subsequent infection associated with the use of antibiotic and steroidal otic therapy. The mainstay of treatment is meticulous cleaning of the ear canal and antifungal therapy. Otic antibiotics must be discontinued, as they may be a causative agent and have no clinical benefit at this time. Carbamide peroxide (Debrox) is used to treat partial or complete earwax obstructions.

10. (4) Amoxicillin has been recommended as a first-line agent in the past because of its narrow spectrum and relatively low cost. However, there is increasing emergence of antimicrobial resistance among respiratory pathogens, including pneumococci and *Haemophilus influenzae.* Amoxicillin-clavulanate rather than amoxicillin is recommended as empiric first-line therapy for nonpenicillin-allergic adults. Doxycycline is a reasonable alternative for first-line therapy and can be used in patients with a penicillin allergy. Azithromycin is not recommended for empiric therapy because of its high rate of resistance of *Streptococcus pneumoniae.*

11. (1) Treatment of mononucleosis includes bed rest while the patient has fever and myalgia (10–14 days), supportive acetaminophen or ibuprofen, warm saline solution gargles, and throat lozenges or analgesic spray. The patient must avoid strenuous exercise and contact sports for 2 months because of the risk of splenic rupture. Splenomegaly is seen in 50% to 60% of all patients with infectious mononucleosis. Corticosteroids are recommended only for patients with impending airway obstruction, and an immediate referral to an otolaryngologist is warranted. Ampicillin is not recommended because of the viral etiology of this disease. Additionally, rashes are common in patients with infectious mononucleosis and are treated with amoxicillin or ampicillin. Approximately 95% of patients with mononucleosis recover uneventfully with supportive treatment.

12. (1) Pen VK is safe to use for strep throat during pregnancy and is one of the most common medications prescribed along with cephalexin and amoxicillin. Pen VK can be used during pregnancy and lactation. The following antibiotics should be avoided during pregnancy: chloramphenicol, aminoglycosides, tetracyclines, and quinolones.

13

Integumentary

Disorders

1. A 65-year-old woman presents to the clinic for evaluation of small rough areas on her face that have increased in size over the past year. She states that she had several similar lesions on her neck removed a few years ago. Physical examination reveals 1 × 1 cm areas of erythematous, scaly sandpaper-like lesions that are yellow to light brown in color above her brow. No discharge is noted. Which of the following should the WHNP/midwife educate the patient regarding lesions of this type?
   1. Risk of squamous cell carcinoma.
   2. Risk of melanoma.
   3. Risk of infection.
   4. The lesions are benign.

2. A 34-year-old female patient presents with an erythematous area of skin on her left buttock. She states that it is painful because it is located along her bikini line. She is worried she may not be able to continue to relax in the hot tub at her apartment community in the evenings. She denies any recent injuries to the area. Which of the following should the WHNP/midwife suspect as the most likely cause?
   1. *Pseudomonas aeruginosa.*
   2. *Staphylococcus aureus.*
   3. *Staphylococcus epidermidis.*
   4. Contact dermatitis.

3. A patient complains of intolerable itching in the pubic hair. On exam, the WHNP/midwife notes erythematous papules and tiny white specks in the pubic hair. The differential diagnosis includes all *except*:
   1. Pediculosis pubis.
   2. Scabies.
   3. Impetigo.
   4. Atopic dermatitis.

4. An adult female presents to the clinic complaining of pain on her left arm. Inspection of the extremity reveals no erythema. Her skin is intact with no evidence of lesions. The patient's past medical history includes herpes zoster. Which clinical diagnosis would the WHNP/midwife make as supported by this patient's presentation and past medical history?
   1. Phantom pain.
   2. Postherpetic neuralgia.
   3. Urinary tract infection.
   4. Tinea infection.

5. What is a chronic skin condition that is sometimes associated with arthritis?
   1. Eczema.
   2. Psoriasis.
   3. Neurodermatitis.
   4. Pityriasis rosea.

6. Which is a true statement about psoriasis?
   1. It is usually worse in the summer.
   2. It is highly contagious.
   3. It can be aggravated by stress.
   4. All patients have accompanying pruritus.

7. What information should be provided to a patient with actinic keratosis?
   1. The affected areas are a normal part of aging and are benign.
   2. These lesions can develop into squamous cell carcinomas.
   3. This is part of an allergic reaction, and the offending allergen needs to be identified.
   4. This skin condition responds well to sunlight, which will help alleviate the symptoms.

8. An older adult woman has an area of vesicles in clusters with an erythematous base that extend from her spine, around and under her arm and breast, to the sternum on her left side. She states that the area was very tender last week and that the vesicles started erupting yesterday. She is complaining of severe pain in the area. What is the probable diagnosis for this condition?
   1. Psoriasis.
   2. Herpes zoster.
   3. Contact dermatitis.
   4. Cellulitis.

9. A patient known to be positive for HIV presents with several painless, persistent, raised purple lesions on the lower arm. What is the most likely diagnosis of the lesions?
   1. Seborrheic dermatitis.
   2. Molluscum contagiosum.
   3. Kaposi sarcoma.
   4. Fungal infection.

10. A middle-aged patient presents for an office visit with a complaint of a symmetrical red rash on her trunk and spreading to her extremities. She was seen several days ago for bronchitis and started on trimethoprim-sulfamethoxazole (TMP-SMX; Septra DS) 1 tab PO bid. What is the recommended action for the WHNP/midwife?
    1. Instruct the patient to continue the medication and see if any change occurs in the rash.
    2. Discontinue TMP-SMX.
    3. Take the patient off medication for 3 days, then restart the drug.
    4. Decrease TMP-SMX to half-dose.

11. A patient complaining of hyperhidrosis should be counseled that:
    1. This is a normal occurrence.
    2. There are no therapies for this complaint.
    3. Bathing in 20% alcohol solution of aluminum chloride hexahydrate (Drysol) may be beneficial.
    4. A history and physical exam need to be completed to rule out any medical etiologies.

12. During the physical exam, the WHNP/midwife assesses a maculopapular skin lesion on a patient's back that is warty, scaly, greasy in appearance, and light tan in color. What would be the probable diagnosis?
    1. Actinic keratosis.
    2. Basal cell carcinoma.
    3. Seborrheic keratosis.
    4. Senile lentigines.

13. The WHNP/midwife is assessing an older patient diagnosed with herpes zoster (shingles) in the prodromal stage. What would the practitioner expect to find on the assessment of this patient?
    1. Erythematous lesions present over four different parts of the body.
    2. Red, pinpoint, painless rash.
    3. Linear burning pain in a line on only half the patient's chest that does not cross the midline.
    4. Painless purulent lesions for 2 days followed by complaints of itching, burning, and nausea.

14. A semiprofessional golfer presents with a dome-shaped, pearly, firm nodule with telangiectasia on her nose. In making a diagnosis, the WHNP/midwife recognizes this to be:
    1. Compound nevus.
    2. Melanoma.
    3. Bullous pemphigoid.
    4. Basal cell carcinoma.

15. An adult female patient presents with an irregular, variegated nevus on her lower left back that has doubled in size in the past 3 months. What would be an appropriate action for the WHNP/midwife?
    1. Do a punch biopsy to confirm the diagnosis.
    2. Take a photograph of the lesion and recheck it in 1 month.
    3. Refer immediately to a dermatologist.
    4. Reassure the patient that these are normal changes related to hormone variations.

16. A young adult female patient presents to the WHNP/midwife's office stating that she has had a red rash over her trunk for 2 weeks that does not itch. She has tried over-the-counter lotions and creams, but the rash is still there. The rash started as a small, round, red patch on her chest and has since spread across her chest, back, arms, and legs. A physical exam reveals a generalized distribution of erythematous and scaly macular lesions that run parallel to each other, creating a "Christmas tree" pattern. The WHNP/midwife should:
    1. Do a thorough medication history, investigate any potential allergens, and send the patient to an allergy specialist.
    2. Prescribe triamcinolone 0.025% cream (Aristocort A) twice a day for 2 weeks.
    3. Teach the patient that the rash is self-limiting, lasting usually 2 to 8 weeks.
    4. Refer the patient to a dermatologist for a biopsy.

17. An adult patient presents to the WHNP/midwife's office complaining of flu-like symptoms, a large red spot in the right groin, headaches, and generalized muscle pain. These symptoms have persisted for approximately 4 to 5 weeks. In taking the history, it would be most important to determine whether the patient:
    1. Was using new skin care products.
    2. Was taking any new medications, such as vitamins or herbal therapies.
    3. Has had a recent insect bite or was potentially exposed to insects, such as ticks.
    4. Has been exposed to a person with tuberculosis.

18. When do bites from insects, spiders, snakes, and bees most often occur?
    1. High humidity months.
    2. Spring to early fall.
    3. Winter.
    4. Any time of the year.

19. Medical management for a brown recluse spider bite includes:
    1. Warm, moist soaks to the affected area.
    2. Ice pack and elevation and immobilization of the area.
    3. Active and passive range of motion to the area.
    4. Avoidance of antihistamines.

20. A Girl Scout leader is explaining about snakes and snake bites, and says to her group about the coral snake, "Red on yellow, kill a fellow; red on black, venom lack." Later, one of the girls is bitten by a snake described as having broad rings of red and black, separated by narrow rings of yellow. The WHNP/midwife understands that this patient will probably experience all the following *except*:
    1. Numbness and change in sensation.
    2. Local swelling at the fang mark site.
    3. Dizziness and diplopia.
    4. No symptoms

21. A young adult reports itching that seems to be worse at night. On exam, the WHNP/midwife notes a rash on the sides of the fingers and inner aspect of the elbows. The rash causes little bumps that often form a line that is approximately 2 to 3 mm long and the width of a hair. What does the WHNP/midwife suspect?
    1. Scabies.
    2. Hives.
    3. Fleas.
    4. Ticks.

22. What are common sites for atopic dermatitis (eczema) in adults?
    1. Cheeks, forehead, and scalp.
    2. Wrists, ankles, and antecubital fossae.
    3. Antecubital fossae, face, neck, and back.
    4. Hands and face.

23. An older adult presents with complaints of a red, greasy scaly rash on her scalp, forehead, and eyebrow. What is the most likely diagnosis?
    1. Seborrheic dermatitis.
    2. Atopic dermatitis.
    3. Psoriasis.
    4. Rosacea.

24. What is a recommended treatment option for actinic keratoses?
    1. Hydrotherapy.
    2. Observation as this is not considered to be a premalignant lesion.
    3. Topical chemotherapy.
    4. Systemic chemotherapy.

Pharmacology

25. What would be the appropriate management for a patient with herpes zoster (shingles)?
    1. Valacyclovir (Valtrex).
    2. Miconazole (Monistat-Derm).
    3. Clotrimazole (Lotrimin).
    4. Corticosteroid (prednisone).

26. An adult patient is diagnosed with seborrheic dermatitis of the face. Which of the following treatments should the WHNP/midwife choose as initial therapy? Select three appropriate therapeutic treatments for seborrheic dermatitis:
    1. Ketoconazole 2% topical.
    2. Chlorhexidine gluconate 4% topical.
    3. Betamethasone topical 0.1%.
    4. Hydrocortisone 2.5%.
    5. Clobetasol ointment 0.5% topical.

27. An obese woman presents to the clinic with complaints of tenderness and irritation under both of her breasts. An exam reveals a very irritated, moist, inflamed area with macules and papules present. What is the best treatment for this woman?
    1. Nystatin cream two or three times a day for 10 days, with thorough drying of the area and exposure to light and air.
    2. Systemic anti-staphylococcal antibiotics (dicloxacillin) and soaking with moist pads of normal saline solution three times daily.
    3. Gentle washing of the area and removal of crusts, then application of antibiotic ointment.
    4. Antiviral treatment (acyclovir) and topical ointment to prevent secondary infection.

28. An adult patient presents to the outpatient health clinic with complaints of pruritus of both hands and axillae. On examination, multiple papules are visualized between the fingers and in both axillae. Small burrows can be appreciated proximal to the papules. Which of the following should the WHNP/midwife choose as treatment?
    1. Hydrocortisone.
    2. Permethrin.
    3. Diphenhydramine.
    4. Ketoconazole.

29. A WHNP/midwife is examining multiple geriatric patients with pediculosis in an assisted living facility. Which of the following treatments should be initiated first?
    1. Lindane shampoo.
    2. Ivermectin oral.
    3. Crisaborole oral.
    4. Pyrethrin shampoo.

30. When treating infections suspicious of methicillin-resistant *Staphylococcus aureus* (MRSA), the WHNP/midwife should be aware that which of the following is true regarding use of bacitracin or mupirocin (Bactroban)?
    1. Both medications are equally effective against MRSA.
    2. Mupirocin is more effective against MRSA.
    3. Bacitracin is more effective against MRSA.
    4. Neither is effective against MRSA.

31. When treating genital warts with topical podophyllin, it is important for the WHNP/midwife to:
    1. Apply the preparation directly to the wart and approximately 5 mm around the base.
    2. Cover with a dressing so that the solution remains moist and caution the patient not to remove the dressing for 24 hours.
    3. Instruct the patient to wash off the medication in 4 to 6 hours.
    4. Treat with liquid nitrogen before applying podophyllin.

32. What is the recommended treatment of rosacea?
    1. Oral hydrocortisone.
    2. Oral ketoconazole.
    3. Low-dose oral tetracycline.
    4. Topical 5-fluorouracil.

33. An adult female patient presents to the health clinic complaining of a pruritic and uncomfortable area under her left arm for 2 days. She states that she has been unable to shave under her arms. Exam of the left axilla reveals multiple follicular pustules. The area is mildly erythematous and painful to touch. Which of the following interventions should the WHNP/midwife initially choose?
    1. Reassurance.
    2. Topical clindamycin.
    3. Penicillin PO.
    4. Trimethoprim/sulfamethoxazole (TMP-SMX) PO.

34. When using lidocaine with epinephrine 1% to 2% as a local anesthetic in the repair of an injury, it is essential to remember that the maximum allowable dose is:
    1. 4.5 mg/kg.
    2. 2.5 mg/kg.
    3. 10 mg/kg.
    4. 15 mg/kg.

35. What therapeutic treatment option would be prescribed by the WHNP/midwife for a frail female patient who presents with several skin tears with no other contributory findings in a physical exam?
    1. Diuretic therapy to prevent fluid accumulation.
    2. Use of topical emollients to hydrate skin.
    3. Baby aspirin to prevent cardiovascular disease.
    4. Antibiotic to prevent infection.

36. A young adult female patient presents several days after being examined and treated for a localized skin infection for which she was prescribed oral antibiotics. Today she complains of a new-onset systemic maculopapular rash. She complains of intense pruritus but is in no acute distress. Her vital signs are within normal limits. A physical exam reveals diffuse small macules and papules. Which of the following should be the priority treatment in this patient?
    1. Prednisone 40 mg intravenously (IV) once, now.
    2. Topical corticosteroid cream.
    3. Diphenhydramine 50 mg IV once, now.
    4. Immediate cessation of antibiotic treatment.

37. On a return visit to the clinic, a patient receiving sulfonamide therapy exhibits generalized rash, mucous membrane lesions, skin sloughing on the palms and feet, high fever, and generalized malaise. These findings would alert the WHNP/midwife to consider:
    1. Hepatitis B.
    2. Stevens-Johnson syndrome.
    3. HIV infection/AIDS.
    4. *Pneumocystis carinii* pneumonia.

38. What is the first-line treatment for tinea versicolor?
    1. Ketoconazole.
    2. Mupirocin.
    3. Prednisone.
    4. Tretinoin.

13 Answers and Rationales

Disorders

1. (1) These lesions are most likely actinic keratosis. Actinic keratosis is a premalignant lesion at high risk of developing into squamous cell carcinoma of the skin. Actinic keratosis is most likely seen in sun-exposed areas and is described as a scaly sandpaper-like lesion of a yellow to light brown coloration that may be erythematous.

2. (1) Hot tub folliculitis caused by *Pseudomonas aeruginosa* is one of the most commonly considered gram-negative aerobic bacilli and should be suspected in any patient presenting with folliculitis and recent exposure to hot tubs. The infected area is most often in an area where wet clothing causes extended close contact with infected water. *Staphylococcus aureus* should be suspected in patients without a known exposure or risk factor because it is the most common cause of folliculitis overall.

3. (3) Intense itching is characteristic of pediculosis pubis, scabies, and atopic dermatitis. Impetigo starts out as a tender erythematous papule and progresses through a vesicular to a honey-crusted stage with no itching.

4. (2) Postherpetic neuralgia refers to pain persisting beyond 4 months from the initial onset of the rash and is a potential complication that can occur following activation of herpes zoster virus. Unlike with acute presentations, there is no evidence of customary lesions associated with shingles leading patients to present with pain presentations classified as allodynia. Phantom pain presents in patients with an amputation. Although most elderly patients present with atypical symptoms in the presence of urinary tract infections, on the basis of this patient's past medical history, it is more likely that she is experiencing a complication of herpes zoster. Tinea infection would present with a skin lesion finding.

5. (2) Approximately 10% to 30% of people with psoriasis develop an accompanying form of arthritis called psoriatic arthritis. Eczema (dermatitis), neurodermatitis (lichen simplex chronicus), and pityriasis rosea are dermatologic conditions that are not directly associated with arthritis.

6. (3) Stress can aggravate psoriasis. Sunlight helps psoriasis, so it is usually better in the summer. It is not contagious, and only approximately 30% of patients with psoriasis have pruritus.

7. (2) Actinic keratoses are potentially precancerous lesions that are commonly found in areas of skin exposed to sunlight.

8. (2) Herpes zoster typically presents with a history of tenderness followed by eruptions and vesicles that follow a dermatome on one side of the body. The condition is very painful. Other symptoms may include fever, headaches, and malaise. Psoriasis is characterized by thick, white, silvery, or red patches of skin. Contact dermatitis is a rash caused by touching something. Cellulitis is a skin infection characterized as red, hot, swollen, and tender skin.

9. (3) Although any of these conditions can affect the skin, particularly of a patient who is HIV-positive, the description relates most closely to Kaposi sarcoma and warrants a biopsy.

10. (2) In case of suspected drug reactions, it is recommended that the drug be eliminated and documented in the patient's record so that it is not reintroduced.

11. (4) Excessive sweating may be normal, but a history and physical exam are needed to rule out underlying causes. Therapies can be offered. Drysol is for use only on the feet and axilla.

12. (3) The assessment describes a seborrheic keratosis. The actinic keratosis is an irregular, rough, scaly, white to erythematous macular lesion found most often on sun-exposed areas, such as on the dorsal surface of the hands, arms, neck, and face. It has malignant potential. The basal cell carcinoma is a smooth, round nodule with a pearly gray border and central induration. Senile lentigines are gray-brown, irregular, macular lesions on sun-exposed areas of the face, arms, and hands.

13. (3) Herpes zoster (shingles) is a vesicular dermatomal eruption related to a reactivation of latent varicella virus. It increases with advanced age and is characterized by burning pain and paresthesia along one or two dermatomes, not crossing the midline, and may be accompanied by fever, malaise, or headache. The vesicular stage lasts 2 to 3 weeks. The vesicles are initially clear or blood filled and become purulent. The area along the dermatome is erythematous, and the vesicles crust and then scab, which may leave hypopigmented scars. The other options discuss painless lesions and are not specific to this prodromal stage.

14. (4) These are classic signs of a basal cell carcinoma, also supported by the patient's employment history. Exposure to ultraviolet radiation from sunlight is the most important environmental cause of basal cell carcinoma. Melanoma would be pigmented; compound nevus would not

be firm or have telangiectasia; and bullous pemphigoid results in bullous lesions.

15. (3) Refer this patient immediately to a dermatologist because the findings are highly suspicious for a melanoma. A punch biopsy should never be done on a suspected melanoma, and any delay could be detrimental to the outcome.

16. (3) The patient presents with a classic case of pityriasis rosea, a benign, self-limiting skin eruption of unknown etiology. Although a medication/allergen history would be warranted, referral to an allergy specialist or dermatologist would not be necessary. Triamcinolone would not be indicated unless there is itching because the treatment is mainly symptomatic. Sunlight in moderate amounts has been shown to hasten healing in some patients. There is one study that suggested having pityriasis rosea during the first trimester, specifically prior to 15 weeks, may lead to adverse pregnancy outcomes, including preterm labor.

17. (3) The signs and symptoms presented are classic for Lyme disease, which is transmitted by ticks. Therefore it would be important to inquire about potential exposure to ticks before the signs and symptoms developed. Exposure to new skin care products would be important if the WHNP/midwife suspected an allergic reaction, which is not consistent with the signs and symptoms. Although always important, a thorough medication history probably will not reveal the cause of the signs and symptoms in this case. Tuberculosis does not present in this manner.

18. (2) Insects reproduce, are more active, and are present in greater numbers in the warm months of spring to early fall.

19. (2) Heat application is contraindicated; ice packs are preferred, as is elevation to decrease the edema. The area should be immobilized. Tdap or Td immunization may be given along with antihistamines to reduce swelling and relieve itching.

20. (4) This was a venomous coral snake bite. The typical symptoms are those listed, as well as nausea, vomiting, and muscle fasciculations.

21. (1) The location and appearance of the lesions are typical of scabies. A rash causes little bumps that often form a line that are approximately 2- to 3-mm long and the width of a hair. The inflammatory lesions are erythematous and pruritic papules most commonly located in the finger webs, flexor surfaces of the wrists, elbows, axillae, buttocks, genitalia, feet, and ankles. The older adult may itch more severely with fewer cutaneous lesions and is at risk for extensive infestations, probably related to a decline in cell-mediated immunity. In addition, there may be back involvement in those who are bedridden.

22. (4) Atopic dermatitis is a chronic, pruritic inflammatory skin disease that occurs most frequently in children but also affects adults. Atopic dermatitis in adults may be generalized; however, it frequently appears in the creases of the elbows or knees, dorsa of the feet, and nape of the neck in adults, and frequently the hands and face are involved in adults. The clinical presentation is typically on the face, scalp, and extensor limb surfaces of infants and toddlers, flexural areas are involved in older children and adolescents. Localized eczema (e.g., chronic hand or foot dermatitis, eyelid dermatitis, or lichen simplex chronicus) may continue throughout adulthood; typically, atopic dermatitis declines with increasing age.

23. (1) Seborrheic dermatitis is usually salmon in color and has a red, greasy appearance with thick adherent crusts and indistinct margins. There is minimal pruritus. In adults, it is most commonly located in hairy skin areas: scalp and scalp margins, eyebrows and eyelid margins, nasolabial folds, ears and retroauricular folds, presternal area, middle to upper back, buttock crease, inguinal area, genitals, and armpits. Rashes in atopic dermatitis and eczema are pink, or red if inflamed, and have a whiter, nongreasy appearance. Scalp psoriasis is more sharply demarcated than seborrheic dermatitis and has crusted, infiltrated plaques rather than mild scaling and erythema. Rosacea is characterized by facial flushing, erythema, papules, pustules, and telangiectasia in a symmetric, central facial distribution and is uncommon in older adults (over 60 years of age).

24. (3) Actinic keratosis is considered to be a precancerous lesion, and topical chemotherapy is indicated for the affected areas. Hydrotherapy is not suggested as a treatment option. Cryotherapy can be used as a treatment option along with photodynamic therapy, scraping, or curettage.

Pharmacology

25. (1) Antiviral therapy with valacyclovir 1000 mg three times daily for 7 days may expedite healing if started within 2 to 3 days of onset, especially in immunocompromised individuals. Miconazole and clotrimazole are antifungal creams. Prednisone would only be used to decrease the incidence of postherpetic neuralgia and may increase the incidence of disseminated infection, so it is not recommended during the acute phase.

26. (1, 3, 4) Initial therapy in treatment of seborrheic dermatitis of the face includes topical low-potency corticosteroids, including hydrocortisone, as well as topical antifungals, including ketoconazole and ciclopirox. Systemic medications and higher-potency topical corticosteroids, such as clobetasol, are not indicated for initial therapy or uncomplicated disease.

27. (1) The description is consistent with intertriginous candidiasis, which is treated with an antifungal ointment or oral medication. It is not a staphylococcal infection; the area needs to be kept dry, not moist. An antibiotic ointment will not relieve the problem. Herpes zoster is treated with antiviral medications; this case is not described as particularly painful, and it is bilateral.

28. (2) The patient in this scenario likely has scabies, caused by the *Sarcoptes scabiei* mite. Treatment is aimed at both symptom relief and prevention of transmission. Treatment should include either permethrin 5% cream or oral ivermectin. For severe cases, combination treatment may be used. Other treatment choices include crotamiton, malathion, or lindane. Lindane is indicated only as an alternative therapy due to risk of serious side effects.

29. (4) Pediculosis is more common in children but can regularly be seen in long-term care facilities and older adults living in close quarters. Pediculosis is caused by the head louse (*Pediculus humanus capitis*). Initial treatments include over-the-counter pyrethrins, such as pyrethrin shampoo and permethrin lotion. Prescription medications include ivermectin lotion, benzyl alcohol lotion, malathion lotion, and spinosad topical suspension. The medication lindane has been restricted to use as a second-line agent because of the risk of serious side effects and has an FDA black box warning of severe neurologic toxicity and should only be used when first-line agents have failed. Additional care, including washing linens and clothing, should be instituted.

30. (2) It is important to note that mupirocin (Bactroban) is a more effective treatment of methicillin-resistant *Staphylococcus aureus* (MRSA) infections. Mupirocin is indicated for use for topical skin infections, as surgical skin prophylaxis, or intranasally to eliminate MRSA colonization. Bacitracin is indicated for skin infections but has been shown to have decreased effectiveness against MRSA infections. Other topical anti-infectious agents include retapamulin (Altabax) and combinations of bacitracin with neomycin and polymyxin B.

31. (3) Patients need to be instructed to wash off podophyllin. It should be applied sparingly, only to the wart and avoiding normal skin, and allowed to dry thoroughly before the patient dresses. No rationale exists to treat with both liquid nitrogen and podophyllin.

32. (3) Systemic treatment with low-dose tetracycline is very effective for rosacea; topical treatment with metronidazole or low-dose hydrocortisone may also be useful. Oral cortisone and antifungal agents are not known to be effective. Topical 5-fluorouracil is used in the treatment of actinic keratosis, a precancerous skin condition.

33. (2) Folliculitis of the axilla without other risk factors or exposures is most likely caused by *Staphylococcus aureus.* Medical treatment is not usually indicated for a single lesion of folliculitis. Patients with multiple sites or moderate skin involvement should first be treated with topical mupirocin and clindamycin. Oral antimicrobials are indicated for refractory or severe cases, including beta-lactam antibiotics, trimethoprim/sulfamethoxazole (TMP-SMX), clindamycin, or doxycycline for 7 to 10 days.

34. (1) The maximum allowable dose for adults is 4.5 mg/kg of lidocaine with epinephrine and 5 mg/kg of lidocaine without epinephrine. Although local anesthetics are often used, the maximum allowable doses are rarely emphasized, and overdose can result in anaphylactic shock.

35. (2) Skin tears are seen in the frail elderly population, and therapeutic treatment should be focused on maintaining hydration of the skin. Diuretic therapy could lead to dehydration. Baby aspirin therapy is unrelated to the appearance of skin tears. Antibiotic therapy would be used only if infection was suspected or identified on exam.

36. (4) The patient most likely has experienced morbilliform (drug-induced) drug eruption, also commonly called an exanthematous drug eruption, which is a type IV hypersensitivity reaction that typically occurs 5 to 14 days after treatment. Many medications can cause reactions, but antibiotics, such as penicillin, cephalosporins, macrolides, quinolones, and TMP-SMX, are some of the most commonly implicated. Treatment priorities involve first stopping the offending agent followed by symptomatic treatment with corticosteroids and/or antihistamines. Immediate treatment with diphenhydramine or systemic corticosteroids would not be indicated because this patient is clearly not experiencing an acute reaction.

37. (2) Stevens-Johnson syndrome is a severe form of erythema multiforme that can be fatal. The clinical picture is mucous membrane lesions, conjunctival and corneal lesions, fever, malaise, arthralgia, and sloughing of the skin of the hands and feet. Distinguishing characteristics of the syndrome are eruption of vesicles, mucosal ulcerations, and sloughing skin.

38. (2) Tinea versicolor (pityriasis versicolor) is a common skin infection caused by the fungal organism *Malassezia furfur.* First-line treatment involves topical antifungals (azoles, ciclopirox, terbinafine) and selenium sulfide. Patients should be educated that treatment may take several months to resolve symptoms. Treatment with corticosteroids or a retinoid would be ineffective. Mupirocin is indicated for bacterial infections.

14

Endocrine

Disorders

1. The etiology of type 1 diabetes can be best described as:
   1. An autosomal dominant genetic disorder.
   2. Autoimmune destruction of the beta cells.
   3. Overnutrition and resulting obesity as the major risk factor.
   4. Prevented by exercise, which increases the concentration of insulin receptors.

2. The WHNP/midwife understands that acromegaly is typically caused by:
   1. Hypersecretion of benign pituitary tumors.
   2. Hyposecretion of pituitary hormones.
   3. Hypersecretion of adrenal cortex hormones.
   4. Metastatic tumors within the pituitary.

3. Hirsutism presenting in a female with normal menstruation and normal plasma androgens is most likely:
   1. An ovarian tumor.
   2. Cushing syndrome.
   3. Idiopathic.
   4. Polycystic ovary disease.

4. QSEN When counseling a patient with diabetes on foot care, it is important to emphasize:
   1. Daily foot soaks in warm, soapy water.
   2. Careful daily foot inspections.
   3. Trimming corns and calluses regularly.
   4. Trimming toenails close to the nail bed.

5. Clinical findings in a patient with hypothyroidism include:
   1. Hyperactive bowel sounds.
   2. Oily skin and acne.
   3. Postural tremors of the hands.
   4. Edema of the face and eyelids.

6. A young adult reports anxiety, tremulousness, headaches, palpitations, and sweating 2 to 4 hours after eating. Physical exam is normal. No lab results are currently available. No medical conditions are noted in the history. What is the most likely diagnosis?
   1. Dumping syndrome.
   2. Hypoglycemia.
   3. Alcohol abuse.
   4. Hyperthyroidism.

7. Which of the following is the most likely etiology for hypercalcemia in the medically well asymptomatic adult?
   1. Hyperthyroidism.
   2. Hyperparathyroidism.
   3. Hyperpituitarism.
   4. Hypothyroidism.

8. A middle-aged adult with no previous medical history presents with a 30-lb. weight gain in 2.5 months. She denies any medication use or allergies. She was recently laid off from a very active job and has been sedentary. Physical exam reveals blood pressure of 172/111 mm Hg, central obesity, and fasting blood sugar of 200 mg/dL. What is the most likely cause of the patient's weight gain?
   1. Cushing syndrome.
   2. Hypothyroidism.
   3. Depression.
   4. Diabetes.

9. A 45-year-old female patient presents to the office complaining of a 6-month history of fatigue, 15-lb. weight gain, lethargy, an inability to tolerate cold temperatures, forgetfulness, hair loss, and constipation. Physical exam findings include dry, coarse skin; periorbital edema and puffy facies; bradycardia; hyporeflexia and muscle weakness; and a smooth, goitrous thyroid. The WHNP/midwife would make the diagnosis of:
   1. Heart failure.
   2. Diabetes mellitus.
   3. Hypothyroidism.
   4. Thyroid cancer.

10. The role of the WHNP/midwife in the initial management of a patient with a thyroid nodule involves:
   1. Referring the patient to an endocrinologist for further evaluation.
   2. Obtaining fine-needle aspiration (FNA) biopsy of the nodule and sending it to cytology.
   3. Ordering an ultrasound and a thyroid panel.
   4. Ordering levothyroxine (Synthroid) to reduce the size of the nodule.

11. When teaching a patient with diabetes about "sick day" guidelines, the WHNP/midwife explains that the patient should:
   1. Stop measuring blood glucose and only check urine for ketones.
   2. Not take the usual dose of insulin at the usual time.
   3. Be sure to take metformin (Glucophage) and acarbose (Precose), even if nausea and vomiting are present.
   4. Administer extra doses of regular insulin according to instructions for blood glucose levels above 240 mg/dL.

12. A young adult female patient presents to the clinic with complaints of nervousness, tremulousness, palpitations, heat intolerance, fatigue, weight loss, and polyphagia. After a complete history and physical, along with thyroid function tests, the WHNP/midwife makes the diagnosis of hyperthyroidism, recognizing that the most common cause of this condition is:
   1. Thyroid cancer.
   2. Graves disease.
   3. Pituitary adenoma.
   4. Postpartum thyroiditis.

13. A young adult patient presents to the office stating that she found a lump in her neck. Physical exam reveals a firm, 2-cm nodule that is fixed, nontender, and located on the right lobe of the thyroid gland. Right posterior cervical lymphadenopathy is also noted. The WHNP/midwife should:
   1. Order a TSH level and ultrasound and refer the patient to a surgeon for a possible fine-needle aspiration (FNA) biopsy of the nodule.
   2. No intervention is necessary at this time; schedule a follow-up visit in 6 months.
   3. Prescribe levothyroxine (Synthroid) 0.1 mg PO daily and schedule a 6-week follow-up visit.
   4. Immediately ablate the patient's thyroid with radioactive iodine and refer her to an endocrinologist.

14. During an evaluation of a patient with prediabetes (glucose intolerance), the WHNP/midwife identifies what finding in the patient's objective data as being associated with the increasing insulin resistance?
   1. Triglycerides more than 150 mg/dL.
   2. High-density lipoprotein more than 40 mg/dL in men and more than 50 mg/dL in women.
   3. Blood pressure less than 130/85 mm Hg.
   4. Fasting blood sugar less than 110 mg/dL.

15. While taking a history on a patient, the WHNP/midwife identifies what finding that may be associated with osteopenia/osteoporosis?
   1. High calcium intake.
   2. Minimal alcohol intake.
   3. Smoking 1 pack per day for 20 years.
   4. Walking 30 minutes 4 days a week.

16. When prescribing a meal plan for a patient with type 2 diabetes, the WHNP/midwife tells the patient that the macronutrient with the most influence on postprandial glucose levels is:
   1. Fiber.
   2. Fat.
   3. Protein.
   4. Carbohydrate.

Pharmacology

17. The WHNP/midwife is very familiar with the precautions about tapering of steroid medications. Which of the following is a true statement about the actual need and/or process of doing so that the WHNP/midwife understands?
   1. All dosing regimens, no matter the dose and the duration of therapy, require tapering of doses.
   2. Patients who have had several steroid prescriptions in the past year are at lessened risk of sustaining a poor outcome if the doses are not tapered.
   3. Dosing regimens lasting longer than 2 weeks require consideration of a tapering schedule.
   4. Pulse doses of steroid (i.e., 3-day bursts) do not require tapering if they occur more than 6 months apart.

18. When prescribing oral medications for an overweight patient with type 2 diabetes who also has a voracious appetite, the WHNP/midwife is likely to prescribe which medication to encourage weight loss and reduce appetite, as an adjunct to improved diet and exercise?
   1. Exenatide (Byetta).
   2. Pioglitazone (Actos).
   3. Metformin (Glucophage).
   4. Glyburide (Micronase).

19. Timing of taking thyroid medication has traditionally been in the morning on an empty stomach. If the patient insists on taking thyroid medication with an evening meal, is this acceptable? What would be two appropriate responses?
    1. No, the circadian rhythm cycles are best supported with AM dosing.
    2. This is acceptable if there is a 2- to 4-hour separation from an ingested full evening meal.
    3. There is no difference between AM and PM dosing guidelines.
    4. This is a feasible option if there are no other medications taken at that time that would cause interactions or absorption issues.

20. Glargine (Lantus) is an insulin analogue that essentially has no peak and is *usually* administered:
    1. Before meals.
    2. With lispro insulin (Humalog) in one injection.
    3. Before breakfast and dinner.
    4. Once daily.

21. Which of the following is the best alternative for treating hyperthyroidism diagnosed during the first trimester of pregnancy?
    1. Radioactive iodine in a smaller than usual dose during first trimester.
    2. Propylthiouracil during first trimester, subtotal thyroidectomy during second trimester, no thyroid replacement.
    3. Propylthiouracil during first trimester, subtotal thyroidectomy during second trimester, thyroid replacement.
    4. No treatment until after delivery.

22. An adult female patient with type 2 diabetes has a creatinine level of 1.8 mg/dL. Which of the following drugs is contraindicated?
    1. Pioglitazone (Actos).
    2. Metformin (Glucophage).
    3. Repaglinide (Prandin).
    4. Acarbose (Precose).

23. Patients started on metformin (Glucophage) need to be monitored closely for what potential side effect?
    1. Significant increase in weight.
    2. Elevation of LDL level.
    3. Lactic acidosis.
    4. Increase in insulin requirements.

24. A patient with type 2 diabetes is taking glipizide (Glucotrol) 10 mg PO bid. In evaluating the medication's effectiveness, the WHNP/midwife knows that glipizide reduces blood glucose by:
    1. Delaying the cellular uptake of potassium and insulin.
    2. Stimulating insulin release from the pancreas.
    3. Decreasing the body's need for and use of insulin at the cellular level.
    4. Interfering with the absorption and metabolism of fats and carbohydrates.

25. The WHNP/midwife would expect which symptom to be a side effect of metformin (Glucophage)?
    1. GI upset.
    2. Photophobia.
    3. Hypoglycemia.
    4. Skin eruptions.

26. A patient is receiving antithyroid medication. The WHNP/midwife understands that:
    1. Lifelong daily treatment is necessary to keep TSH levels within the normal range.
    2. Antithyroid medications do not cross the placenta.
    3. The drugs are somewhat expensive and have serious cardiac and hematologic side effects.
    4. Patients remain on drug therapy for 1 to 2 years, and then the medication is gradually withdrawn.

27. When prescribing an antihypertensive medication for a patient with type 2 diabetes, the drug classifications that would tend to reduce insulin sensitivity are:
    1. Diuretics and calcium channel blockers.
    2. Diuretics and beta blockers.
    3. Calcium channel blockers and angiotensin-converting enzyme (ACE) inhibitors.
    4. Alpha blockers and ACE inhibitors.

28. A 35-year-old female sees the WHNP/midwife with a complaint of cold intolerance, fatigue, dry skin, weight gain, and heavy menstrual periods. Physical exam reveals a pulse of 58 beats per minute; a "waxy," sallow complexion; and a firm goiter. Her TSH level is 176 mU/L. What is the best treatment choice for this patient?
    1. Begin levothyroxine (Synthroid) at 25 mcg (0.025 mg) PO daily and repeat TSH in 2 weeks.
    2. Administer loading dose of PO levothyroxine and start full replacement dose.
    3. Administer loading dose of intravenous (IV) levothyroxine and start on half replacement dose.
    4. Begin levothyroxine at 100 mcg (0.1 mg) PO daily and recheck TSH in 6 weeks.

29. The WHNP/midwife is seeing an obese, middle-aged female patient for a follow-up visit. She was diagnosed with type 2 diabetes 3 months ago and started on a regimen of diet and exercise. Today, her fasting plasma glucose is 200 mg/dL and A1C is 10%. She has lost 2 lbs. She reports her home glucose monitoring has ranged from 180 to 300 mg/dL. The rest of her chemistry profile is within normal limits. What is the best treatment choice for the patient?
    1. Review her diet and exercise plan, increase exercise regimen, and reduce caloric intake. Schedule her for another follow-up in 3 months.
    2. Start her on sliding-scale insulin and instruct her on recording glucose and insulin requirements. Schedule her to return in 1 week for reevaluation regarding long-acting insulin.
    3. Initiate treatment with metformin (Glucophage).
    4. Initiate treatment with an oral sulfonylurea agent (e.g., glyburide).

30. What is associated with chronic overtreatment with levothyroxine (Synthroid)?
    1. Tachycardia.
    2. Osteoporosis.
    3. Insomnia.
    4. Sweating.

31. A patient on antithyroid drug therapy for hyperthyroidism presents with complaints of palpitations and dry mouth for the past 2 days. She has had a cough and cold symptoms for the past 3 days, which she has been treating with over-the-counter medications. Which medication would the WHNP/midwife encourage the patient to avoid?
    1. Benzocaine (Chloraseptic) lozenges.
    2. Guaifenesin (Robitussin).
    3. Ibuprofen (Advil).
    4. Pseudoephedrine (Sudafed).

32. What is the most frequent complaint of patients who use insulin pumps?
    1. Problems with elevated glucose after changing the catheter-type (nonneedle) infusion set.
    2. Skin and site problems with dressing adhesive not sticking; redness and pain at infusion site.
    3. Mechanical problems with the pump's digital readout.
    4. Understanding "sick day" management modifications.

33. The WHNP/midwife understands that pioglitazone (Actos) or rosiglitazone (Avandia) is indicated for:
    1. Prenatal patients with gestational diabetes.
    2. "Brittle" patients with type 1 diabetes.
    3. Patients with type 2 diabetes requiring insulin who have poor glycemic control and insulin resistance.
    4. Patients with type 2 diabetes to prevent the rapid postprandial blood glucose surges by delaying carbohydrate absorption.

34. A patient is newly diagnosed as being hypothyroid and is placed on levothyroxine (Synthroid) 100 mcg (0.1 mg) PO daily. What should be the WHNP/midwife's approach to follow-up?
    1. No follow-up visits are necessary.
    2. The patient should return to the clinic in 4 to 6 weeks for TSH measurement and determination of any symptomatic improvement.
    3. The patient should have weekly levothyroxine levels measured.
    4. The patient should have monthly complete blood counts while on levothyroxine (Synthroid) because the medication has been found to be myelosuppressive.

35. Classes of medications typically used to treat hyperthyroid conditions include:
    1. Antibiotics and corticosteroids.
    2. ACE inhibitors, anxiolytics, and antithyroid medications.
    3. Beta blockers, nonsteroidal antiinflammatory drugs, and antithyroid medications.
    4. Calcium channel blockers and corticosteroids.

36. A patient with hypothyroidism receiving daily levothyroxine (Synthroid) for 3 weeks presents to the clinic with complaints of intermittent chest pain. What is the appropriate therapeutic response?
    1. Discontinue levothyroxine because chest pain is a contraindication to its continuance.
    2. Schedule the patient for a stress test.
    3. Decrease dose of levothyroxine, order an electrocardiogram, and consult immediately with endocrine and/or cardiology health team members.
    4. Prescribe an anxiolytic agent for the patient.

37. The WHNP/midwife understands that lispro insulin (Humalog):
    1. Can be injected just before eating.
    2. Is less costly than regular insulin.
    3. Increases the likelihood of late postprandial hypoglycemia due to its length of action.
    4. Causes teratogenic effects.

38. When prescribing sulfonylureas, the WHNP/midwife educates the patient that the most common side effect of therapy is:
    1. Upset stomach.
    2. Diarrhea.
    3. Angina.
    4. Hypoglycemia.

39. The primary action of pioglitazone (Actos) and rosiglitazone (Avandia) is to:
    1. Decrease hepatic glucose output.
    2. Increase secretion of insulin from the pancreas.
    3. Increase glucose uptake into the muscle and fat.
    4. Increase postprandial uptake of glucose into the intestine.

40. Which of the following osteoporosis medications does not carry the critical warning that the patient must take the medication with a full glass of water and remain upright 30 to 60 minutes after dosing?
    1. Alendronate (Fosamax).
    2. Ibandronate (Boniva).
    3. Risedronate (Actonel).
    4. Zoledronic acid (Zometa).

41. Education concerning home blood sugar testing with a personal glucometer includes the following key point:
    1. Use the matching test strips designed for the particular glucometer because different brands are not interchangeable.
    2. When opening a new canister of test strips, recalibration or setting control codes are no longer needed.
    3. The values obtained from self-monitoring glucometers match serum blood values.
    4. Remember to cleanse the fingertip or alternative testing site with alcohol prior to using the lancing-type device.

42. Which group of antihypertensive agents have some positive impact on the development of diabetic nephropathy?
    1. Alpha blockers.
    2. Beta blockers.
    3. Calcium channel blockers.
    4. ACE inhibitors.

14 Answers and Rationales

Disorders

1. (2) Type 1 diabetes is caused by destruction of the beta cells mediated through the immune system. The other three choices refer to type 2 diabetes.

2. (1) Pituitary masses associated with acromegaly are usually benign tumors that create a disruption in normal feedback mechanisms. Symptoms noted on physical exam result from the effects of growth hormone excess or from the secreting tissue effect of the pituitary mass on surrounding brain structures. This is not typically an adrenal cortex dysfunction. Although tumors can cause acromegaly symptoms, pituitary masses associated with acromegaly are typically noncancerous lesions.

3. (3) Hirsutism is due to increased androgenic (male) hormones, either from increased peripheral binding (idiopathic) or increased production from the ovaries, adrenals, or body fat. In this patient situation it is most likely idiopathic. There are iatrogenic causes (i.e., medications). Diseases related to the ovaries would cause changes in the menstrual cycle and, with Cushing syndrome, would be associated with adrenal androgen overproduction.

4. (2) It is important for patients with diabetes to have their feet inspected daily either by self-exam or by a family member. Feet should be washed daily but never soaked. Soaking feet can cause skin breakdown and increase risk of infection. Corns and calluses should receive a professional's care. Nails should be trimmed straight across to avoid injury to the nail beds.

5. (4) Accumulation of hyaluronic acid in interstitial tissues increases capillary permeability to albumin and causes the interstitial edema of the face and eyelids in patients with hypothyroidism.

6. (2) Although alcohol abuse may be a cause of hypoglycemia, the patient is presenting with classic symptoms of postprandial hypoglycemia. Assessment for alcohol abuse as the etiology of the hypoglycemia would be advisable. Increased circulating thyroid hormones increase beta-cell sensitivity and increase insulin release. This does not typically manifest as hypoglycemia; instead, most patients with hyperthyroidism develop glucose intolerance due to an antagonism of the peripheral action of insulin on cells.

7. (2) Hyperparathyroidism accounts for more than 60% of patients with hypercalcemia and is likely to be the explanation for elevated serum calcium levels.

8. (1) Although depression may explain the weight gain, Cushing syndrome is the correct diagnosis for the constellation of symptoms of rapid weight gain, hypertension, and elevated blood sugar. These symptoms suggest adrenal dysfunction. Serum cortisol and adrenocorticotropic hormone (ACTH) levels should be checked.

9. (3) The symptoms (weight gain, lethargy, inability to tolerate cold temperatures, forgetfulness, hair loss, and constipation) describe the classic presentation of a patient with hypothyroidism. A patient with heart failure would have jugular venous distention, rales, and peripheral edema. The criteria for diagnosing diabetes mellitus are polydipsia, polyphagia, polyuria, and weight loss. Thyroid cancer typically presents without many physical symptoms other than hoarseness and dysphagia, and often the only physical finding is a hard, fixed nodule on the thyroid gland.

10. (3) The WHNP/midwife's role in primary care for a patient with a thyroid nodule initially involves the early identification of the thyroid nodule on physical exam and ordering an ultrasound and thyroid panel, then referring the patient to an endocrinologist for further evaluation, and possibly obtaining some preliminary thyroid-stimulating hormone (TSH) and antibody testing. The endocrinologist performs the fine-needle aspiration (FNA) if the nodule is less than 1 cm with normal TSH level. Levothyroxine may or may not be used to diminish the size of the nodule, based on the findings derived from the FNA and the endocrinologist's chosen treatment plan.

11. (4) Patients with diabetes must understand that when they are sick, blood glucose levels will probably increase, even when they are not eating. They need to monitor blood glucose levels every 2 to 4 hours. The medications metformin and acarbose should not be given until the patient's nausea and vomiting have subsided and the patient has resumed a normal diet; blood glucose monitoring is important during this time. Dehydration will increase the risk of metabolic acidosis for patients on metformin.

12. (2) Graves disease, an autoimmune condition also known as "diffuse toxic goiter," is the most common cause of hyperthyroidism in this age group. Much less common

causes include cancer of the thyroid, adenoma of the pituitary gland, and postpartum (or silent) thyroiditis.

13. (1) The thyroid-stimulating hormone (TSH) level should be ordered to determine whether the patient is euthyroid, hypothyroid, or hyperthyroid, along with an ultrasound. The patient should also be sent to an endocrinologist or surgeon because all nodules of the thyroid should be biopsied to rule out malignancy. "Watching and waiting" is inappropriate without having a biopsy performed. Thyroid hormone replacement therapy would be indicated only for patients found to be hypothyroid and in whom thyroid cancer has been ruled out. Thyroid ablation may be indicated in patients whose fine-needle aspiration (FNA) biopsy results are positive for thyroid cancer, but this cannot be determined without an endocrinologist's intervention.

14. (1) Glucose intolerance increases the release of free fatty acids, which elevates triglycerides. The other values are still within normal limits.

15. (3) Smoking causes thinning of the bones and can lead to osteopenia/osteoporosis. A diet high in calcium with minimal alcohol intake and walking are all self-care practices that may prevent or delay the onset of osteopenia/osteoporosis.

16. (4) Carbohydrate is the macronutrient with the greatest impact on the postprandial glucose levels. Ingested protein has minimal effect on the blood glucose levels. A diet high in fat may be associated with cardiovascular disease. Fiber has little effect on the plasma glucose response, but it may result in decreased low-density lipoprotein (LDL) cholesterol.

Pharmacology

17. (3) Continuous dosing of steroid medication conditions the adrenal feedback system to become less sensitive to discontinuation of the exogenous hormone supply, which normally would trigger a natural ramp-up of innate steroid production. Duration longer than 2 or 3 weeks and moderate to high doses trigger the need to evaluate current values and prepare for a gradual reduction in dosage before the patient stops taking the steroid medication.

18. (1) Incretin mimetic medications, such as exenatide, are associated with weight loss. Metformin is associated with weight neutrality and appetite suppression. Glyburide is considered a second-generation sulfonylurea, which tends to stimulate insulin secretion from the pancreas, thus causing a slight weight gain. Pioglitazone is an insulin sensitizer and increases glucose uptake in the muscle and fat. Common side effects include fluid retention and an increase in central adiposity.

19. (3, 4) There is no change in thyroid function and hormone levels in patients who take evening doses, as long as there is a separation of meals and the standard medication review to avoid drug-to-drug interactions. It is also recommended to take medications, such as levothyroxine, in the evening, typically due to side effect profiles, such as insomnia, rather than efficacy.

20. (4) Glargine is a long-acting basal insulin usually given once daily and lasts almost 24 hours without a peak. This clear insulin must be given alone and not mixed with other insulins in the same syringe. Lispro insulin is a rapid-acting insulin usually given three times daily with meals. A basal insulin can be used at the same time with a different injection. In rare cases, basal insulins are given more than once per day, but this is not usual practice.

21. (3) Low-dose antithyroid drugs are considered a good alternative to prevent the effects of hyperthyroidism on the mother and developing fetus until surgery can be performed. Another option is using an antithyroid drug until after delivery, and then having surgery. Removal of the thyroid during the second trimester can be performed safely and is the usual recommendation. Replacement is essential after removal of the gland.

22. (2) Metformin should not be given to women with a serum creatinine level ≥1.4 mg/dL, because it can predispose the patient to lactic acidosis. Pioglitazone and repaglinide are metabolized primarily in the liver and require monitoring of liver function tests. Acarbose is metabolized mainly in the gastrointestinal (GI) tract.

23. (3) Lactic acidosis is a potentially severe and fatal reaction to metformin. Metformin does not contribute to weight gain; it often helps with weight loss and decreases LDL, triglyceride levels, and insulin requirements.

24. (2) Sulfonylureas reduce blood glucose by stimulating insulin release from the pancreas. Over time, these drugs also may actually increase insulin effects at the cellular level and decrease glucose production by the liver, which is why sulfonylureas are used in patients with type 2 diabetes who still have a functioning pancreas.

25. (1) Anorexia, nausea, and a metallic taste in the mouth are common side effects. Over time, gastrointestinal (GI) symptoms subside and can be relieved by taking the medication with food or by starting at a lower dose. Metformin has a safety profile that does not include hypoglycemia unless mixed with other agents that trigger it.

26. (4) Antithyroid medications or thionamides (propylthiouracil; methimazole) are relatively inexpensive and do cross the placenta. The patient remains on the medications for 1 to 2 years with the hope of a permanent remission of symptoms when the medications are withdrawn.

27. (2) Both of these drug classifications (diuretics and beta blockers) tend to reduce insulin sensitivity and can cause hyperglycemia. Angiotensin-converting enzyme (ACE) inhibitors, calcium channel blockers, and selective alpha blockers are metabolically neutral; some may actually have a beneficial effect.

28. (4) The patient's symptoms indicate hypothyroidism, as does the elevated thyroid-stimulating hormone (TSH) level (normal levels are 0.5–4.7 mU/L). A full replacement dose of levothyroxine should be the goal for the patient with a standard starting dose of 100 to 125 mcg (0.1–0.125 mg) for a 70-kg person. The TSH level should be checked in 6 weeks, which is the time it may take for a given dose to become effective. Loading doses should never be given, except for coma, which is treated by IV medication in the hospital.

29. (3) Metformin is a better option in an obese patient because it is frequently associated with weight neutrality or even some weight loss, whereas sulfonylureas may actually cause weight gain. Insulin is now considered an option, but the use of a sliding scale is no longer current practice. Diet and exercise were unsuccessful, and the longer the patient's blood sugar remains elevated, the greater her risk for end-organ damage. An A1C level in this range (10%) requires aggressive treatment to decrease vascular complications.

30. (2) Chronic overtreatment is associated with osteoporosis; the other options are related to acute overdose of levothyroxine and can be relieved by omitting the dose for 3 days and then starting on a lower dose.

31. (4) Pseudoephedrine and other decongestant medications that contain sympathomimetics lead to adverse reactions of central nervous system (CNS) overstimulation, palpitations, headache, hypertension, and nervousness. Guaifenesin in combination with dextromethorphan and phenylpropanolamine (Robitussin-CF) or pseudoephedrine (Robitussin-PE) can also cause palpitations and CNS overstimulation. Guaifenesin with dextromethorphan (Robitussin-DM) may cause gastrointestinal (GI) upset, drowsiness, headache, and rash. Many over-the-counter (OTC) medications also have an iodine component that may alter thyroid levels.

32. (2) Infusion site problems and skin irritation are by far the most frequent complaints of patients who use an insulin pump and often are the reason why the pump is discontinued. Patients also find it is more time-consuming and costly. However, the Diabetes Control and Complications Trial (DCCT, 1993) researchers reported a reduced risk of microvascular complications when insulin pumps and multiple daily injections were used.

33. (3) Pioglitazone and rosiglitazone act by decreasing peripheral insulin resistance in skeletal muscle and adipose tissue without enhancing insulin secretion and improving glucose tolerance in patients with type 2 diabetes. Prenatal patients are managed with insulin or metformin, not an insulin sensitizer. The action of alpha-glucosidase inhibitors, such as acarbose (Precose) and miglitol (Glyset), prevents the rapid postprandial blood glucose surges by delaying carbohydrate absorption (known as "starch blockers").

34. (2) The response to therapy is based on a clinical symptomatology and a thyroid-stimulating hormone (TSH) assay approximately 4 to 6 weeks after the initiation of therapy. This is continued until a stable dose is obtained. TSH and a free T_4 level are the two standard tests that can be used to monitor the status of the thyroid; a levothyroxine level cannot be measured. Levothyroxine is not a myelosuppressive.

35. (3) Beta blockers are initially prescribed to reduce the signs and symptoms of the condition and to reduce the peripheral conversion of T_4 to triiodothyronine (T_3); nonsteroidal antiinflammatory drugs are indicated for reducing inflammation associated with thyroiditis; and antithyroid medications (propylthiouracil; methimazole) are used to treat severe hyperthyroidism. Corticosteroids are sometimes used in the treatment of thyroiditis, but the remaining classes (antibiotics, ACE inhibitors, calcium channel blockers, and anxiolytics) are not routinely used in the management of hyperthyroidism.

36. (3) Monitoring TSH is the most accurate way to assess thyroid function in a patient taking levothyroxine. Decreasing the dose of levothyroxine and evaluating the patient's cardiac status are the appropriate interventions in this situation, in addition to quickly involving the other health care team members. Discontinuing the thyroid replacement would be inappropriate because the patient remains hypothyroid and requires therapy for life. An anxiolytic may be a helpful adjunct, but it is not appropriate as the sole intervention because it ignores the cardiac symptoms.

37. (1) Lispro (Humalog) was the first analogue of human insulin and has several advantages over regular insulin, including more rapid onset and shorter duration of action. It reaches peak activity in 1 to 2 hours and has a 4-hour duration versus 6 to 8 hours for regular insulin. It is convenient because it can be injected immediately

before eating (10–15 minutes). It is also more expensive than regular insulin, and some third-party payers may not reimburse patients.

38. (4) Hypoglycemia and weight gain are the most common side effects of sulfonylurea therapy.

39. (3) Pioglitazone and rosiglitazone decrease insulin resistance, which increases the glucose uptake in the muscle and fat. Metformin decreases hepatic glucose output. Oral sulfonylureas increase insulin secretion in the pancreas. The alpha-glucosidase inhibitors increase postprandial glucose uptake in the intestine.

40. (4) Zoledronic acid (Zometa) is administered as an intravenous (IV) infusion. The others are all oral medications that carry the need to remain sitting upright to decrease the risk for esophageal irritation. The IV medication does require good hydration to decrease renal risks.

41. (1) Test strips are proprietary to the specific monitor. Test strips are frequently not interchangeable, even in monitors from the same manufacturer. Similarly, lancets are specific to the device used to provide a skin puncture. Some newer monitors do not require frequent calibrations or a code number. Handwashing must be completed with soap and water. Alcohol is not used to cleanse the digits, unless medically indicated. Serum, capillary, and deeper puncture glucose values do vary, especially over time.

42. (4) Although the reduction of hypertension is important to renal health, the angiotensin-converting enzyme (ACE) inhibitors and some selected angiotensin II receptor blocker (ARB) agents have a "renal protective" effect apart from the vascular tension issue. This does not extend to their direct renin inhibitor "cousins." There may be some positive impact from the sodium glucose cotransporter (SGLT-2) group, but more research is needed.

15

Musculoskeletal

Disorders

1. Which observation by the WHNP/midwife would lead to inclusion of a differential diagnosis of osteoporosis in a 78-year-old female patient who is complaining of bone and joint pain?
   1. Decrease in skin turgor.
   2. Low vitamin D level.
   3. Bilateral swelling of the feet.
   4. Temperature elevation.

2. A 45-year-old female patient complains of knee pain when kneeling and a "clicking" noise when walking up steps. The WHNP/midwife notes slight knee effusion and tenderness when palpating the patella against the condyles. The diagnosis for this patient is:
   1. Anterior cruciate tear.
   2. Dislocated patella.
   3. Chondromalacia patella.
   4. Patellar tendonitis.

3. A patient has been diagnosed with polymyalgia rheumatica (PMR). The WHNP/midwife understands that this disorder is:
   1. An autoimmune, multisystem problem in which the body makes antibodies to its own proteins.
   2. A degenerative disorder with no inflammatory changes in which joint cartilage wears away with age and eventually causes bone spurs.
   3. An inflammatory disorder involving the axial skeleton and large peripheral joints.
   4. An inflammatory rheumatic condition disorder that affects primarily older women and is associated with giant cell (temporal) arteritis.

4. The WHNP/midwife is talking with an older adult who is obese. The patient is complaining of knee and hip pain. What would be an appropriate goal for this patient to reduce the knee and hip pain?
   1. Prescribe tramadol (Ultram).
   2. Have the patient avoid lower leg exercises.
   3. Reduce body weight.
   4. Prescribe daily naproxen (Aleve).

5. The WHNP/midwife is examining a patient who is complaining of pain in her hips and knees. She has a history of osteoarthritis. On exam, the joints are painful to movement and are warm to touch. The best immediate therapy for this patient is:
   1. Physical therapy for range of motion of affected areas.
   2. Decreased physical activity and immobilizing splints for affected joints.
   3. Moist heat and/or cold therapy on painful joints.
   4. ESR to determine level of activity.

6. The history of a patient who may have contracted Lyme disease may include what characteristic?
   1. Erythematous rash on the bridge of the nose and on the cheeks with discoid patches on the trunk.
   2. Immediate development of arthritis symptoms, especially in the knees.
   3. Expanding rash with central clearing within 1 month of being bitten by a tick.
   4. Early symptoms of meningitis and myocarditis.

7. The WHNP/midwife is explaining to a patient who has osteoarthritis about the importance of stretching and flexibility. How does this improve joint function?
   1. Increases exercise intensity.
   2. Increases muscle mass.
   3. Increases joint laxity.
   4. Increases range of motion.

8. Pain in a lumbosacral strain typically begins:
   1. Immediately with the injury.
   2. 1 to 2 hours after injury.
   3. 6 to 8 hours after injury.
   4. 12 to 36 hours after injury.

9. An acute onset of pain that descends down to the lower leg and foot of a 25-year-old obese adult is likely to be a symptom of:
   1. Lumbosacral strain.
   2. Herniated intervertebral disc injury.
   3. Osteomyelitis.
   4. Osteoporosis.

10. A patient with rheumatoid arthritis presents for follow-up. What is the best evaluative question the WHNP/midwife can ask that will help determine the severity of the disease?
    1. "Were you able to drive the car to your appointment today?"
    2. "Were you able to fix your dinner last night?"
    3. "How long does it take for your joints to loosen up after you get up in the morning?"
    4. "How many pounds can you carry?"

11. When counseling a postmenopausal 60-year-old female patient on prevention of osteoporosis, all of the following are therapeutic recommendations *except*:
    1. Cessation of smoking.
    2. Daily intake of 200 mg of calcium and 40 IU of vitamin D.
    3. Continue hormone replacement therapy (HRT).
    4. Monitor bone loss by dual-energy x-ray absorptiometry (DEXA) every 1 to 2 years.

12. A patient tells the WHNP/midwife that she has "whiplash." The WHNP/midwife understands that this is:
    1. Cervical facet joint dysfunction.
    2. Cervical disc injury.
    3. Zygapophyseal joint injury.
    4. Cervical strain.

13. Which of the diet selections indicate that the older patient understands health education regarding the prevention of osteoporosis?
    1. Chicken and baked potato.
    2. Glass of skim milk and toasted cheese sandwich.
    3. Hamburger and salad.
    4. Ice cream sundae with whipped cream.

14. Primary treatment of joint injury involves:
    1. Rest, ice, compression, and elevation.
    2. Narcotic pain control and radiograph.
    3. Specialist referral and magnetic resonance imaging.
    4. Nonsteroidal antiinflammatory drugs (NSAIDs) and exercise.

15. The most common complaint in a patient with back injury who has cauda equina syndrome, a surgical emergency, is:
    1. Urinary retention.
    2. Numbness below the level of injury.
    3. Weakness in the lower extremities.
    4. Leg pain.

16. Which patient is at highest risk for osteoporosis?
    1. A 55-year-old male smoker and retired athlete.
    2. A 60-year-old, 105-lb., postmenopausal white female switchboard operator.
    3. A 42-year-old black female intensive care unit nurse who is lactose intolerant.
    4. A 50-year-old obese white woman with three children living on a farm.

17. A patient, who has hypovitaminosis D, asks the WHNP/midwife if she should spend more time sunbathing without using sunscreen because she heard that your skin can manufacture vitamin D. What would be an appropriate response by the WHNP/midwife?
    1. Continue to use sunscreen, take vitamin D supplements, and choose foods high in vitamin D.
    2. The more ways to get vitamin D the better, so sunbathing is okay on a weekly basis.
    3. Avoid sunlight exposure and take vitamin D 50,000 IU supplements twice a day.
    4. Leave sunscreen off of a sun-exposed area of the body and sunbathe for 20 minutes a day until the skin appears slightly red and tingles.

18. What would be an appropriate schedule for the WHNP/midwife to teach the older adult patient when to do strength training exercises?
    1. Every other week along with aerobic exercise.
    2. Every day for 20 minutes, lift weights.
    3. Every other day walk or ride the bicycle for 30 minutes.
    4. Focus one day on upper body exercises and the next day on lower body exercises.

Pharmacology

19. A 65-year-old postmenopausal female patient has been treated with alendronate (Fosamax) for 6 years. Current screening indicates no increase in risk factors. Based on clinical guidelines, which treatment option would the WHNP/midwife suggest to the patient?
    1. Discontinue medication at this time.
    2. Switch medication from oral to intravenous route to maintain adequate coverage.
    3. Add vitamin D 500 IU/day to the treatment regimen.
    4. Increase calcium supplementation to 1500 mg per day.

20. The WHNP/midwife is seeing a middle-aged, severely arthritic woman who has been receiving maintenance therapy of prednisone 10 mg per day for the past 6 weeks. She now presents as acutely ill with signs and symptoms of acute pneumonia. She is fatigued and weak with loss of appetite, and her blood pressure is lower than at previous visits. Which action should be taken in regard to prednisone?
    1. Immediately discontinue the medication.
    2. Increase the dosage to 60 mg per day, then taper back to 10 mg per day.
    3. Gradually taper from 10 to 1 mg per day.
    4. Maintain the dosage at 10 mg per day.

21. What is the initial drug of choice for a patient with active rheumatoid arthritis (RA)?
    1. Tramadol.
    2. Cyclobenzaprine.
    3. Methotrexate.
    4. Hydrocortisone.

22. A patient with rheumatoid arthritis (RA) is placed on prednisone 5 mg PO qd. In teaching the patient about her medication, it would be important for the WHNP/midwife to include what information?
    1. When the symptoms of arthritis subside, she will be able to quit taking her medication.
    2. It is important to take the medication as prescribed, even after the redness and swelling decrease.
    3. Increased fluid intake is important to prevent renal damage by the steroids.
    4. The medication should be taken approximately 30 minutes before eating.

23. Disease-modifying drugs for rheumatoid arthritis in adults include:
    1. Ibuprofen (Motrin, Advil), sulindac (Clinoril), and salicylates (aspirin, Disalcid).
    2. Corticosteroids (prednisone, methylprednisolone).
    3. Misoprostol (Cytotec).
    4. Hydroxychloroquine (Plaquenil), sulfasalazine (Azulfidine), methotrexate, and gold sodium thiomalate (Myochrysine).

24. The WHNP/midwife, in using best practice, would prescribe which dosage for vitamin D supplementation for the elderly patient to prevent osteoporosis?
    1. 1500 mg of vitamin D every other day.
    2. 400 IU on a daily basis.
    3. 800 to 1000 IU on a daily basis.
    4. 600 mg of vitamin D on a daily basis.

25. The most appropriate medication used to control pain for a patient with osteoarthritis would be:
    1. Acetaminophen.
    2. Systemic corticosteroids.
    3. Gold salts.
    4. Misoprostol.

26. What is a serious side effect of ibuprofen in the older adult patient?
    1. Rebound headaches.
    2. Impairment of renal function.
    3. Neuropathy.
    4. Pancreatic failure.

27. An older adult woman comes into the clinic complaining of "sores" in her mouth. The WHNP/midwife observes several inflamed ulcers on her gums and lips. Which medication would the nurse identify as most likely to cause this problem?
    1. Propranolol (Inderal).
    2. Spironolactone (Aldactone).
    3. Fexofenadine (Allegra).
    4. Alendronate (Fosamax).

28. A patient has a history of mild hypertension and osteopenia. The WHNP/midwife orders a thiazide diuretic. What is the mechanism of action and effect of a thiazide diuretic on the bones?
    1. Increases both calcium and magnesium retention by the kidneys.
    2. Decreases bone mineral density (BMD).
    3. Decreases calcium excretion by the kidneys and stimulates osteoblast production.
    4. Increase in osteoclast and osteoblast activity.

29. What information should the WHNP/midwife include when teaching a patient about taking alendronate (Fosamax)?
    1. Take it midmorning.
    2. Take with food.
    3. Take with a full glass of orange juice.
    4. Remain upright after taking medication.

15 Answers and Rationales

Disorders

1. (2) Low vitamin D level may be associated with a clinical diagnosis of osteoporosis. A decrease in skin turgor is a normal consequence of the aging process. Bilateral swelling of the feet may be due to vascular insufficiency and/or a consequence of standing. An elevation in temperature is typically not associated with osteoporosis.

2. (3) These are common symptoms of chondromalacia patella. With anterior cruciate tears, the patient generally cannot bear weight on the extremity without it buckling or giving way. With a dislocated patella, the patient would have severe pain associated with considerable effusion (loss of normal knee hollow on sides of patella) and possible patellofemoral compartment. Patellar tendonitis, or jumper's knee, causes pain, weakness, and swelling of the knee joint, but no "clicking" noises.

3. (4) PMR is an inflammatory rheumatic condition disorder that affects primarily older women and is associated with giant cell (temporal) arteritis. Anemia is common in PMR, along with an elevated erythrocyte sedimentation rate (ESR). There is a common complaint of morning stiffness; rheumatoid factor is negative. An autoimmune, multisystem disorder is characteristic of systemic lupus erythematosus. A degenerative joint disorder is characteristic of osteoarthritis. An inflammatory disorder involving the axial skeleton and large peripheral joints is characteristic of ankylosing spondylitis.

4. (3) Obesity and overweight are modifiable risk factors that adversely affect the knee and hip joints of older adults. The primary goal for the patient would be reduction of body weight. Exercise is encouraged because it improves fitness level, reduces friction in the joint over time, and reduces body mass, which then reduces the total force on the joint. Naproxen (Aleve) is useful for short-term pain reduction in osteoarthritis. Long-term daily use is not recommended due to side effects and the older adult is more susceptible to side effects, including serious gastrointestinal effects—bleeding, ulceration, intestinal perforation—and with prolonged use there is increased risk of adverse cardiovascular events. Tramadol is an opioid analgesic and would not be indicated because of the risk for addiction and dependence. The older adult may be especially prone to side effects with tramadol due to lowered liver or kidney function and reduced metabolism or excretion.

5. (3) Moist heat or cold, whichever relieves the pain more effectively, is appropriate to use on acutely affected joints. Physical therapy is recommended after the acute involvement of the joint; care must be taken to decrease repetitive movements. Immobilization is avoided because it tends to increase the stiffness of the joint. The erythrocyte sedimentation rate (ESR) is not an appropriate indicator to determine the level of activity in patients with osteoarthritis.

6. (3) Expanding rash with central clearing may also be described as the "bull's-eye rash," which is associated with Lyme disease. An erythematous rash on the bridge of the nose and on the cheeks describes the malar or "butterfly" rash of systemic lupus erythematosus (SLE). The arthritis symptoms and other complications (meningitis and myocarditis) occur later in the disease process, especially if the patient is not treated with antibiotics, usually tetracycline, doxycycline, or amoxicillin.

7. (4) Stretching can help improve flexibility, and consequently range of motion of the joints. Joint laxity or hypermobility is a connective tissue problem characterized by excessive flexibility of the ligaments and tendons. Exercise intensity is how difficult or hard the person is exercising, usually associated with aerobic exercise activity (e.g., swimming, running, walking, etc.). Muscle mass is increased by diet and intense compound muscle group exercises.

8. (4) As the soft tissue swells, pain onset usually occurs approximately 12 to 36 hours after injury.

9. (2) Herniated intervertebral disc pain typically descends to the lower leg and foot. Lumbosacral strain causes pain in the back, buttock, and sometimes thigh. Osteomyelitis must be preceded by an event that permits an infectious agent to enter the bone. Osteoporosis occurs most often in postmenopausal women.

10. (3) Morning stiffness or activity and the length of time required for maximal improvement are American Rheumatism Association Classification criteria for rheumatoid arthritis, and useful, measurable tools for effects of treatment. The other questions are good indicators of quality of activities of daily living but do not give a full, overall, measurable picture of the patient's joint discomfort.

11. (2) This is a subtherapeutic amount of calcium and vitamin D. Recommended calcium for women ages 51 years and older is 1200 mg daily and 800 to 1000 IU daily of vitamin D. The other choices are recommendations for prevention of osteoporosis.

12. (4) Most whiplash injuries are associated with a cervical neck strain related to spasm of the cervical and upper back muscles from injury.

13. (2) Calcium intake is important in minimizing the development of osteoporosis. Both these foods contain calcium. The other options are not focused on calcium intake.

14. (1) The RICE principle is used for initial treatment: **R**est, **I**ce, **C**ompression, and **E**levation. All other treatments mentioned may be appropriate, but not as the primary treatment.

15. (1) Although all symptoms may be associated with cauda equina syndrome, urinary retention and loss of bowel or bladder control are important clues to the immediate need for surgery.

16. (2) The five risk factors for osteoporosis include being of female gender, white or Asian, over age 45 years, low body weight, postmenopausal, sedentary lifestyle, low calcium intake, and a smoker.

17. (1) Although the skin can manufacture vitamin D from sunlight exposure, the majority of people can get their vitamin D from nutritional supplements and from vitamin D–fortified foods. Food sources include wild-caught salmon, mackerel, tuna and sardines, beef liver, eggs, cod liver oil, and mushrooms, along with fortified milk and foods, such as breakfast cereals, yogurt, and orange juice. Exposure to sunlight (UVB light) causes skin cancer and it is important to teach patients to use sunscreen and protect their skin from excessive sunlight exposure. The American Cancer Society does not support sun exposure for increasing vitamin D. There are patients with specific issues who might need a prescription for high levels of vitamin D, but for most people, 50,000 IU daily will raise the vitamin D level too high. High levels of vitamin D can be toxic (signs of hypercalcemia) because it is stored in fat.

18. (4) Different exercises should be performed at a minimum of 2 or more nonconsecutive days each week using major muscle groups. An easy schedule to explain to the patient is to make 1 day focused on upper body muscles and the next day would focus on lower body muscles. A third day could be rest to provide a sufficient recovery period from the strength training exercises and then repeat the schedule again.

Pharmacology

19. (1) Patients who have low fracture risk after being treated with alendronate (Fosamax) for at least 5 years qualify for a drug holiday because the effects of the medication are still present. There is no need to switch the route of medication. Vitamin D supplementation should be within 800 to 1000 IU/day. Calcium supplementation greater than 1200 mg per day may be associated with an increased risk of complications ranging from kidney stones to cardiac events.

20. (2) Patients on chronic steroid therapy should be evaluated for adrenal insufficiency during an acute illness, which increases stress. Signs and symptoms indicate subtle clinical manifestations of adrenal insufficiency. Recommended treatment is to treat the patient empirically with stress-dose corticosteroids during acute illness. Stopping the medication or maintaining the same dose may precipitate acute adrenal insufficiency.

21. (3) Methotrexate is the first-line disease-modifying antirheumatic drug (DMARD) in patients with active RA. Early DMARD therapy to slow disease progression and induce remission is the standard of care. Nonsteroidal antiinflammatory drugs (NSAIDs) can be used for symptomatic pain relief. Steroids (prednisone) may be given but are not the drug of choice and are administered when response is poor to other therapies. Tramadol is effective in RA pain but is not a first-line therapy. Cyclobenzaprine is a muscle relaxant.

22. (2) The patient needs to understand the importance of maintaining the prescribed steroid dose. When symptoms decrease, the medication is effective. It is not influenced by fluids and should be taken with food.

23. (4) These drugs modify rheumatoid arthritis when nonsteroidal antiinflammatory drugs (NSAIDs), such as ibuprofen, sulindac, and salicylates, have not worked. Corticosteroids can be used until the disease-modifying agents begin to work. Misoprostol is used to prevent ulcer development related to long-term medication use.

24. (3) Recommendations for vitamin D for patients ages 50 years and older are 800 to 1000 IU on a daily basis. Vitamin D is measured in IU as opposed to the metric system of weights. For individuals who are younger than age 50 years, the recommendation is between 400 and 800 IU.

25. (1) Acetaminophen or nonsteroidal antiinflammatory drugs (NSAIDs) are generally used for pain relief in patients with osteoarthritis. Systemic corticosteroids are not indicated in osteoarthritis. Gold salts may be one of several pharmacologic approaches to the treatment of rheumatoid arthritis. Misoprostol is used to minimize the development of NSAID-induced gastric ulcers.

26. (2) Renal function may already be reduced in older adults, and ibuprofen can further impair renal function,

which in turn can result in nephrosis, cirrhosis, and congestive heart failure.

27. (4) Gastritis and oral ulcers are common complications of alendronate (Fosamax). Alendronate is used to increase calcium absorption in patients with osteoporosis. If these effects occur, the medication should be discontinued. The medications in the other options do not cause this problem.

28. (3) This positive side effect of thiazides results in a decrease in calcium bone loss and an increase in bone mineral density with a resultant reduction in the risk of hip fracture. Thiazide diuretics lower whereas loop diuretics promote calcium excretion by the kidney. The mechanisms by which thiazides promote preservation of the bones are uncertain. The beneficial bone effects may result from a decrease in parathyroid hormone–stimulated bone resorption and an associated reduction in the bone turn-over rate. Osteoclasts break down bone (bone resorption), releasing the minerals, resulting in a transfer of calcium from bone fluid to the blood. Osteoblasts are mature bone cells responsible for bone formation and ossification.

29. (4) Patients taking alendronate are instructed to take the medication on awakening, 30 minutes before eating, and with a full glass of water. Patients should be instructed to remain upright to prevent esophageal irritation. Taking medication with food (reduces bioavailability by 40%), coffee, orange juice (decreases bioavailability by 60%), or after eating significantly reduces absorption.

16

Neurology

Disorders

1. The WHNP/midwife is seeing a 65-year-old patient with a presenting concern of headache. Which question would be most valuable in developing differentials for this patient?
   1. Do you have a family history of headaches?
   2. How old were you when the headaches began?
   3. When did this headache begin?
   4. Where is your headache located?

2. The WHNP/midwife understands that the most common form of facial paralysis in the adult patient is:
   1. Facial nerve fasciitis.
   2. Trigeminal neuralgia.
   3. Bell palsy.
   4. Herpes zoster.

3. Many patients who suffer from recurrent headaches have similar symptoms with each episode. Which is a sign that a headache may be from a more serious cause?
   1. It occurs on the right side.
   2. Rhinorrhea occurs with the headache.
   3. It becomes more and more painful.
   4. It increases when the patient bends over.

4. The WHNP/midwife understands that benign paroxysmal positional vertigo:
   1. Is described as vertigo and nystagmus with positional change and occurs most often in older adults.
   2. Is more common in young persons and occurs suddenly and in episodes that include vertigo, tinnitus, hearing loss, feeling of fullness in the ears, and nausea and vomiting.
   3. Follows a viral syndrome (upper respiratory or gastrointestinal) with exacerbation of the vertigo with position change without hearing loss or tinnitus.
   4. Involves gradual hearing loss and tinnitus along with vertigo, eventually with facial numbness and weakness.

5. A 52-year-old patient presents with "funny feeling in my feet and calves, like I can't feel them." The sensation has been continuous over the past 2 days and seems to be worsening. The patient is otherwise healthy except for a recent upper respiratory infection. Your primary differential based on the history is:
   1. Amyotrophic lateral sclerosis.
   2. Guillain-Barré syndrome.
   3. Multiple sclerosis.
   4. Muscular dystrophy.

6. What would be appropriate to include in the health promotion plan for a patient with a diagnosis of multiple sclerosis?
   1. Avoid aerobic exercise due to muscle weakness.
   2. Keep warm (especially extremities) to improve neurologic function.
   3. Avoid antioxidants (vitamins C and E, beta-carotene); they contribute to loss of myelin sheath.
   4. Consume a low-fat, high-fiber diet with daily cranberry juice and calcium supplement.

7. A patient has had a stroke and is incontinent of urine. The family should be taught to:
   1. Restrict fluid intake.
   2. Insert a Foley catheter.
   3. Establish a scheduled voiding pattern.
   4. Reposition the patient often to reduce the discomfort of urgency.

8. What is the best approach to test the hearing of a patient with Bell palsy?
   1. Stand out of sight of the patient and ask the patient to move or do something.
   2. Use a tuning fork to test for lateralization of sound.
   3. Stand in front of the patient and whisper "Raise your hand."
   4. Snap your fingers next to the patient's ear and ask if the sound was heard.

9. Inflammation and swelling of the seventh cranial nerve with resultant unilateral facial muscle paralysis is called:
   1. Bell palsy.
   2. Temporal (giant cell) arteritis.
   3. Facial droop.
   4. Trigeminal neuralgia.

10. The WHNP/midwife understands that the following trigger helps differentiate a migraine from a tension headache:
    1. Alcohol.
    2. Bright lighting and noxious stimuli.
    3. Stressful situations.
    4. Sleep pattern disturbances.

11. Many visits to emergency departments by adults are prompted by headaches. Which symptom may help the WHNP/midwife differentiate a migraine headache from a headache that may indicate severe problems?
    1. It is preceded by an "aura."
    2. It occurs mainly behind one eye and tends to be grouped.
    3. Onset is sudden and accompanied by nuchal rigidity.
    4. It occurs mainly on awakening.

12. An adult patient presents with a complaint of facial paralysis that started suddenly. In making a diagnosis, the WHNP/midwife considers which of the following symptoms of Bell palsy?
    1. Concurrent paralysis of the opposite arm and leg.
    2. Pain in the (ipsilateral) ear that accompanied or preceded the paralysis.
    3. Loss of bowel control.
    4. Loss of hearing on the opposite side.

13. A patient recently diagnosed with multiple sclerosis asks the WHNP/midwife about the disease process. The WHNP/midwife knows that:
    1. 90% of patients have a quickly progressive form of the disease.
    2. 90% of patients, after the first onset of symptoms, have relapses and remissions.
    3. 10% of patients will respond to corticosteroids.
    4. 10% of patients have problems with optic neuritis and sensory loss.

14. A 30-year-old female patient has had several episodes of incontinence, weakness, visual loss, and some ataxia. Physical exam reveals slight swelling of the optic disc on fundoscopy, difficulty with heel-to-toe walking, lower extremity weakness, and 2+ deep tendon reflexes. Which condition does the WHNP/midwife suspect?
    1. Multiple sclerosis.
    2. Parkinson disease.
    3. Amyotrophic lateral sclerosis.
    4. Myasthenia gravis.

15. A patient has a 3-year history of recurrent headaches once or twice a month lasting 12 to 18 hours. When the patient presents at the clinic, she has taken 6 g of acetaminophen in the past 12 hours with no relief. The WHNP/midwife would:
    1. Recommend a parenteral narcotic analgesic, as well as prescribe opioids for prn use.
    2. Consider an analgesic rebound relative to the dose of acetaminophen taken.
    3. Order naproxen (Anaprox) for prophylactic treatment of the headaches.
    4. Order an EEG and MRI to rule out pathology.

16. A patient presents to the emergency department, stating it is the "worst headache of my life." The patient reports that the headaches have not responded to the usual over-the-counter headache remedies. What is a priority differential?
    1. Brain tumor.
    2. Migraine.
    3. Onset of newly diagnosed seizure disorder.
    4. Subarachnoid hemorrhage.

17. A patient with a recent history of a left hemisphere stroke returns to the clinic for a checkup. What symptoms would the WHNP/midwife anticipate the patient to exhibit?
    1. Left-sided weakness.
    2. Bilateral weakness of lower extremities.
    3. Difficulty with speech.
    4. Left visual field deficit.

18. The WHNP/midwife is evaluating a group of older adult patients for risk factors of an embolic stroke. Which condition would be least likely to precipitate this type of stroke?
    1. Mitral valve disease.
    2. Atrial fibrillation.
    3. Endocarditis.
    4. Diabetes mellitus.

19. A patient returns to the clinic for a follow-up visit. She has a history of simple partial seizures. When questioning the patient, the WHNP/midwife would identify recurrence of this seizure activity if the patient reported:
    1. Short episodes when she loses consciousness but does not fall.
    2. No loss of consciousness, but jerking and tingling of her right leg, and then right hand.
    3. Auditory hallucinations, unconsciousness, and urinary incontinence.
    4. Short period of unconsciousness, followed by period of confusion.

20. A patient with a history of myasthenia gravis presents with ptosis, facial weakness, dysphagia, and generalized weakness. What is important for the WHNP/midwife to ask on initial assessment?
    1. When did the symptoms first begin, and have they increased in severity?
    2. What medications is the patient taking, and when did she last take them?
    3. What activity was the patient participating in when the symptoms began?
    4. Has the patient experienced any seizure activity with the increase in symptoms?

21. A patient presents with miosis, ptosis, and anhidrosis of the ipsilateral face and neck. The initial diagnosis would be:
    1. Horner syndrome.
    2. Damage to cranial nerves III and IV.
    3. Ménière disease.
    4. Mycotic aneurysm.

22. The WHNP/midwife is seeing a patient for new-onset headaches. Which statement by the patient would cause the most concern?
    1. "This headache makes me sick to my stomach."
    2. "This headache is behind my right eye and is giving me stabbing pain."
    3. "This headache has awakened me from sleep for the past week."
    4. "I have needed to wear dark glasses for the past 3 days in a row."

23. The WHNP/midwife is treating a patient with Parkinson disease. What finding should the WHNP/midwife anticipate?
    1. Visual hallucinations and paranoia.
    2. Bowel and bladder dysfunction.
    3. Disorders in extraocular movements.
    4. Pulmonary hypertension associated with left ventricular failure.

24. Which of the following statements is correct concerning brain tumors?
    1. Meningiomas are the most frequent type of primary malignant tumors.
    2. A history of breast cancer has no associated risk for brain tumor.
    3. New-onset seizures are a common clinical finding.
    4. Increased intracranial pressure is a classic early finding in meningioma.

25. The WHNP/midwife suspects a patient has Parkinson disease. Which assessment would be least helpful in supporting this diagnosis?
    1. Observing the gait for center of gravity.
    2. Performing passive flexion/extension of the forearm.
    3. Pulling the patient's shoulders from behind.
    4. Testing for hyperactive deep tendon reflexes.

26. Historically, pain has been appropriately treated in which population?
    1. Pediatric patients.
    2. Middle-aged adults.
    3. Older-aged adults.
    4. Patient from a minority group.

Pharmacology

27. **QSEN** Which product would be the safest choice for an 81-year-old patient with insomnia?
    1. Diphenhydramine (Benadryl).
    2. Doxepin (Silenor).
    3. Oxazepam (Serax).
    4. Ramelteon (Rozerem).

28. A patient is taking an antiepileptic medication. The WHNP/midwife understands that the antiepileptic medication:
    1. Must be taken indefinitely.
    2. Is usually discontinued after 4 years of no seizure activity, and EEG confirms lack of seizure activity.
    3. Is usually given in combination with other antiepileptics or sedatives to reduce the seizure threshold.
    4. Must be given to all patients who experience a seizure.

29. A 67-year-old patient presents with the concern of right-sided facial pain. She describes the pain as burning and sharp. The pain has not awakened her from sleep. She explains she has to "press on it" when it starts, and she does not talk or move her mouth because it worsens the pain. The WHNP/midwife will consider what management based on the symptoms:
    1. Carbamazepine (Tegretol).
    2. Indomethacin (Indocin).
    3. Prednisone.
    4. Valacyclovir (Valtrex).

30. Which product would reduce essential tremors?
    1. Alcohol.
    2. Caffeine (over-the-counter).
    3. Pseudoephedrine (Sudafed).
    4. Enalapril (Vasotec).

31. The WHNP/midwife is seeing a 56-year-old patient with a history of hypertension, dyslipidemia, and Barrett esophagitis. The patient has experienced headaches since playing volleyball in high school. Which product would you discourage the patient from continuing based on her chronic illnesses?
    1. Acetaminophen (Tylenol).
    2. Amlodipine (Norvasc).
    3. Sumatriptan (Imitrex).
    4. Prochlorperazine (Compazine).

32. Which medication class is recognized for the treatment of moderate to severe dementia?
    1. Cholinesterase inhibitors.
    2. N-methyl-D-aspartate (NMDA) receptor antagonists.
    3. Selective serotonin reuptake inhibitors (SSRIs).
    4. Central alpha$_2$ agonists.

33. QSEN Before prescribing an abortive agent for migraines, a priority question to ask the patient would be:
    1. "Do you have a history of gastric colic?"
    2. "Do you have a history of panic episodes?"
    3. "Do you have a history of cardiac disease?"
    4. "Do you have a history of seizure disorder?"

34. What would be a priority to teach in a newly diagnosed patient initially using an anticonvulsant?
    1. Contact sports pose no risk to persons with epilepsy.
    2. The anticonvulsant medication will cause drowsiness.
    3. Avoid solitary activities.
    4. Medical alert bracelets are unhelpful.

35. Which factor demonstrates the best evidence in patient outcomes when initially treating ischemic stroke?
    1. Cardiac rhythm control.
    2. Blood pressure control.
    3. Timely use of thrombolytics.
    4. Renal protection, including fluid support.

36. The WHNP/midwife recognizes that which antibiotic class can interfere with the metabolism of first-generation antiepileptic drugs, such as carbamazepine?
    1. Cephalosporins.
    2. Quinolones.
    3. Sulfonamides.
    4. Macrolides.

37. The WHNP/midwife is discussing the worth of the herpes zoster vaccination with a 52-year-old patient. What would be an accurate statement in promoting the vaccine?
    1. Postherpetic neuralgia is not a reason to accept the vaccine.
    2. A severe case of zoster increases the risk of postherpetic neuralgia.
    3. Age is not correlated with risk for postherpetic neuralgia.
    4. Herpes zoster cannot affect the central or peripheral nervous systems.

38. What information is important for the WHNP/midwife to teach the patient regarding the use of medications to treat trigeminal neuralgia?
    1. Medications may cause seizure-like activity.
    2. Therapeutic levels of the drug may take up to 1 month to be reached.
    3. Relief of the symptoms should occur within 24 hours of starting the medication.
    4. Permanent side effects are not a concern of this condition.

16 Answers and Rationales

Disorders

1. (2) Headaches should decrease in frequency and severity with age. New onset of headaches after age 50 years is considered a dangerous sign. Other dangerous signs include asymmetric responses to light in pupils, change in the patient's level of consciousness, headache described as "worst pain in my life," a "different" type of headache, headaches awakening the patient during sleep, painful temporal arteries, or behavioral changes.

2. (3) The most common form of facial paralysis is Bell palsy, a disorder affecting the facial nerve characterized by muscle flaccidity of the affected side of the face. Trigeminal neuralgia is a disorder of cranial nerve V that is characterized by an abrupt onset of pain in the lower and upper jaw, cheek, and lips. Herpes zoster affects the dermatomes and does not cause a paralysis, but rather pain, herpetic grouped skin vesicles, and possibly postherpetic neuralgia.

3. (3) If a headache becomes more and more severe, if there is new onset of severe headache in a patient over 35 years old, if the headache's character or progression is different from other headaches, or if there is vomiting, but no nausea, there could be a new and serious cause for the headache. The side on which the headache occurs, and accompanying rhinorrhea, may or may not be significant. Increasing pain when bending over is characteristic of sinus pressure or infection.

4. (1) Benign paroxysmal positional vertigo usually occurs in older patients. Younger persons who experience a sudden episode of vertigo, tinnitus, hearing loss, sensation of fullness, and nausea and vomiting typically have Ménière disease. Peripheral vestibulopathy usually follows upper respiratory or gastrointestinal viral illness and involves nearly incapacitating vertigo that increases with positional changes, but not hearing loss or tinnitus. The WHNP/midwife should suspect acoustic neuroma if gradual hearing loss, tinnitus, and vertigo occur before the development of facial numbness and weakness.

5. (2) Guillain-Barré syndrome presents with progressive paresthesias and weakness most commonly in the lower extremities. It can occur following a recent illness. The symptoms are bilateral. Amyotrophic lateral sclerosis typically presents with unilateral paresthesias in one of the upper extremities, as does multiple sclerosis in a lower extremity. Muscular dystrophy commonly presents in younger patients and with pain and stiffness.

6. (4) In addition to the factors listed, keeping cool, not warm, is associated with improvement of neurologic function. A regular exercise program is encouraged, along with daily intake of a multivitamin, antioxidants, and low-dose aspirin (81 mg). Maintaining ideal body weight, having rest periods or naps daily, and becoming informed about the disease process are important aspects of promoting health.

7. (3) Reestablishing regularity will assist in maintaining bladder control. A catheter exposes the patient to infection. Fluids should not be restricted.

8. (1) Bell palsy involves a sensorineural hearing loss. In contrast to being able to read lips, this patient must be able to hear the direction of sound without any visual prompting. The tuning fork assists in differentiating between air and bone conduction of sound.

9. (1) The symptoms describe Bell palsy, which is thought to be caused by a virus. This sudden onset of unilateral facial paralysis usually resolves within 2 weeks but can endure for months. A few patients may have residual problems. Temporal or giant cell arteritis is a generalized, large-vessel vasculitis commonly affecting the branches of the proximal aorta that supply the neck and the extracranial structures of the head. Facial droop occurs with Bell palsy because of paralysis of the muscles innervated by the facial (seventh cranial) nerve. Trigeminal neuralgia is sudden pain along the fifth cranial nerve.

10. (4) Sleep pattern disturbances, either too little or too much, may trigger a migraine headache. Lighting and noxious stimuli, along with alcohol use and stress, may trigger both tension and migraine headaches.

11. (3) A sudden onset headache and nuchal rigidity may indicate a subarachnoid hemorrhage. Migraine headache without aura is the most common; however, migraine with aura occurs before the onset of pain. Cluster headaches occur behind one eye and are grouped. Headaches associated with hypertension occur mainly on awakening.

12. (2) Bell palsy is typically preceded or accompanied by pain in the ear on the paralyzed side often 1 to 2 days before the onset of facial paralysis. The paralysis is confined to the face, and there is no bowel involvement. Postauricular pain, tinnitus, and a mild hearing deficit may occur on the affected side.

13. (2) Multiple sclerosis (MS) is characterized by exacerbations and remissions of the symptoms. Only 10% of patients with MS have a progressive form of the disease from the onset. Many patients (35%–40%) have problems of optic neuritis, sensory loss, and weakness, and do respond to corticosteroids.

14. (1) Involvement of more than one central nervous system area, age 15 to 60 years, two or more separate episodes of symptoms involving different sites, or gradual progression over at least 6 months meet the criteria for multiple sclerosis.

15. (2) The recommended dose for acetaminophen is no more than 4 g per day. This patient may be experiencing an analgesic rebound headache. Appropriate prophylactic medications for migraine include beta blockers (propranolol), tricyclic antidepressants (amitriptyline), selective serotonin reuptake inhibitors (paroxetine), anticonvulsants (topiramate), and calcium channel blockers (verapamil). It is not necessary to order expensive tests for patients with migraine or tension headache. Usually a careful, thorough history is sufficient.

16. (4) This is a common patient complaint ("worst headache of my life") with a subarachnoid hemorrhage. This patient should have an emergent noncontrast CT scan of the brain and lumbar puncture with immediate referral to a neurologic surgeon, if either is positive.

17. (3) The speech center (Broca area) is most often located in the left cerebral hemisphere. The patient would experience weakness of the right side of the body and a right-sided visual deficit as well.

18. (4) Mitral valve disease, atrial fibrillation, and endocarditis all precipitate the development of an embolus that can result in an embolic stroke. Diabetes will precipitate occlusive disease of the cerebral arteries and the possible development of a thrombotic stroke, not an embolic stroke.

19. (2) A simple partial seizure is characterized by unilateral paresthesia, numbness and tingling, and spastic movement of the extremities. The patient has no loss of consciousness or incontinence of the bowel or bladder.

20. (2) It is important to determine first whether the patient has stayed on the medication schedule. The symptoms may be the result of missed medication or overmedication, especially with pyridostigmine (Mestinon). The symptoms may also be exacerbated by exercise and heat.

21. (1) The clinical presentation is classic for Horner syndrome, especially the lack of sweating (anhidrosis) on the ipsilateral (same) side of the face and neck as the eye symptoms. The patient needs to be referred for further neurologic workup.

22. (3) Headaches that awaken the patient from sleep are associated with intracranial tumors. Although nausea can also be present with increased intracranial pressure, intracranial tumors are associated with vomiting. Headache behind one eye is associated with cluster headaches, and photosensitivity is a common finding in migraine headaches.

23. (1) Psychosis is a common comorbidity of Parkinson disease (PD), with up to 40% of patients experiencing hallucinations. Bowel/bladder dysfunction, extraocular movement disorders, and cardiac complications, including left-ventricular pathology, are not associated with PD.

24. (3) Approximately one-half of patients with brain tumors have a seizure. A history of breast, lung, melanoma, renal, and colon cancer increases risk for brain metastases. Gliomas are the most common type of primary malignant brain tumors. Increased intracranial pressure is a late finding in slow-growing tumors.

25. (4) Hyperactive deep tendon reflexes are not an expected finding of Parkinson disease. Asymmetric deep tendon reflexes may be present. Observing for flexed posture is a cardinal sign in the attempt to maintain a secure center of gravity with quick, short steps. Passive flexion/extension of the forearm with rigidity and cogwheeling is an expected finding, as well as imbalance with sudden pulling of the shoulders from behind the patient.

26. (2) Pain has been studied primarily in middle-aged patients. Pediatric patients, older adults, and patients from minority groups have historically not received adequate management of their pain.

Pharmacology

27. (4) Ramelteon (Rozerem) is a melatonin-receptor agonist, which has the lowest side effect profile for the elderly. Ramelteon should be avoided in severe hepatic impairment. Diphenhydramine (first-generation antihistamine), doxepin (tricyclic antidepressant), and oxazepam (benzodiazepine) have anticholinergic properties, including risk for sedation, confusion, falls, and urinary retention in the elderly patient.

28. (2) Although most medication is discontinued after 4 years of no seizure activity a confirmatory EEG should be obtained. Not all patients with seizure require medication; referral to and monitoring by a neurologist are appropriate.

29. (1) The patient's symptoms are diagnostic of trigeminal neuralgia. This disorder responds well to anticonvulsant therapy (carbamazepine). Indomethacin and prednisone reduce inflammation but are not considered first-line therapy in trigeminal neuralgia. Valacyclovir is an antiviral used to treat herpes zoster. This patient's pain has several similarities with herpes zoster, but herpes zoster has more continuous pain, including while trying to sleep.

30. (1) Patients with essential tremors are at higher risk for alcohol abuse as alcohol reduces the tremor. Caffeine products (tea, soda, coffee, chocolate) and over-the-counter cold/cough medications worsen tremor. Beta blockers are used to reduce tremors, not ACE-inhibitors.

31. (3) Sumatriptan targets 5-hydroxytryptamine receptors in the brain that are associated with headaches. Triptans cause vasoconstriction, which can place patients at risk for cardiac and cerebral ischemia, especially with a medical history of preexisting cardiac and vascular disease. Acetaminophen, amlodipine, and prochlorperazine do not place the patient at risk for vasoconstriction.

32. (2) NMDA receptor antagonists (e.g., memantine) are recognized as the class for management of moderate to severe Alzheimer dementia. This group of medications controls the effects of glutamate (the major excitatory transmitter in the central nervous system) at NMDA receptors, which are believed to play a critical role in learning and memory. The NMDA receptor regulates calcium entry into the neuron. Selective serotonin reuptake inhibitors (SSRIs) are antidepressants used in the treatment of depression and anxiety. Central alpha$_2$ agonists are used in the treatment of hypertension.

33. (3) Abortive medications for migraines cause cranial vasoconstriction, which will be generalized to all vessels, including cardiac. A history of cardiac disease, especially ischemia, increases risk for cardiac event.

34. (2) Patients should be aware that all antiseizure medications can cause drowsiness, so driving, bathing, swimming, using machinery, climbing, and others, are all risky behaviors, especially when starting new medications. Contact sports would not be encouraged because the patient would be at risk of worsening seizure control should a head injury occur. Avoiding solitary activities is not discouraged, providing machinery and high areas are not involved. Medical alert bracelets or necklaces allow expedient information should the patient be injured and unconscious following a seizure.

35. (3) Timely intervention with thrombolytics has the best evidence for patient outcomes. The goal from onset of symptoms to thrombolytics is 180 minutes. The risk of disability is greatly reduced with thrombolytic use, and the benefits outweigh the risk of a bleed.

36. (4) Macrolide antibiotics, such as erythromycin and clarithromycin, can increase the plasma concentration of carbamazepine; therefore when these medications are used together, carbamazepine levels must be closely monitored.

37. (2) The risk for postherpetic neuralgia increases with age, as well as zoster severity. Postherpetic neuralgia can be a chronic, life-altering condition and is associated with increased risks of suicide. Zoster targets the peripheral nervous system (individual dermatomes), but can also infect the central nervous system, causing myelitis and encephalitis.

38. (3) Onset of drug action and relief of trigeminal neuralgia symptoms occur in 24 hours, usually in 4 to 6 hours. Laboratory tests are usually monitored based on the specific medication, not a peak and trough. These medications may be given to treat seizures.

17

Gastrointestinal and Liver

Disorders

1. A 20-year-old female patient in her third year of college presents with altered stool consistency and frequency for the past 6 months. She notes there is no pattern, and she cannot predict when she will have diarrhea. She notes increased stress as she prepares for final exams. The WHNP/midwife suspects irritable bowel syndrome (IBS). What other history would assist in a diagnosis of IBS?
   1. Weight loss of 15 lbs.
   2. Lower abdominal cramping that is associated with a bowel movement.
   3. Symptoms occur frequently after she has cereal with milk in the morning.
   4. Stomach upsets in high school.

2. A sudden onset of diarrhea that consists of 5 to 6 loose stools per day and awakens the patient at night with cramping, but without blood in the stools, would most likely be caused by:
   1. Infection.
   2. Irritable bowel syndrome (IBS).
   3. Ischemic colitis.
   4. Lactose intolerance.

3. The WHNP/midwife suspects peritonitis in a patient. What assessment finding is most indicative of peritonitis?
   1. Palpate and watch for a positive Murphy sign.
   2. Perform a rectal exam and test the stool for blood.
   3. Auscultate the abdomen for increased bowel sounds.
   4. Palpate for rebound tenderness.

4. An older adult woman is noted to have iron-deficiency anemia. She has no pain or rectal bleeding. What history would raise the suspicion of a gastric ulcer?
   1. Symptoms of acid reflux for the past 2 years, occurring at least 3 times a week.
   2. Postmenopausal with no recent history of vaginal bleeding.
   3. Weight loss of 10 lbs. in the past 2 months.
   4. An ankle sprain requiring 800 mg of ibuprofen three times a day for the past 6 weeks.

5. A 45-year-old woman is seen for anal itching and a rash. Symptoms have been present for 3 months and are worse after a bowel movement and at night. She uses medicated wipes to clean her perianal area several times a day. She notes intense itching, burning, and pain around the anus. She has no comorbidities and is otherwise healthy. She has tried hemorrhoid cream with no relief. The WHNP/midwife suspects pruritus ani. What would be the best treatment for her?
   1. Topical hydrocortisone cream applied to the perianal area three times a day for 6 weeks.
   2. Antifungal cream applied twice a day for 2 weeks.
   3. Keep the perianal skin dry and clean with water and avoid severe rubbing.
   4. Sitz baths four times a day and apply a moisture barrier cream, such as zinc oxide, daily for 3 weeks.

6. A patient with a chief complaint of diarrhea alternating with constipation, intermittent cramping, and bloating and relieved by a bowel movement is most likely:
   1. Antibiotic-induced diarrhea.
   2. Inflammatory bowel disease (IBD).
   3. Gastroenteritis.
   4. Irritable bowel syndrome (IBS).

7. Which problem would most likely worsen the symptoms of gastroesophageal reflux disease (GERD)?
   1. Small sliding hiatal hernia.
   2. An empty stomach when lying down.
   3. Gaining 10 lbs. over a period of months.
   4. Gastroparesis.

8. Which finding most likely indicates a need for an endoscopy in patients with heartburn?
   1. Any new onset of heartburn.
   2. Symptoms persisting after 8 to 12 weeks of empiric therapy.
   3. Negative *Helicobacter pylori* test.
   4. Good response to empiric treatment after 7 to 10 days.

9. Irritable bowel syndrome (IBS) affects:
   1. Men more than women.
   2. Children more than young adults.
   3. Women more than men.
   4. Elderly persons more than young adults.

10. The WHNP/midwife understands that hepatitis B can be transmitted through blood and blood products. Another mode of transmission of hepatitis B is:
    1. Respiratory contact.
    2. Arthropod vectors.
    3. Fecal-oral route.
    4. Perinatal exposure.

11. A rare but emergent potential complication of a hernia includes:
    1. Infection.
    2. Incarceration.
    3. Bowel obstruction.
    4. Testicular torsion.

12. A 54-year-old woman complains of intermittent crampy abdominal pain over the past 18 hours, loss of appetite, vomiting, abdominal bloating, and inability to have a bowel movement. She has a history of hysterectomy 20 years ago, cholecystectomy 5 years ago, and 2 laparoscopies for abdominal pain over the past 4 years. The WHNP/midwife sends her to the emergency room because she suspects:
    1. Appendicitis.
    2. Small bowel obstruction.
    3. Biliary ductal obstruction.
    4. Gastroenteritis.

13. The WHNP/midwife sees a 65-year-old woman with constipation. She reports a history of "slow bowels" for most of her life and has taken laxatives on a regular basis. She has had worsening symptoms requiring her to increase bisacodyl (Correctol) from every other day to daily over the past 3 months. She still has a stool every 3 to 4 days and can have no stool for 7 days or more at times. She has no abdominal pain and never feels that she has a "good bowel movement." What is her most likely diagnosis?
    1. Loss of bowel function related to chronic stimulant laxative use.
    2. Pelvic floor dyssynergia.
    3. Colonic inertia.
    4. Irritable bowel syndrome—constipation predominant.

14. Which is true about enterobiasis (pinworm infection)?
    1. The parasite is in the soil and enters the body through the feet. It can cause anemia.
    2. The parasite causes pruritus around the anus because the gravid females exit through the anus at night and lay eggs on the skin. The human is the only host of this parasite.
    3. The eggs of this parasite enter the body by ingestion of dirt (pica) or dirt on unwashed vegetables that contain the eggs, or through water containing the eggs.
    4. This parasite is a protozoan. The source is usually contaminated water, but it is spread from person-to-person by fecal-oral contamination.

15. When a patient complains of chronic constipation with no alarm symptoms, what should be the first step?
    1. Colonoscopy to rule out blockage from colon cancer.
    2. Defecography to rule out rectocele.
    3. Increasing fiber intake to 30 to 35 g per day.
    4. Physical therapy to strengthen pelvic floor muscles.

16. An organism associated with etiology of peptic ulcer disease (PUD) is:
    1. *Streptococcus pneumoniae.*
    2. *Helicobacter pylori.*
    3. *Moraxella catarrhalis.*
    4. *Staphylococcus aureus.*

17. A common cause of cirrhosis and need for liver transplantation in the United States is:
    1. Hepatitis A.
    2. Nonalcoholic fatty liver disease (NAFLD).
    3. Chronic hepatitis B.
    4. Alcohol ingestion.

18. An acute illness with jaundice, anorexia, malaise, arthralgias, an incubation period of 2 to 6 months, a chronic and acute form, and that is transmitted by parenteral, sexual, and perinatal routes describes:
    1. Hepatitis A.
    2. Hepatitis B.
    3. Hepatitis C.
    4. Hepatitis E.

19. A patient with a history of cholelithiasis presents to the office complaining of increased right upper quadrant abdominal pain. The WHNP/midwife would arrange immediate hospital admission for possible, prompt intervention if the history also showed that the patient is:
    1. 40 years old and having diarrhea.
    2. 75 years old and diabetic.
    3. 5 weeks pregnant.
    4. 23 years old and obese.

20. A 70-year-old woman complains of increased gas and bloating over the past 6 months. She has difficulty controlling the gas and expels it frequently. She also notes intermittent diarrhea after eating. The WHNP/midwife had seen the patient 6 months ago for bronchitis but had not treated her with antibiotics. She notes symptoms are worse when she has cheese and ice cream. She denies lactose intolerance. The following lab tests were normal: complete blood count (CBC), comprehensive metabolic panel (CMP), and urinalysis (UA). Her thyroid stimulating hormone (TSH) was 5.2, with upper limit of normal 4.5, and a *Helicobacter pylori* immunoglobulin G antibody was elevated. What is the most likely cause of her symptoms?
    1. Lactose intolerance.
    2. Celiac disease.
    3. Hyperthyroidism.
    4. *Helicobacter pylori* infection.

21. A 66-year-old woman was sent to the WHNP/midwife after an evaluation for a cough by pulmonary function test. Her pulmonary function test was normal, and she is not responding to fluticasone propionate HFA or albuterol (Proventil HFA). She has had a dry cough for the past year that is worse after eating. Occasionally she wakens at night coughing. She denies chest pain, dyspnea, fever, or signs of an upper respiratory illness. She has type 2 diabetes and hyperlipidemia and is taking metformin and atorvastatin. She has no history of heart disease and had a negative ECG. She had gained 20 lbs. but her weight has been stable for the past year. What is the likely cause of her cough?
    1. Environmental allergies including pollen.
    2. Exposure to fumes at her job.
    3. Sinusitis and postnasal drainage.
    4. Gastroesophageal reflux disease (GERD).

22. A 19-year-old woman presents to the WHNP/midwife for evaluation of 2 days of increasing crampy abdominal pain. She states that she also has some mild nausea, anorexia, and a low-grade fever. The patient states that the pain is periumbilical. Her STAT complete blood count (CBC) reveals a slightly elevated white blood count but is otherwise normal. What is the WHNP/midwifes next step in the care of this patient?
    1. Refer to a gynecologist for evaluation of possible ectopic pregnancy.
    2. Order a CT scan of the abdomen and refer to surgeon for evaluation of possible appendicitis.
    3. Observe overnight and reassess the next day.
    4. Place on a clear liquid diet and have patient watch for increasing symptoms.

23. A 54-year-old woman has early alcoholic cirrhosis diagnosed by a liver biopsy. While teaching the patient to manage her symptoms, the WHNP/midwife instructs that it is most important that the patient:
    1. Take daily vitamin E supplement.
    2. Decrease her alcohol intake to less than two drinks a day.
    3. Abstain from alcohol.
    4. Maintain a nutritious diet.

24. A 72-year-old woman presents with fever, leukocytosis, and a sudden onset of lower left quadrant pain for the past 12 hours. She has not had a bowel movement since the pain began. The WHNP/midwife's top differential diagnosis would be:
    1. Appendicitis.
    2. Diverticulitis.
    3. Irritable bowel syndrome (IBS).
    4. Ruptured ovarian cyst.

25. Which patient would be at **lowest** risk for developing diverticular disease?
    1. A vegetarian on a high-fiber diet.
    2. A patient with chronic constipation for 10 years.
    3. An older patient on a six small meals per day diet.
    4. A patient on a low carbohydrate diabetic diet.

26. The WHNP/midwife knows that in patients with ulcerative colitis that involves the entire colon (universal or pancolitis), careful surveillance of the colon is required because of an increased risk of:
    1. Colon cancer.
    2. Diverticulosis.
    3. Ischemic colitis.
    4. Irritable bowel syndrome.

27. Which is true of peptic ulcer disease (PUD) in older adult patients over the age of 65 years?
    1. Smoking does not increase the risk of PUD.
    2. Duodenal ulcers are more common in older adults.
    3. Perforation is a common complication.
    4. Weight loss and anorexia are often the only symptoms.

28. A patient has a history of colon polyps. The WHNP/midwife knows:
    1. A history of polyps increases the risk of colon cancer, and more frequent screening is required.
    2. Hyperplastic polyps are a concern for malignancy.
    3. Small polyps <1 cm are not a concern.
    4. A colonoscopy is 100% accurate for finding colon polyps and cancer.

29. A 32-year-old patient presents with a complaint of intermittent diarrhea and cramping for the past 2 years. Screening blood tests reveal iron-deficiency anemia and elevated liver transaminases. The WHNP/midwife suspects:
    1. Hepatitis B.
    2. Celiac sprue.
    3. *Salmonella* infection.
    4. Bleeding peptic ulcer.

30. Irritable bowel syndrome (IBS) can produce which of the following symptoms?
    1. Abdominal cramping, rectal bleeding, and diarrhea.
    2. Diarrhea alternating with constipation, but no pain.
    3. Abdominal cramping, diarrhea, and fecal incontinence.
    4. Abdominal cramping, diarrhea, and bloating.

31. When discussing diet with a patient with irritable bowel syndrome (IBS), the WHNP/midwife tells the patient to avoid:
    1. Simple sugars.
    2. Dairy products.
    3. Red meat.
    4. Vegetables.

32. Patient education for nonalcoholic fatty liver disease (NAFLD) should include:
    1. Working on lowering cholesterol intake.
    2. Discontinuing any statin medication.
    3. Beginning exercise and working on weight loss with diet.
    4. Taking vitamin A 15,000 IU daily.

33. This viral strain that can cause gastroenteritis is seen in adolescents and adults. It has a short incubation period (18–72 hours) and short duration of symptoms (24–48 hours). It is characterized by an abrupt onset of nausea and abdominal cramps, followed by vomiting and diarrhea, and is often accompanied by headache and myalgia. What is the most likely cause?
    1. *Campylobacter.*
    2. Norovirus (Norwalk).
    3. Rotavirus.
    4. Cytomegalovirus.

34. When evaluating acute abdominal pain, what would be characteristics that would require emergent care?
    1. 3-week history of bloating, nausea, and upper abdominal fullness.
    2. 3-month history of nonspecific upper abdominal discomfort.
    3. 1-year history of worsening rising retrosternal burning pain occurring daily.
    4. Sudden knife-like epigastric pain.

35. A patient complains of melena-black, tarry stools. The WHNP/midwife knows that this:
    1. Has no pathologic significance.
    2. Involves a loss of blood less than 30 mL.
    3. Is likely bleeding from the colon.
    4. May likely be bleeding from the esophagus or stomach.

36. Which is not a risk factor for cholelithiasis (gallstones)?
    1. Male gender.
    2. Obesity.
    3. Rapid weight loss.
    4. Pregnancy.

37. Management of nausea and vomiting is based on the underlying cause. Which of the following is the most common cause of nausea and vomiting in adults and children?
    1. Food poisoning.
    2. Peptic ulcer disease.
    3. Gastroenteritis.
    4. Cholecystitis.

38. A 54-year-old woman complains of right upper quadrant (RUQ) abdominal pain, nausea, and vomiting that began last night approximately 4 hours after eating a rich, fatty meal. She has a temperature of 100°F and a palpable RUQ mass. The most likely diagnosis is:
    1. Cholecystitis.
    2. Acute pancreatitis.
    3. Acute hepatitis A.
    4. Appendicitis.

39. A 21-year-old white college student complains of fatigue, RLQ abdominal pain, and diarrhea for the past 2 months. She has lost 10 lbs. and notes chills periodically. She denies rectal bleeding. She notes that she is stressed about final exams. The WHNP/midwife would be most concerned about:
    1. Irritable bowel syndrome.
    2. Intestinal infection.
    3. Crohn disease.
    4. Ulcerative colitis.

Pharmacology

40. The WHNP/midwife is examining a 30-year-old obese woman with a body mass index (BMI) of 35 who complains of almost daily indigestion and heartburn for the past year, with a strong acid taste in the mouth approximately 1 hour after meals, and frequent belching and awakening at night with choking. The history is negative for chronic illnesses and alarm symptoms. A diagnosis of gastroesophageal reflux disease (GERD) is made. What is the best initial treatment for the patient?
    1. Lansoprazole (Prevacid) 15 mg with breakfast daily.
    2. Hyoscyamine (Levsin) 0.125 mg tid 15 minutes before eating.
    3. Famotidine (Pepcid) 20 mg bid.
    4. Omeprazole (Prilosec) 20 mg every morning 30 to 60 minutes before breakfast.

41. A 42-year-old woman complains of rectal pain after a bowel movement that persists for an hour. This began 10 weeks ago, after a particularly hard, large stool. Since then she has had pain with every stool and has noted a slight amount of bleeding on the tissue paper. The WHNP/midwife suspects an anal fissure. What would be the most appropriate treatment for a chronic anal fissure?
   1. Sitz baths, psyllium fiber, and bulking agents.
   2. Topical lidocaine gel.
   3. Pramoxine-hydrocortisone cream (Analpram-HC singles rectal).
   4. Topical nitrate ointment 0.2%.

42. Which of the following would be prescribed by the WHNP/midwife as initial treatment for a 72-year-old woman with uncomplicated peptic ulcer disease (PUD) and negative *Helicobacter pylori* (*H. pylori*) by stool antigen?
   1. Clarithromycin.
   2. Tetracycline and metronidazole and a histamine 2 receptor antagonist (H_2RA).
   3. Pantoprazole (Protonix).
   4. Bismuth (Pepto-Bismol).

43. After percutaneous or permucosal exposure to a hepatitis B source, what is the appropriate treatment for the patient?
   1. In an unvaccinated patient, begin the hepatitis B series.
   2. In a person with a positive hepatitis B surface antibody, no treatment is necessary.
   3. In a vaccinated person with a negative antihepatitis B surface antigen, give hepatitis B immune globulin (HBIG), and initiate a new hepatitis B vaccine series.
   4. In a patient with a positive antihepatitis B surface antibody who completed the entire hepatitis B vaccine series, give a hepatitis B booster.

44. Successful treatment for an adult patient with *Helicobacter pylori (H. pylori)*–induced peptic ulcer disease requires therapy with which regimen?
   1. Clarithromycin, amoxicillin, and omeprazole (Prilosec) for 14 days.
   2. Bismuth (Pepto-Bismol), cephalexin (Keflex), and metronidazole (Flagyl) for 10 days.
   3. Amoxicillin, bismuth (Pepto-Bismol), metronidazole (Flagyl), and cimetidine (Tagamet) for 10 days.
   4. Clarithromycin, tetracycline, cephalexin (Keflex), and lansoprazole for 14 days.

45. A primary therapy for patients with mild ulcerative colitis is:
   1. Metronidazole (Flagyl).
   2. Mesalamine (Asacol).
   3. Ciprofloxacin (Cipro).
   4. Prednisone (Deltasone).

46. For a patient exposed to household or sexual contacts with hepatitis A, the WHNP/midwife would:
   1. Give immunoglobulin 0.02 mL/kg as soon as possible but no later than 2 weeks after exposure.
   2. Give one dose of HBIG and immunoglobulin 0.02 mL/kg as soon as possible.
   3. Give immunoglobulin 0.02 mL/kg and two doses of HBIG.
   4. Understand that no injections are needed.

47. A young woman presents with a history of recent unprotected sexual activity (in the past 2 weeks) with a partner now diagnosed with hepatitis B. She is currently asymptomatic and does not recall having a vaccine in the past. What is the best action for the WHNP/midwife?
   1. Obtain a hepatitis B e antibody test (anti-HBe).
   2. Administer one dose of hepatitis B immune globin (HBIG).
   3. Obtain a viral load for hepatitis B.
   4. Administer one dose of HBIG and initiate vaccination.

48. What condition is a contraindication for the administration of the hepatitis B vaccine?
   1. Pregnancy.
   2. Lactation.
   3. Severe hypersensitivity.
   4. Age older than 60 years.

49. A patient takes bismuth subsalicylate (Pepto-Bismol). The patient calls the WHNP/midwife to report that her stools are unusually dark. She is not experiencing any gastric discomfort, orthostatic hypotension, or increased lethargy. How would the WHNP/midwife interpret the information?
   1. She is probably bleeding and should come in immediately.
   2. She ate something to affect the color of her stool.
   3. Her stools are dark, secondary to Pepto-Bismol.
   4. The stool discoloration is caused by metronidazole.

17 Answers and Rationales

Disorders

1. (2) IBS is the most common disorder of gut–brain interaction, formerly known as a functional gastrointestinal disorder. Newly revised diagnostic criteria include abdominal pain at least 1 day a week for the past 3 months with onset at least 6 months prior, and/or associated with a change in stool frequency and/or stool appearance. An unexplained weight loss is an alarm symptom that requires further investigation and is not associated with IBS. Symptoms with dairy intake may be lactose intolerance, whereby the lack of the enzyme lactase inhibits the breakdown of mild sugar. A history of stomach upsets is nonspecific and could be related to gastroesophageal reflux, IBS, or other conditions.

2. (1) Diarrhea is a common symptom with a wide differential. Clues include awakening at night and cramping without blood. A sudden onset that awakens a patient suggests pathology, which could be inflammation or infection. Obtaining a travel history, exposure to infection, and medication history may suggest infection. Irritable bowel syndrome is a functional disorder that does not awaken the patient. Ischemic colitis presents with rectal bleeding, as well as pain and diarrhea. Lactose intolerance and other dietary triggers cause functional diarrhea and cramping.

3. (4) Rebound tenderness is found with placing pressure on the abdomen and quickly lifting the hand. Patients will complain of more pain with release of the pressure on the abdomen rather than the pressure itself. This suggests parietal peritoneal irritation and inflammation. Other signs include a positive cough test, guarding, and rigidity. Murphy sign is indicative of gallbladder inflammation and occurs with complaints of right upper quadrant (RUQ) pain and tenderness. Stool for occult blood is not a test for peritonitis as it would indicate gastrointestinal bleeding. Increased bowel sounds, also known as borborygmi, are more associated with the gastrocolic reflex and hyperactivity in intestines and would not be present with peritonitis. However, decreased bowel sounds may be present with peritonitis.

4. (4) Nonsteroidal antiinflammatory drugs (NSAIDs), such as ibuprofen, carry a high risk of gastrointestinal erosion and ulcers. There may be no symptoms until anemia is noted. Gastroesophageal reflux does not contribute to anemia, unless there is gastritis with erosions or other signs of bleeding. Postmenopausal history is significant because it rules out a cause of anemia, but not a concern for ulcer development. Weight loss of 5 lbs. per month is a nonspecific symptom that needs further exploration.

5. (3) Pruritus ani is an uncomfortable sensation around the anal orifice. It is common and may be associated with hemorrhoids. The main symptom is intolerable impulse to scratch the perianal region, most often after a bowel movement and at bedtime. Hydrocortisone cream could relieve the symptoms but should be used for only a short period, 2 weeks or less. Long-term corticosteroid use can lead to atrophy, infections, and contact dermatitis. Antifungal cream would not be helpful unless there was secondary infection. The skin needs to be kept clean and dry and not vigorously rubbed. Moisture and creams are not helpful as the symptoms will continue. Some food and drink can exacerbate the symptoms and should be avoided, such as coffee, tea, cola, chocolate, and beer. Regular bowel habits are also important.

6. (4) Irritable bowel syndrome (IBS) presents with abdominal pain and altered bowel habits that can be erratic and unpredictable. The symptoms can be aggravated by stress and food triggers. Diarrhea should not occur during sleep, but abdominal pain can occur at any time. Antibiotic-induced diarrhea occurs in association with a recent course of antibiotics, especially in the previous 3 months. Antibiotics may trigger *Clostridium difficile* colitis. Bacterial or viral gastroenteritis presents with a sudden onset of diarrhea and does not alternate with constipation. Inflammatory bowel disease (IBD) presents with more consistent symptoms of diarrhea and pain and possibly rectal bleeding. In fact, the symptoms of IBD can be present for months to years before diagnosis. Extraintestinal manifestations, such as arthritis and skin lesions, may be present, and nocturnal diarrhea and fecal incontinence can be present if rectal inflammation is present.

7. (4) Gastroparesis can be a significant complication for patients with reflux. The lingering contents in the stomach contain acid, and the frequency of reflux will be increased. Persons with a small sliding hiatal hernia are not likely to have a significant change in their symptoms. Reflux is less likely to occur after lying down with an empty stomach. Weight gain may worsen symptoms, but usually it is noted with a significant change in weight, not just 10 lbs.

8. (2) An endoscopy is needed for patients with no/minimal response to therapy, indicated by persistent symptoms after 8 to 12 weeks of therapy. Heartburn may be

characterized by burning substernal chest pain and may have gastroesophageal reflux. The factors that would raise a red flag would be long-term history of reflux, dysphagia, or weight loss. It is not recommended to test with endoscopy for all patients with heartburn. A negative *H. pylori* test lessens the chance of inflammation and ulceration. Response to treatment within 2 weeks is a positive indication that the patient has gastroesophageal reflux and can continue treatment and be followed in the office.

9. (3) Most epidemiologic studies demonstrate that IBS is up to 50% more common in women than in men, appears to be familial, and is estimated to affect 10% to 30% of the adult population in Western countries. A disease of young and middle-aged adults, IBS peak prevalence occurs in the third and fourth decades of life, and the condition is usually diagnosed before age 50 years.

10. (4) A means of hepatitis B (HBV) transmission is from an infected mother to baby, perinatally. Before the hepatitis B vaccine, it was estimated that 30% to 40% of chronic HBV infections were transmitted perinatally. Since the widespread use of the vaccine and guidelines of vaccinating newborns, this rate has dropped dramatically. The main routes of transmission are contact with an infected person, including sexual; transfusions; sharing razors or toothbrushes; sharing needles, syringes, and other drug-injecting equipment; blood and open sores; and needle sticks or other sharp instruments. HBV is not spread by food, water, sharing eating utensils, breastfeeding, hugging, kissing, coughing, sneezing, or the fecal-oral route.

11. (2) Symptoms of an incarcerated hernia that has strangulated include acute pain, redness, nausea, and vomiting, and is considered a surgical emergency and requires immediate referral to a surgeon. Strangulated hernias should be surgically repaired as early as possible to prevent complications, such as necrosis and viscus perforation. Bowel obstruction and testicular torsion are emergent conditions but are not associated with an incarcerated hernia.

12. (2) The patient's symptoms most likely represent a small bowel obstruction (SBO). The history of multiple abdominal surgeries provides a possible cause, as adhesions commonly develop after surgery and are one of the most common causes of SBO. Appendicitis would be documented on a CT scan, which would likely be done at the emergency room. Appendicitis can present with these symptoms, but the pain is usually progressive and not intermittent. Biliary ductal obstruction is unlikely as the patient's gallbladder has been removed and although stones can reform it takes many years, usually more than 5 years. Another cause of biliary obstruction is a neoplasm, but the patients usually do not have pain, and bowels are not generally affected. Gastroenteritis is usually accompanied by diarrhea, not constipation.

13. (1) Chronic long-term use of stimulant laxatives, such as bisacodyl, can worsen constipation as the bowels become dependent and develop a resistance to the stimulants. Pelvic floor dyssynergia can cause fecal incontinence, diarrhea, or constipation; however, stimulant laxatives would cause diarrhea because the colon motility is not the problem. Colonic inertia is an infrequent cause of constipation and can be severe, it may be a differential diagnosis, but not the most likely. Irritable bowel syndrome has pain as a major symptom, which is not present with this patient's symptoms.

14. (2) The pinworm parasites reside in the intestine. Females lay eggs on the skin outside the anus, resulting in extreme pruritus. The only host is humans and it is transmitted by the fecal-oral route, easily spreading among households, daycares, and schools. Hookworm larvae reside in the soil, enter the body through the feet, and can cause anemia. When dirt containing roundworm eggs are ingested through pica or unwashed vegetables, or if contaminated water is consumed, an intestinal infestation occurs. Giardiasis results from ingestion of the protozoan *Giardia lamblia* through contaminated water or oral-fecal transmission.

15. (3) Lifestyle modifications should be the first step in managing constipation. Most patients do not have enough fiber in their diet. Thirty to thirty-five grams per day is recommended, most of which should come from the diet. Fiber supplements can help but do not add a significant amount of fiber. Patients need to read food labels to determine their fiber amount. Increasing fluids and exercise are also useful to maintain regular bowel function. In the absence of alarm symptoms, such as weight loss, rectal bleeding, or significant abdominal pain, conservative therapy should be tried before considering testing. It is rare that colon cancer causes constipation and blockages as this would be an advanced cancer. Rectocele can be a cause of constipation and should be considered if lifestyle modifications are not improving bowel function.

16. (2) *Helicobacter pylori* has been shown to be responsible for most duodenal and gastric ulcers. The other common cause of ulcers is from use of nonsteroidal antiinflammatory drugs (NSAIDs) at regular and/or high doses. The other organisms listed are implicated in other types of infections (e.g., acute otitis media; skin infections). *Streptococcus pneumoniae* and *Moraxella catarrhalis* have been implicated as causative agents in pneumonia.

17. (2) Hepatitis A never becomes chronic and is not a cause of cirrhosis. Nonalcoholic fatty liver disease (NAFLD)

is common, affecting 25% to 30% of the general population, and is related to the metabolic syndrome. Excess fat deposits, partially due to insulin resistance, can cause inflammation and scarring that lead to cirrhosis. NAFLD has been increasing in incidence and severity and is becoming the number one reason for liver transplant in the United States. Chronic hepatitis B is not a major cause of cirrhosis in the United States but is a worldwide epidemic and responsible for hepatocellular cancer. Alcohol in large and/or daily amounts can cause cirrhosis.

18. (2) These characteristics describe hepatitis B, which affects less than 1% of the US population and is a much less common cause of cirrhosis. Hepatitis A has symptoms of fever and jaundice (up to 50%), but the incubation period is 15 to 50 days (average 30 days) and does not have a chronic form. Hepatitis C infection causes jaundice up to 25% of the time and can cause arthralgia, but there is no fever. The incubation period is 14 to 18 days (average 42–49 days). Up to 75% of those infected with hepatitis C will develop chronic infection. Hepatitis E is characterized by oral-fecal transmission that is associated with contaminated food and water and has an incubation period of 14 to 60 days and no chronic disease state.

19. (2) Although some patients need eventual intervention including a cholecystectomy, those who are older adults and diabetic are at increased risk for complications and should be hospitalized for prompt diagnosis, which could include a right upper quadrant (RUQ) abdominal ultrasound, and possibly a magnetic resonance cholangiopancreatography (MRCP). The MRCP is very sensitive at documenting a gallstone lodged in the bile duct. Abnormally elevated transaminases and possibly pancreatic enzymes would be present with bile duct blockage, and the patient may have secondary pancreatitis. Intravenous fluids, pain control, and surgical consultation would also be warranted.

20. (1) Intermittent diarrhea, gas, and bloating can occur after ingestion of dairy if the patient is lactose intolerant. This can occur at any time and can present after a viral illness. The decrease or loss of the enzyme lactase that breaks down lactose in dairy results in colonic bacteria breaking down the lactose and producing gas and diarrhea. Some patients can be extremely sensitive to all dairy, including butter. Patients with celiac disease are usually anemic and may have elevated liver enzymes. Hyperthyroidism can cause diarrhea, but the patient's TSH is high meaning she has hypothyroidism. *Helicobacter pylori* infection can cause abdominal pain and bloating but would not necessarily cause diarrhea and the elevated antibody is not confirmatory of infection.

21. (4) GERD can present with a variety of symptoms, including atypical extraesophageal symptoms, such as cough. Acid in the esophagus can trigger a bronchospasm resulting in a cough and other pulmonary symptoms. Her weight gain coincides with the onset of the cough, which can worsen reflux. The timing of the cough, after meals and at night, correlates with when reflux is likely to be occurring. Not everyone who has GERD is aware of it and has no classic heartburn on regurgitation. Environmental allergies can contribute but her symptoms would likely be more seasonal and not continuous the entire year, depending on her location. Exposure to fumes would trigger a cough, but pulmonary workup was negative, and she did not respond to treatment. Sinusitis and postnasal drainage can cause a cough, but likely would be seasonal and not necessarily occurring after meals.

22. (2) Increasing crampy abdominal pain that starts as periumbilical pain, anorexia, and fever are classic symptoms of appendicitis. A surgeon should evaluate the patient to decrease the risk of rupture. An abdominal CT scan has a high sensitivity to document appendicitis. Although ectopic pregnancy should always be a consideration in young women with abdominal pain, the characteristics of the pain and other symptoms are not typical of an ectopic pregnancy. However, a good gynecologic history would be needed. The patient should not be sent home unless the CT scan was negative, and then follow-up within 24 hours would be warranted.

23. (3) Abstinence from alcohol, the most important treatment for cirrhosis, can halt progression of cirrhosis and reverse the damage if the liver is minimally scarred. Continuing to drink even occasionally can be detrimental and rapidly increase the disease process. It is known that an average of 1 to 2 drinks a day for a woman raises her risk of cirrhosis up to four times the risk of the general population (2–3 drinks a day for men). A standard drink is considered 14 g of pure alcohol, which translates to 12 ounces of beer, 5 ounces of wine, or 1.5 ounces of distilled spirits. Recent research shows that current drinking may be more of a factor than a lifetime amount. The patient's diet should be nutritious, and she should avoid herbal and other supplements because some have been known to cause liver toxicity. There is no recommendation for vitamin E supplementation.

24. (2) Diverticulitis is defined as clinically evident macroscopic inflammation of a diverticulum or diverticula. It occurs in 4% of patients with diverticulosis. Patients usually present with a sudden onset of abdominal pain in the left lower quadrant. The patient may have a low-grade fever and leukocytosis. Patients with diverticulitis can have a range of mild to severe inflammation and 15% will develop complications. Nausea and vomiting may accompany severe pain. Appendicitis may present with pain in the periumbilical region that eventually travels to the right lower quadrant (RLQ) and may not be

severe for several hours after onset. Other signs, including nausea and vomiting, leukocytosis, and fever, may or may not be present. Irritable bowel syndrome (IBS) may present with aching or cramping in the periumbilical or lower abdominal regions, often precipitated by meals and relieved by defecation. The pain can be severe occasionally, and there is an altered frequency and consistency of the stools. Fever, leukocytosis, and awakening at night are not indicative of IBS. A ruptured ovarian cyst would not be a differential in an older adult woman, as the ovaries shrink and stop functioning with menopause.

25. (1) A high-fiber diet is important for preventing and treating for diverticular disease, and vegetarians who eat increased amounts of fruits, vegetables, grains, and cereals with high fiber are in the lowest risk category. Chronic constipation causes chronic increased pressure in the sigmoid colon, which can increase the likelihood of bowel wall weakening and diverticula (out-pouches) developing. Small meals and low-fiber diets (low carbohydrate with low intake of grains) would also increase the risk of constipation.

26. (1) Colorectal cancer (CRC) risk in patients with left-sided and universal ulcerative colitis increases by 0.5% to 1% per year after the eighth year of disease. Ulcerative colitis limited to the proctosigmoid region carries less of a risk. Crohn disease, which can affect any part of the gastrointestinal tract from the mouth to the rectum, carries a higher risk if the colon is involved. Colonoscopy with random biopsies every 1 to 2 years is recommended beginning 8 to 10 years after the IBD began. Diverticulosis is common in the general population but is less common in ulcerative colitis and is not a risk factor for CRC. Ischemic colitis occurs when a mesenteric artery is temporarily blocked and the colon at the splenic flexure develops ischemia from lack of blood flow. There is not a higher risk of ischemic colitis for patients with ulcerative colitis. Irritable bowel syndrome is common in the general population and in patients with ulcerative colitis, but it is a disorder of brain–gut interaction and does not increase risk of colon cancer.

27. (4) Patients with a gastric ulcer may not have any symptoms, especially in the older adult. Weight loss and anorexia may be present, but the patient may attribute this to "getting older." The patient may not realize an ulcer is present until it bleeds and causes significant anemia. Smoking does increase the risk, and perforation can occur, but is not common. Gastric ulcers are thought to be more common than duodenal ulcers in older adult patients.

28. (1) A history of polyps does increase the risk of colon cancer, and on average patients will need a repeat colonoscopy in 3 to 5 years, rather than the recommended 10 years if there are no polyps and no family history. Hyperplastic polyps, in general, are not a concern and do not develop into cancer. Adenomatous polyps can develop into cancer. Small polyps may be adenomas and will be removed during the colonoscopy. Histologic analysis is required to identify adenomatous polyps. A colonoscopy is the most sensitive and specific test for polyps and cancer, but there are factors that affect the efficacy contributing to a variable miss rate for polyps and cancer.

29. (2) Celiac sprue is a genetic disease of the small bowel that is caused by gluten intolerance. The diarrhea and cramping are related to the effects of malabsorption of gluten. Because of malabsorption, many patients have iron-deficiency anemia and can have elevated liver enzymes. Hepatitis B would produce elevated liver enzymes, but not the other listed symptoms. *Salmonella* infection could produce diarrhea and cramping, but not anemia. A bleeding ulcer could produce anemia, but not the other symptoms.

30. (4) The symptoms of cramping, diarrhea, and bloating are classic for irritable bowel syndrome (IBS) with diarrhea predominant. Abdominal pain is a symptom of IBS but is not associated with rectal bleeding or fecal incontinence.

31. (1) People with irritable bowel syndrome (IBS) can have many food triggers. The challenge is to identify the foods without having them avoid entire food groups. Simple sugars, specifically fermentable oligo-, di-, and mono-saccharides and polyols (FODMAPS) can cause symptoms of cramping, gas, bloating, and diarrhea. Rather than avoiding all fruits and vegetables, patients need to be aware of the most offending foods and carefully avoid those that cause a problem. Dairy products have lactose, which is not able to be broken down when someone is lacking some or all lactase, the enzyme needed for digestion of lactose. Although people can have IBS and lactose intolerance, it should not be assumed the patient has both. Red meat and saturated fat can cause some problems but are not prime offenders.

32. (3) One of the ways patients can decrease the fat in the liver is to lose weight with exercise. It is important to treat hyperlipidemia because this is associated with fatty liver, and statins should not be discontinued. Lowering cholesterol is not as effective as lowering saturated fats in the diet. Adding vitamin A as a supplement is controversial, and excessive doses over 10,000 IU of vitamin A daily can cause or worsen liver damage.

33. (2) Norovirus (Norwalk) can cause vomiting and diarrhea in adolescents and adults. The incubation period is short (18–72 hours) and the duration of symptoms is short, usually 24 to 48 hours. Cytomegalovirus rarely

causes diarrhea and is commonly reactivated in patients after bone marrow transplant, late stages of HIV infection, and other immunocompromised situations. *Campylobacter* enteritis is the most common cause of bacterial diarrhea, especially in traveler's diarrhea and food poisoning. Rotavirus mainly affects infants 3 to 15 months of age in the winter months, causing excessive watery diarrhea.

34. (4) Sudden knife-like epigastric pain occurs with gallstone pancreatitis and would require immediate evaluation and intervention. Bloating, nausea, and abdominal fullness may be dyspepsia or gastroparesis. Nonspecific abdominal pain can be functional dyspepsia. Retrosternal burning pain is indicative of heartburn. However, all of the above can also represent more serious conditions and require further testing, but not necessarily emergently. Keep in mind the duration can be a key to chronicity, but it is important to always consider and may be misleading when evaluating a history.

35. (4) Black stools without a tarry, shiny, sticky appearance is likely of no concern. Tarry stools indicate passage of blood and usually from the upper gastrointestinal tract, involving a loss of at least 60 mL of blood.

36. (1) Female gender is a risk factor. A well-known mnemonic of the typical cholelithiasis patient is the "six Fs": fat, female, forty (age), flatulent, fertile, and fat-intolerant.

37. (3) All listed are common causes of nausea and vomiting but gastroenteritis is the most common.

38. (1) Patients with an acute attack of inflammation of the gallbladder usually have a gallstone obstructing the gallbladder-cystic duct junction. This is a typical presentation. Acute pancreatitis usually presents with a sudden onset of severe, deep epigastric pain that can radiate into the back. Acute hepatitis A will present with general symptoms of malaise, fever, jaundice, and fatigue. The patient with hepatitis can have RUQ pain and liver enlargement, but not a defined mass. Appendicitis presents initially with abdominal pain, usually severe and throughout the entire abdomen before localizing to the RLQ. No mass is noted. All of these conditions can also present with fever and nausea and vomiting. The history of the onset after a high fatty meal is key to considering the top diagnosis of gallbladder origin. Lab testing and radiology can quickly differentiate the conditions.

39. (3) Crohn disease is a chronic, progressive inflammation of the intestinal tract, most commonly, the small intestine. The peak age of onset is 15 to 25 years, with women and white race more often affected. Her symptoms are a classic presentation. Irritable bowel syndrome is common but there should not be weight loss or fever (chills). Infection should always be ruled out with chronic diarrhea, and a history of exposure to possible causes (travel, antibiotics, food poisoning) would increase suspicion. Ulcerative colitis usually presents with rectal bleeding and is less likely to have fever, and pain would more likely be in the RLQ.

Pharmacology

40. (4) Omeprazole is a proton pump inhibitor (PPI) that blocks all three pathways of acid production: histamine, gastrin, and acetylcholine, for up to 24 hours. Treatment with a PPI is recommended for patients who have frequent symptoms, at least several times a week. It is important to take the PPI on an empty stomach, and then eat 30 to 60 minutes after for maximum pH control. PPIs need food to work, and, if a second dose is required, it should be taken before the evening dose. Anticholinergics (hyoscyamine and others) will likely increase her symptoms by lowering the lower esophageal sphincter pressure. Anticholinergics are effective for the cramping of IBS. Famotidine is a histamine 2 receptor antagonist (H_2RA), which blocks one pathway for acid secretion, histamine, but there are two other pathways that continue to secrete hydrochloric acid. An H_2RA can be effective for occasional symptoms, a few times a week or less, or as a short trial for new onset of symptoms.

41. (4) Topical nitrate ointment applied twice daily for 6 to 8 weeks has been associated with healing of chronic anal fissure at least 50% of the time. It can also decrease rectal pain. The most commonly occurring side effect is headache in 20% to 30% of the patients. Topical calcium channel blockers are also utilized but the data are insufficient to conclude healing superior to placebo. Sitz baths, psyllium, and bulking agents are first-line therapy for acute anal fissure and can be helpful for symptomatic relief. Topical lidocaine gel can provide some relief of pain but does not affect healing. Analpram-HC is used to treat of symptoms of hemorrhoids, including pain, itching, and swelling. An anal fissure is a longitudinal tear in the midline of the anal canal, distal to the dentate line. An acute fissure looks like a simple tear in the anoderm, whereas a chronic fissure is defined as lasting 8 to 12 weeks and has edema and fibrosis associated with it.

42. (3) Goals of PUD treatment include removal of offending agent, relief of pain, healing of ulcer, and cost effectiveness. In this case, the likely cause of her ulcer would be use of nonsteroidal antiinflammatory drugs (NSAIDs). It is estimated that up to 25% of patients taking NSAIDs chronically will develop ulcer disease, and 2% to 4% will develop bleeding or perforation. Risk factors for NSAID-induced ulcers include age greater than 65 years, high

doses of NSAIDs, daily use, use of aspirin or anticoagulants, or antiplatelet medications. Proton pump inhibitors (PPIs) heal 90% of duodenal ulcers after 4 weeks and 90% of gastric ulcers after 8 weeks if *H. pylori* is negative. PPIs, such as pantoprazole, are recommended for ulcers because these drugs provide faster pain relief and more rapid healing than H_2RA because of their ability to decrease acid production. Clarithromycin, tetracycline, metronidazole, and bismuth (Pepto-Bismol) are some of the accepted treatments against active *H. pylori*–associated ulcers. Eradication of *H. pylori* requires a recommended regimen of acid blockers, antibiotics, and possibly bismuth in various combinations.

43. (2) If a person exposed to a patient known to be positive for hepatitis B has sufficient immunity to hepatitis B, no treatment is necessary. If this same person had not been vaccinated, in addition to initiation of the hepatitis B vaccine series, HBIG 0.06 mL/kg IM is also administered. If an exposed person has had an inadequate immune response to the hepatitis B vaccine series (negative anti-hepatitis surface antibody), a hepatitis B booster should be given.

44. (1) Patients with gastric or duodenal ulcers due to *H. pylori* can be successfully treated with triple-drug therapy: a PPI (bid for all except esomeprazole which is qd), clarithromycin, and amoxicillin or metronidazole for 14 days (eradication rates 70%–85%). An alternative US Food and Drug Administration–approved regimen is a quadruple regimen (qd or bid) or H_2RA (bid), metronidazole, bismuth, and tetracycline for 10 to 14 days (eradication rates 75%–90%). Treatment should continue with a proton pump inhibitor (PPI) for at least 2 to 4 weeks after to promote healing of the ulcer. After completion of *H. pylori* therapy, it is recommended that testing be done with the stool antigen for *H. pylori* at 8 weeks to assure eradication of the infection. The PPI would need to be stopped for 2 weeks before testing the stool, as there can be false-negative results. Other treatment regimens have been suggested but eradication rates can vary. Cephalosporins are not included in any recommended regimens for *H. pylori*.

45. (2) Mesalamine (5-aminosalicylic acid) therapy for patients with mild ulcerative colitis has been shown to improve symptoms and induce and maintain remission. It is an antiinflammatory compound similar to aspirin, without the effects on platelets. There are several mesalamine products available, including rectal suspension and suppositories, that can be very helpful for left-sided colitis. If no response is seen after 2 to 4 weeks, the addition of corticosteroids (prednisone) can be helpful, but they are not first-line therapy. Ciprofloxacin and metronidazole are typically used for gastrointestinal infections, including *Clostridium difficile*, which is common with ulcerative colitis.

46. (1) To minimize the risk of a contact developing hepatitis A, which is spread by fecal-oral transmission, immunoglobulin 0.02 mL/kg should be given as soon as possible after exposure. It has not been shown to be effective if administered more than 2 weeks after exposure. Hepatitis B immune globulin (HBIG) is for hepatitis B.

47. (4) For unvaccinated patients with exposure to hepatitis B, one dose of HBIG is administered and the hepatitis B series initiated. HBIG may be protective or may attenuate the severity of the illness if given within 7 days of exposure (adult dose of 0.06 mL/kg). If the patient thinks the individual may have been vaccinated, but does not know whether there was a response, the WHNP/midwife can test antihepatitis B surface antibody. Neither the HBe antibody nor the viral load would be a first-line test. Because of the timing of appearance of the antibodies to hepatitis B, testing would need to be delayed.

48. (3) The only contraindication to the hepatitis B vaccine is prior anaphylaxis or severe hypersensitivity to the vaccine or components of the vaccine.

49. (3) This is a common observation for a patient taking Pepto-Bismol. The patient may also experience a problem with discoloration of her tongue. The stool discoloration is not related to bleeding. Certain foods can affect the stool color, but bismuth is more likely the cause.

18

Hematology

Disorders

1. Sickle cell anemia is caused by:
   1. Exposure to ionizing radiation.
   2. Genetically induced production of abnormal hemoglobin S.
   3. Deficiency of dietary folic acid.
   4. Long-term use of thiazide diuretics.

2. An adult patient presents to the WHNP/midwife with a history of erythrocytosis. One common complaint that could cause a serious complication for the patient is:
   1. A laceration.
   2. Vomiting and diarrhea.
   3. Coughing.
   4. Dizziness.

3. After the loss of her husband 5 months ago, a 67-year-old female patient began abusing alcohol. She has no prior medical problems and no history of alcoholism. Which of the following would be the most likely cause of new-onset anemia development in this patient?
   1. Liver cirrhosis.
   2. Thiamine deficiency.
   3. Folate deficiency.
   4. Cyanocobalamin deficiency.

4. A patient has a folic-acid-deficiency anemia. The WHNP/midwife teaches the patient to eat foods rich in folic acid, such as:
   1. Green leafy vegetables, nuts, and liver.
   2. Carrots, salmon, and avocados.
   3. Cottage cheese, yogurt, and skim milk.
   4. Lima beans, brussels sprouts, and potatoes.

5. Which of the following changes occurs in the red blood cell (RBC) indices for pernicious anemia?
   1. Microcytic, normochromic.
   2. Microcytic, hypochromic.
   3. Normocytic, normochromic.
   4. Macrocytic, normochromic.

6. Which statement is true concerning thalassemia?
   1. It is characterized by defective lymphocyte synthesis.
   2. Thalassemia minor does not require pharmacologic treatment.
   3. Thalassemia major is associated with high RBC counts and elevated serum iron.
   4. It is characterized by an acute onset of symptoms leading to leukocytosis.

7. Iron-deficiency anemia is an example of:
   1. Macrocytic, normochromic anemia.
   2. Macrocytic, hypochromic anemia.
   3. Microcytic, hypochromic anemia.
   4. Normocytic, normochromic anemia.

8. An adult patient with pernicious anemia may present with which signs and symptoms?
   1. Peripheral neuropathy, ataxia, lethargy, and fatigue.
   2. Hepatomegaly, jaundice, and right upper quadrant pain.
   3. Hypertension, angina, and peripheral edema.
   4. Blurred vision, diplopia, and decreased vibratory sensation.

9. In teaching a patient with anemia to include foods rich in iron in the diet, the WHNP/midwife encourages the patient to eat:
   1. Cheese, milk, and yogurt.
   2. Red beans, whole-grain bread, and bran cereal.
   3. Tomatoes, cabbage, and citrus fruits.
   4. Beef, spinach, and peanut butter.

10. Anemia of chronic disease is associated with:
    1. Malnutrition and vitamin B_{12} deficiency.
    2. Infections, inflammation, and neoplasms.
    3. Traumatic injuries and folate deficiency.
    4. Excessive menstrual flow, trauma, and heredity.

11. The WHNP/midwife understands that most adult patients with Hodgkin lymphoma present with:
    1. Nausea, vomiting, and diarrhea.
    2. Night sweats, weight loss, and fever.
    3. Painless, movable mass in the neck, axilla, or groin.
    4. Hepatosplenomegaly with a painful mass in the mediastinum.

12. What is the most common leukemia found in the older adult, typically asymptomatic and characterized by median survival of approximately 10 years?
    1. Acute myelogenous.
    2. Chronic myelogenous.
    3. Acute lymphocytic.
    4. Chronic lymphocytic.

13. Folic-acid deficiency most often results from:
    1. Lead exposure.
    2. Poor dietary habits.
    3. Gastrointestinal bleeding.
    4. Genetic defect.

14. The WHNP/midwife is teaching a client who has pernicious anemia to select which foods?
    1. Rice, bread, and cereals.
    2. Green leafy vegetables.
    3. Beef, chicken, clams, and oysters.
    4. Fresh citrus fruits.

15. What type of anemia is associated with lead poisoning?
    1. Normocytic anemia.
    2. Microcytic anemia.
    3. Macrocytic anemia.
    4. Aplastic anemia.

16. The WHNP/midwife understands the following regarding von Willebrand disease (vWD):
    1. It is a bleeding disorder caused by an excess of platelets.
    2. Common symptoms are ecchymosis and epistaxis.
    3. Has only one inherited type unlike hemophilia, which has different types.
    4. Has a lowered life expectancy of all the coagulation disorders.

17. The WHNP/midwife suspects aplastic anemia in an adult patient with a long history of rheumatoid arthritis. What findings are associated with this diagnosis?
    1. History of taking gold medications.
    2. Short stature with skeletal or nail changes.
    3. Lack of bruising and fever.
    4. Pancytopenia.
    5. History of taking immunosuppressive medications.

Pharmacology

18. A 65-year-old woman is being discharged after a successful hip replacement. What is the minimum duration of therapy the WHNP/midwife would expect for postoperative deep vein thrombosis (DVT) thromboprophylaxis with rivaroxaban (Xarelto)?
    1. 3 to 5 days.
    2. 5 to 7 days.
    3. 10 to 14 days.
    4. 14 to 21 days.

19. The WHNP/midwife determines that an adult female patient has an iron deficiency anemia and has ruled out gastrointestinal (GI) bleeding as the cause. The WHNP/midwife:
    1. Refers the patient to a hematologist.
    2. Orders iron dextran 50 mg IM weekly for 4 weeks and schedules the patient for weekly office visits for the injection.
    3. Prescribes ferrous sulfate 325 mg PO tid and schedules the patient to return in 1 month for a repeat complete blood count, serum iron, and total iron-binding capacity.
    4. Schedules the patient to return in 6 months for additional stool guaiac testing.

20. What information would the WHNP/midwife include in teaching a patient about the treatment of vitamin B_{12} deficiency following a total gastrectomy?
    1. The patient will be taking vitamin B_{12} tablets twice daily for 1 year.
    2. The patient will be taking oral folic acid supplements daily for life.
    3. The patient will receive monthly cyanocobalamin (vitamin B_{12}) injections for life (after being given daily injections for 7 days followed by weekly injections for the first month).
    4. The patient will require iron supplementation and monthly blood transfusions until the deficiency is corrected.

21. Which of the following would most likely need to be given to a patient with sickle cell anemia?
    1. Cyanocobalamin.
    2. Niacin.
    3. Thiamine.
    4. Folate.

22. After initiating vitamin B_{12} therapy, the WHNP/midwife would expect which of the following at a 4-week follow-up visit to the clinic?
    1. Ferritin level of 40 ng/mL.
    2. Reduced RBCs, white blood cells, and platelets.
    3. Increased macrocytosis and anisocytosis.
    4. Increased hemoglobin/hematocrit and reticulocyte count.

23. It is recommended to administer a 0.5 mL (25 mg) test dose of which medication?
    1. Nascobal (intranasal B_{12} gel).
    2. Folic acid.
    3. Iron dextran.
    4. Ferrous sulfate (Feosol).

24. A patient who has been prescribed oral ferrous sulfate reports taking extra doses for the past few months. The patient's serum iron level is 560 mcg/dL. What should the WHNP/midwife order for this patient?
   1. Parenteral deferoxamine (Desferal).
   2. Recheck the iron level in 2 weeks.
   3. Gastric lavage and treatment for acidosis and shock.
   4. Oral deferasirox (Exjade).

25. The WHNP/midwife understands that patients who take both folic acid and vitamin B_{12} that folic acid can:
   1. Reverse the hematologic effects of vitamin B_{12} deficiency.
   2. Cause fetal malformation with high doses.
   3. Improve the neurologic effects of B_{12} deficiency.
   4. Cause a microcytic, normochromic anemia.

26. A patient is receiving oral ferrous sulfate (Feosol) for iron deficiency anemia. The WHNP/midwife is considering placing the patient on an antibiotic drug. Which medication, if taken concurrently with iron, would decrease the absorption of the iron supplement?
   1. Cefixime.
   2. Metronidazole.
   3. Amoxicillin.
   4. Tetracycline.

27. A patient with hemophilia A is undergoing a tooth extraction at the dentist's office. As an adjunct to factor VIII, what other drug would the WHNP/midwife order for the patient?
   1. Desmopressin (Stimate).
   2. Vitamin K.
   3. Tranexamic acid (Cyklokapron).
   4. Ibuprofen (Advil).

18 Answers and Rationales

Disorders

1. (2) Sickle cell anemia is a genetic disorder characterized by the production of hemoglobin S, an anemia secondary to shortened erythrocyte survival, microvascular occlusion by sickle-shaped erythrocytes, and increased susceptibility to certain infections. Exposure to ionizing radiation has been associated with the development of certain malignancies, especially leukemia. A deficiency of dietary folic acid does not cause sickle cell anemia, although folic acid is used in the treatment of these patients to help increase hematopoiesis and aid in recovery from aplastic events. Long-term use of thiazide diuretics has been implicated in the development of hemolytic or aplastic anemias in rare cases.

2. (2) Erythrocytosis (or polycythemia) can be worsened by dehydration from any cause, for example, vomiting and diarrhea. Coughing and dizziness will have no effect on the condition, and a laceration may actually improve the symptoms because of the blood loss.

3. (3) Patients who abuse alcohol often develop macrocytosis (mean cell volume [MCV] >100 fL). Specifically, alcoholic patients often develop macrocytic anemia due to folate (vitamin B_9) and cyanocobalamin (vitamin B_{12}) deficiencies. Folate deficiency manifests within a few months due to relatively lower stores in the liver compared with cyanocobalamin. Additionally, older adults are at a higher risk for development of folate and cyanocobalamin deficiency related to food malabsorption.

4. (1) Green leafy vegetables, oranges and orange juice, and nuts are excellent sources of folic acid. Also, cereals and breads are now fortified with folic acid. Be sure to stress that folate is heat labile and rapidly destroyed by prolonged cooking or food processing. The other foods are not significant sources of folic acid.

5. (4) A macrocytic (MCV >100 fL), normochromic anemia resulting from atrophic gastric mucosa not secreting intrinsic factor is the definition of pernicious anemia. These indices could also include folic-acid-deficiency anemia. Microcytic normochromic or hypochromic could include iron-deficiency anemia or anemia of chronic disease. Normocytic and normochromic could also include anemia of chronic disease.

6. (2) Thalassemias are chronic, inherited anemias characterized by defective hemoglobin synthesis leading to a decreased RBC count, hypochromia (mean corpuscular hemoglobin <20 pg), microcytosis (MCV <70 fL), normal serum iron, and normal RBC distribution width (RDW) in thalassemia minor, which does not require pharmacologic treatment. It should be noted that although the RDW is usually normal, it can be elevated in approximately 50% of patients with thalassemia trait, which is in contrast to iron-deficiency anemia, in which the RDW is almost always elevated (90%). Patients with thalassemia minor should not be given iron supplements to resolve anemia. Patients with thalassemia major are usually managed by a hematologist.

7. (3) Iron-deficiency anemia is a microcytic, hypochromic anemia. The RBCs are smaller (microcytic) because of the decrease in hemoglobin production caused by inadequate amounts of iron, which also makes the cell appear pale (hypochromic). The other selections describe other types of anemia, which would be determined by the peripheral smear.

8. (1) Vitamin B_{12} deficiency may result in neurologic signs and symptoms, including peripheral neuropathy, paresthesias, unsteady gait (ataxia), loss of proprioception, decreased vibratory sensation, lethargy, and fatigue. In the later stages of severe B_{12} deficiency, spasticity, hyperactive reflexes, and presence of Romberg sign are noted because of the formation of a demyelinating lesion of the neurons of the spinal cord and cerebral cortex and presence of a beefy-red tongue. These findings are specific to pernicious anemia and must be assessed in all patients who present with anemia. The other signs and symptoms are not characteristic of pernicious anemia.

9. (4) Beef, spinach, and peanut butter are iron-rich foods. The other options are examples of foods rich in calcium, fiber, and vitamin C, respectively.

10. (2) Anemia or chronic disease is associated with infections (e.g., tuberculosis), chronic inflammatory conditions (e.g., systemic lupus erythematosus, rheumatoid arthritis), and malignancies. Excessive blood loss from menstrual flow or traumatic injuries would more likely cause an iron-deficiency anemia. Malnutrition can contribute to iron, vitamin B_{12}, and folate deficiencies.

11. (3) Most patients with Hodgkin lymphoma present with a painless, movable mass in the neck, axilla, or groin. Constitutional symptoms may also occur, which include weight loss, persistent fever, and night sweats. Often the patient may experience pruritus and pain in the lymph node area after consuming alcohol (an unexplained

finding). Hepatosplenomegaly presents with advanced disease.

12. (4) Chronic lymphocytic leukemia (CLL) is found primarily in middle-aged and older adults (<10% of patients under age 50 years). Median age of diagnosis of CLL is 70 years, affecting more men than women. Acute myelogenous leukemia incidence increases with age, with median age older than 70 years. Chronic myelogenous leukemia occurs between ages 50 and 60 years. Acute lymphocytic leukemia is most common in children and gradually increases in frequency in later life, with the median age of 35 to 40 years.

13. (2) Folic-acid deficiency most often results from dietary deficits and frequently affects the older adult, chronically ill, alcoholic patients, and food faddists (poor food selections). Pregnancy requires an increase in folic acid, as do disease states such as cancer, chronic inflammation, Crohn disease, rheumatoid arthritis, and malabsorption syndromes.

14. (3) The best food sources for vitamin B_{12} are of animal origin, including the following richest sources: beef and chicken liver, lean meat, clams, oysters, herring, and crab.

15. (2) Lead poisoning can cause a microcytic anemia. Lead circulates through the body attached to erythrocytes. It affects heme production, competes with calcium in any calcium-mediated process, alters certain enzyme functions in the bone marrow, and damages the nervous system. Lead poisoning may be associated with a hypochromic, microcytic anemia because most patients have concomitant iron deficiency. Diseases included in the differential diagnoses of microcytic anemia include thalassemia, anemia of chronic disease, sideroblastic anemia, lead poisoning, and aluminum toxicity.

16. (2) Epistaxis, menorrhagia, ecchymosis, and prolonged bleeding with cuts or dental extractions and in the intraoperative or immediate postoperative period are common symptoms of vWD. vWD is a bleeding disorder caused by deficiency or a defect of von Willebrand factor (vWF) protein, and is the most common congenital bleeding disorder, occurring in up to 1% of the general population. There are three major types of vWD, all of which exhibit an autosomal inheritance pattern, thus affecting both male and female sex. vWF is critical to the initial stages of blood clotting, acting as a bridge for platelet adhesion; it also acts as a carrier for factor VIII. Life expectancy is not lower than other disorders of coagulation; actually, it is better with treatment.

17. (1, 4) Aplastic anemia is a condition in which the bone marrow failure syndrome is characterized by immune-mediated bone marrow destruction and peripheral blood pancytopenia. Fatigue, pallor, exertional shortness of breath, or palpitations are seen secondary to anemia. Mucosal bleeding, easy bruising, petechiae, or heavy menstrual bleeding are seen secondary to thrombocytopenia. Infection is uncommon at clinical presentation, but severe neutropenia may lead to fever and sore throat. Short stature with skeletal or nail change findings are associated with congenital-acquired aplastic anemia. Drugs, such as felbamate, cimetidine, nonsteroidal antiinflammatory drugs, antiepileptics, gold salts, chloramphenicol, sulfonamides, trimethadione, quinacrine, and phenylbutazone, are common etiologic factors in acquired aplastic anemia. The treatment for aplastic anemia includes hematopoietic stem cell transplantation and immunosuppressive therapy with antithymocyte globulin and cyclosporine or high-dose cyclophosphamide.

Pharmacology

18. (3) The anticoagulant rivaroxaban (Xarelto) is a factor Xa inhibitor and is recommended for postoperative DVT thromboprophylaxis in hip and knee replacements. It should be started immediately after homeostasis has been achieved postoperatively for a minimum of 10 to 14 days. Therapy in some patients may be extended up to 35 days.

19. (3) Treatment with iron orally for at least 6 months is necessary to correct both the anemia and the depleted body iron stores. Ferrous sulfate should be taken on an empty stomach 1 hour before meals. If the patient experiences GI symptoms, the dose can be reduced or the patient can take the iron with the meal; however, taking it with meals will reduce the delivery and absorption of the iron by 50%. Iron dextran (parenteral) may be used if the patient is unable to take PO medications or if the hemoglobin is less than 6 g/dL. The patient should have hemoglobin/hematocrit, iron, and total iron-binding capacity rechecked after 1 month on iron supplementation. If there is no improvement in all parameters, most notably a rise in the hemoglobin by 1 g/dL, the patient should be referred to a hematologist. Referral to a GI specialist or repeat of stool guaiac testing is unnecessary because there is no indication that this patient's condition is caused by bleeding.

20. (3) If the deficiency is not caused by inadequate intake, the patient will require lifetime supplementation of vitamin B_{12} (1000 mcg of cyanocobalamin) by intramuscular injection to ensure absorption. In patients with irreversible malabsorption (total gastrectomy) and severe neurologic symptoms, parenteral therapy is indicated: 1000 mcg/day for 7 days, and then 1000 mcg weekly for 4 weeks, followed by 1000 mcg monthly for

life. The WHNP/midwife should keep in mind that high-dose, daily oral cyanocobalamin (1000–2000 mcg) is as effective as monthly intramuscular injection and is the preferred route of initial therapy in most circumstances because it is cost-effective and convenient. Oral folic acid, iron, and blood transfusions would not treat the cause of the deficiency, and therefore the resulting anemia would not be corrected.

21. (4) Due to increased RBC turnover, folate supplementation is often required in patients with sickle cell anemia due to relatively low stores of the vitamin in the liver. Other supplementations may be indicated if dietary intake is insufficient but are given without iron. Deferoxamine or other iron chelators may be required in these patients due to a buildup of iron related to transfusions.

22. (4) In addition to a sense of well-being, improved appetite, and decreased neurologic symptoms (gait disturbances, peripheral neuropathy, paresthesias [numbness/tingling in fingers], and extreme weakness), the hemoglobin/hematocrit and reticulocyte count should increase with vitamin B_{12} therapy.

23. (3) The use of intramuscular or intravenous iron dextran is for patients who cannot tolerate oral supplementation or who have GI disease that limits oral absorption. Therapy should be initiated with an intravenous test dose of 0.5 mL (25 mg) to observe for anaphylaxis. It should be administered gradually over at least 30 seconds.

24. (1) Iron is toxic in large amounts. If the plasma level of iron is elevated (>500 mcg/dL), an iron-chelating agent, such as parenteral deferoxamine (Desferal), should be prescribed to immediately lower the iron level. Although gastric lavage may be ordered, it will only remove unabsorbed tablets that are present in the stomach. Oral deferasirox (Exjade) is used for chronic iron overload caused by blood transfusions.

25. (1) Folic acid can reverse the hematologic effects of vitamin B_{12} deficiency, but it does not reverse the neurologic effects, so it is important to determine the degree of B_{12} deficiency to treat it. Folic acid does not cause fetal malformation; but is administered prenatally to prevent neural tube defects. Folic acid causes a megaloblastic anemia.

26. (4) Coadministration of tetracycline and iron reduces absorption of both iron and tetracycline. In addition, antacids reduce the absorption of iron. Cephalosporins (cefixime), metronidazole, and penicillin (amoxicillin) have no significant drug-to-drug interaction with iron.

27. (3) Antifibrinolytic drugs (e.g., aminocaproic acid and tranexamic acid) can be used as adjuncts to factors VIII and IX in special situations, such as a tooth extraction. Nonsteroidal antiinflammatory drugs (ibuprofen) and aspirin should be avoided. Desmopressin is used as replacement therapy but is not used specifically for tooth extractions but indicated for minor procedures. Vitamin K is not indicated in this situation.

19

Urinary

Disorders

1. A 68-year-old multiparous woman returns for ongoing evaluation of stress incontinence that was thought to be associated with chronic urinary tract infections (UTIs). She has been on low-dose trimethoprim-sulfamethoxazole (TMP-SMX, Bactrim) 40/200 mg for 6 months without resolution of her symptoms. This patient should be evaluated for:
   1. Pelvic organ prolapse.
   2. Dementia or a neuromuscular disorder.
   3. Environmental barriers in the home.
   4. Addition of a tricyclic antidepressant.

2. A 65-year-old woman explains to the WHNP/midwife that she has been having frequent and painful urination. A clean-catch urine specimen for routine urinalysis (UA) with culture and sensitivity is ordered. Laboratory results show 10^5 colony-forming units (CFU)/mL of *Escherichia coli (E. coli)* and 10^4 CFU/mL of *Staphylococcus epidermidis (S. epidermidis).* The WHNP/midwife's next step would be:
   1. Treat the *E. coli.*
   2. Order amoxicillin.
   3. Treat the *S. epidermidis.*
   4. Encourage citric fruit juices.

3. A young adult comes to the college student health clinic complaining of severe abdominal discomfort and bloody urine. An initial priority in the diagnostic workup would include:
   1. Intravenous pyelography to rule out a kidney stone.
   2. Straining all urine.
   3. Microscopic urine exam.
   4. 24-hour urine culture.

4. An older adult female client who is incontinent is in an extended care facility and is found to have a red and excoriated perianal area on exam. What would the WHNP/midwife advise the caregiver to **avoid** using on the skin in the perineal area?
   1. Petrolatum.
   2. Moisture-barrier films.
   3. Mild soap and water.
   4. Zinc oxide ointment.

5. Which plan would be most appropriate for an older patient with functional incontinence?
   1. Evaluate need for incontinence pads.
   2. Limit fluid intake in the evenings.
   3. Perform the Credé maneuver.
   4. Provide a bedside commode.

6. A 78-year-old woman returns to the office after a 6-day stay in the hospital for new-onset heart failure. Her chief complaint is urinary incontinence. Which of the following is a possible cause for her new-onset urinary incontinence?
   1. Poor pelvic support causing hypermobility of the base of the female bladder.
   2. Lower urinary tract problems, such as carcinoma.
   3. Cystocele or uterine prolapse.
   4. Ingestion of certain medications, such as sedatives, diuretics, anticholinergics, and α-adrenergic agents.

7. Which statement characterizes functional incontinence?
   1. Leakage of urine during activities that increase abdominal pressure, such as coughing, sneezing, and laughing.
   2. Mainly caused by factors outside the urinary tract, especially immobility, that prohibit proper toileting habits.
   3. Characterized by the inability to delay urination, with an abrupt and strong desire to void.
   4. Occurrence of incontinence with overdistention of bladder.

8. What is the most common pathogen in community-acquired UTIs?
   1. *Klebsiella pneumoniae.*
   2. *Proteus mirabilis.*
   3. *Escherichia coli.*

9. A healthy adult female patient presents with cystitis. The WHNP/midwife would expect which of the following findings?
   1. No symptoms noted.
   2. Acute onset of chills, fever, flank pain, headache, malaise, and costovertebral angle tenderness.
   3. Complaints of dysuria, urgency, frequency, nocturia, and suprapubic heaviness.
   4. Signs and symptoms of fever, irritability, decreased appetite, vomiting, diarrhea, constipation, dehydration, and jaundice.

10. Fifteen days after completion of a course of antibiotics for a UTI, a 66-year-old woman returns to the clinic with reoccurring symptoms. Recurrent UTIs in women are caused by relapse or reinfection. The WHNP/midwife understands the following regarding relapse:
    1. It is less common than reinfection and occurs within 2 weeks of completing drug therapy for the infection.
    2. It is responsible for most recurrent UTIs in women.
    3. May result from residual urine after voiding due to prolapsed uterus or bladder or lack of estrogen.
    4. Can be treated with the same medication regimen used for the original infection.

11. The WHNP/midwife understands the following regarding pyelonephritis:
    1. Young adults with severe illness may present with altered mental state and absence of fever.
    2. Patients complain of localized flank/back pain combined with systemic symptoms, such as fever, chills, and nausea.
    3. Requires hospitalization for most cases, including parenteral antibiotic therapy.
    4. Requires no follow-up.

12. What is the term given to the type of urinary incontinence associated with conditions such as Parkinson disease or Alzheimer disease?
    1. Stress incontinence.
    2. Urge incontinence.
    3. Mixed incontinence.
    4. Overflow incontinence.

13. A 40-year-old woman presents to the clinic with a uric acid renal calculus. Knowing that the alkaline-ash, low-purine diet may be difficult for patients to adhere to, which other option should the WHNP/midwife consider?
    1. Monitor the patient for another episode.
    2. Discuss the alkaline-ash, low-purine diet in detail with the patient.
    3. Start the patient on a xanthine oxidase inhibitor and monitor serum uric acid level.
    4. Refer the patient to a urologist.

14. A 60-year-old female patient presents with complaints of blood in her urine; she denies dysuria or abdominal pain. The WHNP/midwife obtains UA to confirm hematuria. There is no evidence of infection. What is the priority diagnosis in the list of differentials?
    1. Prerenal failure.
    2. Renal calculi.
    3. Renal cell carcinoma.

15. The WHNP/midwife is taking the history of a patient who has been diagnosed with renal calculi. What would be a precipitating factor in the development of renal calculi?
    1. Increased incidence of urinary tract infections (UTIs) over the past 3 years.
    2. Drinking 6 to 8 ounces of milk daily.
    3. History of fractured femur and prolonged bed rest.
    4. High intake of citrus fruit and high-fiber carbohydrates.

16. A 47-year-old female patient complains of frequent urination. Physical exam reveals no abnormalities. She has a history of bipolar disorder controlled with lithium and states she "takes her medications somewhat regularly." Which of the following should the WHNP/midwife suspect?
    1. Central diabetes insipidus.
    2. Nephrogenic diabetes insipidus.
    3. Diabetes mellitus.
    4. Primary polydipsia.

17. A 75-year-old white female patient presents to the clinic with her husband, her primary caregiver. She has a history of multiinfarct dementia, likely from a long history of untreated hypertension. Her husband reports that for the past 2 days she has been agitated and increasingly confused, and he has not been able to redirect her. He denies the addition of new medications or over-the-counter herbal supplements. What would the WHNP/midwife suspect?
    1. New infarct.
    2. Worsening of dementia.
    3. Urinary tract infection.
    4. Underlying stress to caregiver.

18. A patient presents to the clinic with complaints of chills, severe flank pain, dysuria, and urinary frequency. Vital signs are temperature of 102.9°F (39.4°C), pulse of 98 beats per minute, respirations of 24 breaths per minute, and a blood pressure of 120/68 mm Hg. Urinalysis reveals pyuria with leukocyte casts, mild proteinuria, and urine leukocyte esterase positive. What is the probable diagnosis?
    1. Urethritis.
    2. Interstitial cystitis.
    3. Pyelonephritis.

19. A patient is diagnosed with interstitial cystitis. What would be the clinical findings?
    1. Bladder pain that lessens as the bladder fills.
    2. Pyuria with urine culture sensitivity of *E. coli* greater than 100,000 colony-forming units (CFU/mL) from a midstream-catch urine sample.
    3. Urinary frequency or urgency, hematuria, and nocturia.
    4. Elevated temperature and severe flank pain.

20. Which patient with a urinary tract infection (UTI) will require hospitalization and intravenous antibiotics?
    1. A newly pregnant woman with bacteriuria, urgency, and frequency.
    2. A young adult with dysuria, suprapubic pain, and recurrent UTI.
    3. An older adult with a low-grade fever, flank pain, and an indwelling catheter.

21. When should the WHNP/midwife refer a patient with renal calculi to a urologist?
    1. Signs of urosepsis.
    2. Dysuria and urgency.
    3. Sudden onset of severe colicky pain.
    4. Appearance of gross hematuria.

22. What are important teaching points the WHNP/midwife should include when discussing urolithiasis to a client with a history of calcium oxalate stones?
    1. Encourage 2 to 3 L/day fluid intake; advise patient to have clear urine rather than yellow.
    2. Have at least 4 to 5 servings a week of green leafy vegetables, rhubarb, nuts, chocolates, and beans.
    3. Increase protein and salt intake.
    4. Decrease calcium intake by not ingesting dairy products.

23. A patient has been diagnosed with an acute lower UTI and prescribed 160 mg TMP/800 mg SMX twice daily for 3 days. The patient calls the clinic stating that it is still painful to urinate and the frequency and urgency have only slightly diminished. What would be a priority in this patient's plan of care?
    1. Renew the 160 mg TMP/800 mg SMX antibiotic for 14 days.
    2. Change the medication to ciprofloxacin 250 mg twice daily for 3 days.
    3. Obtain a urinalysis and urine for culture and sensitivity.
    4. Have the patient increase fluids and encourage more frequent urination.

24. Which physiologic factor of aging contributes to incontinence in older adults?
    1. Decreased vascularity of the bladder mucosa.
    2. Increased urethral closing pressure.
    3. Increased ability to concentrate urine.
    4. Decreased bladder capacity.

25. A 57-year-old woman complains of fecal leakage intermittently and one episode of incontinence over the past 2 months. The WHNP/midwife elicits the following history: 3 vaginal childbirths, 8-lb. babies, 1 forceps delivery. Why was this history important?
    1. It is routine aspect of past medical history that is elicited at each female patient visit.
    2. It may provide a clue to possible etiology of fecal leakage and incontinence.
    3. It indicates that the patient now has adult children and may be dealing with stress of the "empty nest."
    4. Vaginal deliveries with large babies can cause a rectocele, which would contribute to her incontinence.

Pharmacology

26. A 67-year-old female patient presents with weakness. Available lab results include leukocytes 5200/mm^3, hemoglobin of 7.6 g/dL, and hematocrit of 22.7%. She has a history of nondialysis-dependent chronic kidney disease (CKD). Which of the following medications would the WHNP/midwife expect to be administered?
    1. Epoetin alfa (Procrit).
    2. Filgrastim (Neupogen).
    3. Sargramostim (Leukine).
    4. Sevelamer (Renvela).

27. A 69-year-old female patient reports worsening stress incontinence. Which one of the following agents would be useful in treating her symptoms?
    1. Propantheline (Pro-Banthine) 15 mg before meals; 30 mg at bedtime.
    2. Oxybutynin 2.5 mg three to four times a day.
    3. Doxepin (Sinequan) 10 to 25 mg once a day initially to maximum total daily dose of 25 to 100 mg.
    4. Conjugated estrogen (Premarin) 0.3 to 1.25 mg/day orally or vaginally, and medroxyprogesterone (progestin) 2.5 to 10 mg/day continuously or intermittently.

28. To decrease the production of uric acid kidney stones, the WHNP/midwife orders which medication?
    1. Allopurinol (Zyloprim).
    2. Indomethacin (Indocin).
    3. Bethanechol (Urecholine).
    4. Colchicine (Colcrys).

29. A 70-year-old woman is treated with oxybutynin for her urinary frequency and urgency. The WHNP/midwife would explain to the patient she will probably experience:
    1. Increased sensitivity to sunlight.
    2. Dizziness on standing.
    3. Dry mouth and increased thirst.
    4. Increased bruising.

30. A patient with recurrent calcium oxalate renal calculi can be treated with which of the following medications to aid in the prevention of stone formation?
    1. Triamterene (Dyrenium).
    2. Furosemide (Lasix).
    3. Hydrochlorothiazide (HCTZ).
    4. Acetazolamide (Diamox).

31. A 72-year-old woman with a history of renal calculi presents with complaints of severe flank pain radiating to her groin area. She is also experiencing nausea and vomiting, and her temperature is 99°F (37.2°C). What is the best initial therapy that the WHNP/midwife can provide?
    1. Ketorolac 30 mg intramuscularly.
    2. Ibuprofen (Advil) 600 mg PO q6h.
    3. Increase fluid intake and strain all urine.
    4. Trimethobenzamide (Tigan) 250 mg PO.

32. The WHNP/midwife is prescribing nitrofurantoin (Macrodantin) for a young woman who is experiencing problems with UTIs. What specific directions should be given to the patient regarding administration of nitrofurantoin?
    1. Take with food and expect brownish discoloration of urine.
    2. Do not take with milk products; take on empty stomach for better absorption.
    3. Take four times a day until symptoms have subsided for at least 24 hours.
    4. Do not take acetaminophen (Tylenol) or ibuprofen (Advil) with nitrofurantoin.

33. An adult woman presents with complaints of burning on urination, frequency, and urgency. Phenazopyridine (Pyridium) is prescribed. What specific directions should the WHNP/midwife provide for the patient regarding phenazopyridine?
    1. May discolor contact lenses; if sclerae begin to turn yellow, return to the office.
    2. Always take on an empty stomach to increase absorption.
    3. Do not take any medication containing aspirin or salicylate.
    4. May interfere with effectiveness of mini-pill for birth control.

34. The WHNP/midwife is reviewing lab results from several patients during inpatient service. On review of a urinalysis of a 67-year-old woman it is discovered that muddy brown granular casts are present. The WHNP/midwife would be most concerned about which of the following medications that can lead to this?
    1. Furosemide (Lasix).
    2. Amphotericin (Ambisome).
    3. Gentamicin (Garamycin).
    4. Ibuprofen (Motrin).

35. When prescribing oxybutynin for the patient with stress incontinence symptoms, which disorder in the patient's medical history must the WHNP/midwife consider before prescribing?
    1. Diabetes.
    2. Cough.
    3. Narrow-angle glaucoma.
    4. Gallstones.

36. A patient with no history of allergies presents with an uncomplicated urinary tract infection. When considering fluoroquinolones for the treatment, the WHNP/midwife correctly understands that:
    1. A fluoroquinolone, such as ciprofloxacin, is the drug of choice for UTIs.
    2. Fluoroquinolones are preferable to both nitrofurantoin and trimethoprim/sulfamethoxazole due to high levels of antibiotic resistance.
    3. Fluoroquinolones are considered safe in pregnancy.
    4. Fluoroquinolones should be used cautiously due to potential serious side effects.

37. Angiotensin-converting enzyme (ACE) inhibitors are recommended for slowing the progression of chronic renal disease, but are contraindicated in the following disorder:
    1. Cardiovascular disease.
    2. Hypertension.
    3. Diabetes.
    4. Renal artery stenosis.

38. A frail older adult female patient presents for annual physical exam. Her comprehensive metabolic panel reveals a GFR of 38; the previous year her GFR was 64. Which of the following medications should be eliminated from her profile?
    1. Ibuprofen (Motrin).
    2. Levothyroxine (Synthroid).
    3. Metoprolol tartrate (Lopressor).
    4. Clopidogrel (Plavix).

39. A 72-year-old female patient is scheduled for a renal angiogram. Her list of medications is as follows. Which should the WHNP/midwife be concerned about?
    1. Glyburide (DiaBeta).
    2. Metformin (Glucophage).
    3. Captopril (Capoten).
    4. Temazepam (Restoril).

40. The WHNP/midwife is prescribing nitrofurantoin for a patient's recurrent lower urinary tract infection. If the patient reported having side effects, which one would require discontinuation of the medication?
    1. Fatigue and drowsiness.
    2. Gastrointestinal upset.
    3. Tingling of the fingers.
    4. Dark, amber colored urine.

41. What is important for the WHNP/midwife to know before prescribing methenamine (Hiprex) to a patient?
    1. Prescribe a sulfonamide to enhance the absorption of methenamine.
    2. Check patient's creatinine and BUN (blood urea nitrogen).
    3. Medication is useful in prevention of catheter-induced urinary tract infections (UTIs).
    4. Medication is indicated for acute upper UTIs only.

42. After completing a 3-day course of trimethoprim-sulfamethoxazole (TMP-SMX 160/800 mg 2 times per day) for a urinary tract infection, the patient continues to have a positive urine culture 1 week after completion of the treatment. Which of the following is an appropriate action for the WHNP/midwife?
    1. Order a one-time intravenous dose of ceftriaxone 1 g.
    2. Start a 2-week course of TMP-SMX 160/800 mg two times per day.
    3. Initiate long-term prophylaxis with TMP-SMX 40/200 mg three times per week at bedtime for 6 months.
    4. Order a voiding cystourethrogram to evaluate for a structural abnormality of the urinary tract.

43. A young adult female patient has suprapubic discomfort, pyuria, dysuria, and bacteriuria greater than 100,000/mL of urine for the past 24 hours. Which is the most likely diagnosis and treatment?
    1. Uncomplicated upper urinary tract infection (UTI) requiring 14 days of oral antibiotics.
    2. Uncomplicated lower UTI treatable with short-course therapy.
    3. Complicated lower UTI treatable with single-dose therapy.
    4. Complicated upper UTI requiring hospitalization and intravenous antibiotics.

44. Which medication is a urinary analgesic?
    1. Nitrofurantoin (Macrodantin).
    2. Phenazopyridine (Pyridium).
    3. Trimethoprim (Primsol).
    4. Methenamine (Hiprex).

19 Answers and Rationales

Disorders

1. (1) Stress incontinence in postmenopausal women is associated with weakness in the pelvic floor that can lead to pelvic organ prolapse; multiparity is a key factor. Dementia is associated with overflow incontinence. Environmental barriers put one at risk for functional incontinence, and the addition of tricyclic antidepressants or any hypnotic or sedative can cause retention leading to overflow incontinence.

2. (1) *Escherichia coli (E. coli)* is the most common organism causing urinary tract infections (UTIs) in women. Counts of 10^5 CFU/mL are diagnostic. Counts of 10^2 to 10^3 CFU/mL should be considered positive and indicate treatment when it is *E. coli*. *E. coli* will likely respond to TMP-SMX (Septra DS) or any suitable, sensitive antiinfective agent, and the patient should also be treated for the UTI. *Staphylococcus epidermidis* is normal skin flora and is likely a contaminant because of an inappropriate clean-catch specimen collection technique.

3. (3) The WHNP/midwife suspects UTI and needs to confirm the diagnosis with microscopic urine exam to identify white blood cells (WBCs) and bacteria. If no WBCs or bacteria are seen, a noncontrast CT or ultrasound should be ordered to rule out a kidney stone, which is also part of the differential diagnosis.

4. (2) Although effective in protecting healthy skin from urine, moisture-barrier films often contain alcohol and can burn and irritate denuded skin, and therefore should be used sparingly. If the perineal area is already red and excoriated, using a moisture-barrier film is contraindicated. Each time the patient is changed, the caregiver should cleanse the perineal area with mild soap and water, and then apply a thin layer of petrolatum or zinc oxide to treat the irritant dermatitis. The addition of vitamin C 250 mg and zinc 220 mg daily will aid the healing process. Once the perineal area is healed, vitamin C and zinc should be discontinued.

5. (4) Functional incontinence is the inability to toilet appropriately because of impaired mobility or deficits in cognition. Ensuring that the patient has the appropriate equipment in the home (bedside commode, walker, wheelchair, accessible bathroom, and clothing that is easily removed) will assist the patient in maintaining independence. The patient may also benefit from scheduled toileting every 2 hours to reduce "accidents." Often these patients become socially isolated and depressed because of their concern about an accident in public. The WHNP/midwife should explore all options available. Evaluating the need for incontinence pads is effective with stress incontinence. Limiting fluid intake in the evenings to reduce nocturnal incontinence is appropriate for urge incontinence. Performing the Credé maneuver is appropriate for overflow incontinence.

6. (4) This patient has transient urinary incontinence most likely due to excessive urine and/or new pharmacologic agents as a result of her recent hospitalization. Reversible transient urinary incontinence can be caused by **D**elirium, **I**nfection, **A**trophic vaginitis or urethritis, **P**harmaceuticals (sedative-hypnotics, diuretics, anticholinergics, α-adrenergic agents, and calcium channel blockers), **P**sychiatric disorders (psychosis, depression), **E**xcessive excretion (urine, hyperglycemia), **R**estricted mobility, and **S**tool impaction (**DIAPPERS** is the acronym). Poor pelvic support is a possible cause of stress incontinence. Urge incontinence, or the inability to delay urination with a sudden and powerful urge to void, is a possible result of lower urinary tract problems. A prolapsed uterus or bladder can cause overflow incontinence with overdistention of the bladder.

7. (2) Functional incontinence is the inability to toilet appropriately because of impaired mobility or deficits in cognition. Stress incontinence is leakage from the bladder during activities that increase intraabdominal pressure, and therefore pressure on the bladder, forcing urine leakage. Urge incontinence is an inability to delay urination, with a strong, abrupt urge to void, caused by bladder hyperactivity or hypersensitive bladder. The patient often has little warning before urine passes out of the bladder. Incontinence with overdistention of the bladder is called overflow incontinence, caused by an underactive or noncontracting detrusor muscle or by bladder outlet or urethral obstruction. It is characterized by frequent urination in small amounts.

8. (3) *Escherichia coli* (*E. coli*) is the pathogen in 80% of community-acquired UTIs. Gram-positive *Staphylococcus saprophyticus* (*S. saprophyticus*) is the second most common pathogen in 15% of community-acquired UTIs. *Klebsiella pneumoniae* (*K. pneumoniae*) and *Proteus mirabilis* (*P. mirabilis*) are also possible pathogens. In hospital settings, *E. coli* is less prevalent.

9. (3) Cystitis in adults usually presents with dysuria, urgency, frequency, nocturia, and suprapubic heaviness. Acute onset of chills, fever, flank pain, headache, malaise,

and costovertebral angle tenderness are common in pyelonephritis in adults.

10. (1) Relapse is an uncommon cause of recurrent UTIs in women and occurs within 2 weeks of completion of antibiotic therapy. It may need to be treated for 2 to 12 weeks. Reinfection is the cause of most UTIs in women and may be caused by residual urine resulting from a prolapsed uterus or bladder or by lack of estrogen in perimenopausal women. If the patient has up to two UTIs a year, single-dose or 3-day antibiotic therapy may be used.

11. (2) Pyelonephritis is characterized by localized flank/back pain, costovertebral angle tenderness, combined with systemic symptoms, such as fever (100.4°F [38°C]), chills, and nausea. In older adults, mental status changes and absence of fever is noted. Suggested follow-up is by telephone contact within 12 to 24 hours of initiation of antibiotic therapy, and at 2 weeks and 3 months for post-treatment urine cultures. Outpatient therapy is usually how the patient is followed for mild to moderate illness (not pregnant, no nausea/vomiting; fever and pain not severe), uncomplicated, and tolerating oral hydration and medications. Most patients can be treated as outpatients. With extremes of age (older adult) and severe illness inpatient treatment is indicated.

12. (2) Urge incontinence, an established incontinence versus transient incontinence, is associated with conditions such as Parkinson disease or Alzheimer disease and involves the central nervous system causing detrusor motor and/or sensory instability. Urge incontinence is the involuntary leakage accompanied by or immediately preceded by urgency.

13. (3) Although discussing the alkaline-ash, low-purine diet with the patient is appropriate, most patients, when they learn how difficult the diet is to follow, will be noncompliant with the diet even though they realize they risk developing another uric acid renal calculus. Increasing fluid intake (2–3 L/day) and alkalinization of urine (with potassium citrate or potassium bicarbonate) is also important in the treatment plan. Starting the patient on a xanthine oxidase inhibitor (allopurinol, febuxostat) and monitoring to ensure that the serum uric acid level remains at normal levels will control the incidence of uric acid stones, while allowing the patient freedom without such strict dietary restrictions. Monitoring the patient for another episode is inappropriate because the serum uric acid is likely elevated, and a repeat incident is likely imminent. Referral to a urologist is inappropriate now, because there is no acute episode and the patient does not have recurrent stone formation.

14. (3) Painless hematuria, flank pain, and a palpable abdominal renal mass are the classic triad of symptoms in the patient with renal cell carcinoma. There is no evidence of renal failure (oliguria; edema). Renal calculi would be characterized by both hematuria and flank pain, but no abdominal mass.

15. (3) A sedentary lifestyle or episodes of immobilization can predispose a patient to the development of renal calculi. Urinary tract infections (UTIs) usually do not precipitate problems with renal calculi; however, the presence of renal calculi will predispose the patient to UTIs. Milk intake of 6 to 8 oz daily is not excessive and will not predispose a patient to renal calculi, and increased intake of citrus and high-fiber carbohydrates is good for the patient's dietary needs. However, excess intake of vitamin C can cause hyperoxaluria and predispose a patient to renal stones.

16. (2) Lithium is a mood stabilizer with an unknown mechanism of action. Toxicity of lithium is measured when serum levels rise above 1.5 mEq/L (1.5 mmol/L). Lithium prevents the ability to concentrate the urine with elevated levels causing central nervous system changes, polyuria, and most severely nephrogenic diabetes insipidus (DI). More frequent urination may be controlled by administering lithium in a once-daily regime, whereas treatment of nephrogenic DI requires immediate intervention, cessation of the medication, and close monitoring of sodium levels.

17. (3) Acute onset of increased confusion, inability to redirect, and increased agitation indicate an infection, likely a urinary tract infection (UTI), in the older adult patient with dementia. The WHNP/midwife should obtain a UA and empirically treat for UTI until the UA results are received. Because the patient has no neurologic symptoms (e.g., weakness, flaccidity), a new infarct is unlikely. Acute confusion is not a sign of worsening dementia because dementia is a gradual process. The caregiver bringing the patient with this acute problem would not indicate underlying caregiver stress, which usually presents when persons complain of stress to their own primary care provider.

18. (3) Pyelonephritis is characterized by fever (≥101.4°F [38.5°C]), costovertebral angle tenderness with patient complaints of chills, severe flank pain, dysuria, urinary urgency, and frequency, with urinalysis findings revealing pyuria with leukocyte casts, mild proteinuria, and urine leukocyte esterase positive. Interstitial cystitis is characterized by frequent, urgent, relentless urination day and night, with more than 8 voids in 24 hours. Patients with urethritis typical have the following complaints of urethral discharge, dysuria, and erythema of the urethral meatus.

19. (3) Interstitial cystitis (urethral syndrome, bladder pain syndrome) is a chronic bladder condition that causes

pain, pressure, and discomfort in the bladder and surrounding structures. It is characterized by urinary frequency or urge to urinate. Bladder pain worsens as the bladder fills then resolves with bladder emptying is a symptom of interstitial cystitis. Acute pyelonephritis is characterized by fever, chills, localized flank or back pain. Pyuria with a positive urine culture is associated with a urinary tract infection (UTI).

20. (3) The patient with an indwelling catheter and signs of acute pyelonephritis requires hospitalization and intravenous antibiotics. The other three patients show signs of uncomplicated urinary tract infections (UTIs) that are not severe and can be treated with oral antibiotics. The WHNP/midwife should consider hospitalization for a UTI if a patient is pregnant, severe nausea/vomiting with dehydration, and any child aged <2 years.

21. (1) Urgent referral to a urologist is indicated if the pain is uncontrollable, urosepsis is present, patient is unable to keep fluids down, or oliguria/anuria is present. A patient with renal calculi who has a history of sudden onset of severe pain in the costovertebral angle, flank, and/or lateral abdomen; colicky or constant pain with patient unable to find a comfortable position (often may pace to relieve the pain); hematuria with gross hematuria noted in one-third of patients; nausea; and vomiting. Most patients can be conservatively managed with pain medications (opioids and nonsteroidal antiinflammatory drugs [NSAIDs]) and increased fluids. The majority of patients pass the stone within 48 hours.

22. (1) Increased fluid intake for life cannot be overemphasized for decreasing recurrence of renal calculi. The WHNP/midwife should encourage 2 to 3 L/day fluid intake; advise patient to have clear urine rather than yellow. When patients form calcium oxalate stones, they should minimize high-oxalate foods, such as green leafy vegetables, rhubarb, peanuts, chocolates, and beans. Other diet considerations are to decrease protein and salt intake and increase phytate-rich foods, such as natural dietary bran, legumes and beans, and whole cereal. It is not advisable to lower calcium intake because it may increase urine calcium excretion. Patients should avoid excessive vitamin C and/or vitamin D supplements.

23. (3) If UTI symptoms persist after 2 to 3 days of medication therapy, obtain a urinalysis and urine culture/sensitivity, and change antibiotic accordingly. Switch to another antibiotic drug class and treat for 7 to 10 days. It would not be prudent to order an additional course of medication without first collecting a urinalysis and culture and sensitivity. Increasing fluids and promoting frequent urination are good bladder health teaching points but do not address the current infection not responding to the prescribed antibiotic.

24. (4) Decreased bladder capacity, decreased ability to concentrate urine, and decreased urethral closing pressure after menopause lead to incontinence. Other factors are depression, decreased mobility, decreased vision, and lack of attention to bladder cues of feelings of fullness.

25. (2) A history of vaginal delivery of large babies and possible complications, such as use of forceps, can indicate that she has weakened pelvic floor muscles and has lost the ability to maintain a closed external anal sphincter to control leakage. Typically, the development of incontinence can occur 20 to 30 years after the delivery. Diagnostic testing would include anorectal manometry, and treatment with physical therapy and biofeedback may be helpful. Although the past medical history should include the childbirth history, it is not necessarily obtained in detail and may not be relevant depending on the reason for the office visit. Stress can play a role in worsening many symptoms, but it is less likely to be affecting her bowel control. A rectocele is a rectal prolapse into the vagina that can occur after delivery when the ligaments and muscles weaken. However, the main complaint with a rectocele is constipation, not stool leakage.

Pharmacology

26. (1) Chronic kidney disease often results in a loss of erythropoietin as glomerular filtration rate (GFR) decreases. This increases the risk of anemia. After evaluating and ensuring iron levels are appropriate, initiation of therapy with an erythropoiesis-stimulating agent is appropriate. Initiation of therapy is typically considered at hemoglobin levels <9 g/dL for nondialysis-dependent patients (<10 g/dL if dialysis dependent), especially if the patient is near transfusion levels. Treatment is at 4-week intervals and should be reduced or stopped if hemoglobin is >11 g/dL due to adverse side effects.

27. (4) Combination hormone replacement therapy using conjugated estrogen (Premarin) 0.3 to 1.25 mg/day orally or vaginally and medroxyprogesterone (progestin) 2.5 to 10 mg/day continuously or intermittently can be useful for management of stress incontinence. Propantheline and oxybutynin may be useful in urge incontinence; research is limited on their use for stress incontinence. Doxepin (Sinequan) is a tricyclic antidepressant and is used infrequently.

28. (1) To decrease the formation of uric acid kidney stones, a urinary alkylating agent, such as allopurinol, is frequently used. As standard practice, the WHNP/midwife should check the patient's serum uric acid level monthly for 3 months to ensure the levels are decreasing to normal ranges, and then annually once serum uric acid levels are normalized. Indomethacin is used for its

antiinflammatory properties in the treatment of gout. Urecholine is a cholinergic agent that stimulates the bladder to contract, which improves urine flow. Colchicine is an antigout medication also used for its antiinflammatory properties.

29. (3) Oxybutynin produces anticholinergic effects, and dry mouth is a common side effect. Because this patient is an older adult, the WHNP/midwife should review the patient's list of medications to verify that no other medications will exacerbate dry mouth. If another medication will increase this side effect (e.g., diuretic), the WHNP/midwife should advise the patient of methods to relieve the dry mouth, such as sugar-free hard candy or chewing gum or the use of artificial saliva. The patient may also be taking other medications with anticholinergic side effects, which could be increased with the addition of oxybutynin to the point the patient could be at risk for falls. Careful review of the patient's medication list is essential before adding a new drug. The other reactions are not consistent with oxybutynin administration.

30. (3) Hydrochlorothiazide (HCTZ) decreases the risk of forming calcium oxalate stones because of decreased renal calcium excretion or hypocalciuria. Hypercalcemia is a possible side effect of this medication. Furosemide, acetazolamide, and triamterene may increase the risk of formation of calcium oxalate stones by causing hypercalciuria. It is important to note that HCTZ may subsequently increase the risk of gout and/or uric acid stone formation due to hyperuricemia.

31. (2) The severe pain of renal calculi should be addressed before other treatments or diagnostics. Narcotics and now nonsteroidal antiinflammatory drugs (NSAIDs) are commonly used for pain relief. In most randomized, blinded studies of NSAIDs versus narcotics, NSAIDs have shown equal or greater efficacy for pain relief, shorter duration to pain relief, with equal or fewer side effects. Ketorolac works at the peripheral site of pain production rather than on the central nervous system, and based on clinical findings has been proven to be as effective as opioid analgesics, with fewer adverse effects. Ketorolac is only indicated for short-term therapy and is contraindicated in patients with renal failure. Due to an increased risk of bleeding, it is not given concurrently with other NSAIDs and should be used with caution in patients older than age 65 years.

32. (1) The most important side effects of nitrofurantoin are gastrointestinal upset, which can be decreased if the medication is taken with food or milk, and brown discoloration of the urine. The patient should continue taking nitrofurantoin for at least 3 days after sterile urine is obtained. If applicable to the patient, the drug may interfere with the efficacy of oral contraceptives.

33. (1) The WHNP/midwife should advise the patient that if she experiences yellow discoloration of the sclerae while taking phenazopyridine, she is to return to the office immediately. This may indicate poor renal excretion and requires a renal workup (renal panel, parathyroid and thyroid-stimulating hormone, serum magnesium/calcium, and a 24-hour urine for creatinine clearance) and possible referral to a nephrologist. Phenazopyridine should be administered with food, and no drug interactions occur with aspirin or oral contraceptives.

34. (3) Muddy brown granular casts are indicative of acute tubular necrosis (ATN). ATN is the most common cause of acute kidney injury and is the result of intrinsic (renal) damage of the tubules most often due to ischemia. Leading causes include sepsis, hypotension, rhabdomyolysis, contrast agents, as well as aminoglycosides. Renal damage due to aminoglycosides, such as gentamicin, are often after administration for 5 to 7 days and are relatively uncommon compared with other causes of ATN. Furosemide, amphotericin, and ibuprofen are often implicated in acute interstitial nephritis, and urinalysis would more likely appear with WBCs and/or WBC casts in addition to other symptoms.

35. (3) Oxybutynin is contraindicated in patients with narrow-angle glaucoma (angle-closure glaucoma). Patients with open-angle glaucoma may take this medication. Anticholinergics may increase the pressure within the eye, which puts the patient at risk for progression of the glaucoma, resulting in blindness.

36. (4) Although fluoroquinolones are a common and generally effective treatment for urinary tract infections, these drugs received a black box warning in 2016 due to potential side effects, such as tendon ruptures, peripheral neuropathy, and central nervous system effects. Therefore fluoroquinolones should not be used for minor infections as a first-line agent. Fluoroquinolones should not be used in pregnancy.

37. (4) Angiotensin-converting enzyme (ACE) inhibitors increase pressure within the kidney in renal artery stenosis, causing an increase in serum creatinine and potassium. ACE inhibitors have protective properties for patients with cardiovascular disease, hypertension, and diabetes.

38. (1) Ibuprofen (Motrin) is a nonsteroidal antiinflammatory agent with risk of renal toxicity and should be avoided in patients with preexisting or renal impairment. Levothyroxine is metabolized predominantly in the liver. Metoprolol is a beta blocker and has little effect on the kidneys, unlike the ACE inhibitors. Clopidogrel works on the liver and also has little effect on the kidneys.

39. (2) Metformin is contraindicated in patients with heart failure, liver failure, and impaired renal function. It

is contraindicated for 2 days prior to and 2 days after receiving intravenous (IV) radiographic contrast. Metformin combined with IV contrast dye puts the patient at risk for fatal lactic acidosis. Baseline glomerular filtration rate (GFR) should be documented. Captopril is an ACE inhibitor that is renal protective until GFR is noted to be worsening. Glyburide and temazepam minimally effect the renal function, and there is no need to hold these medications prior to the study.

40. (3) Peripheral neuropathy is most likely to occur in patients with renal impairment and those taking the medication chronically. Symptoms of tingling of the fingers, muscle weakness, and numbness can indicate peripheral neuropathy, which can be an irreversible side effect of nitrofurantoin. The WHNP/midwife would discontinue the medication. The other side effects are not serious and can be reversed by reducing the dosage or following treatment.

41. (2) Methenamine is eliminated by the kidneys and should not be given to patients with renal impairment because crystalluria can occur. The medication is not useful in prevention of catheter-induced UTIs and is indicated for chronic infections of the lower urinary tract. Methenamine should not be combined with sulfonamides because the drug interaction forms an insoluble complex, which poses a risk of urinary tract injury from crystalluria.

42. (2) If a patient continues to have a positive urine culture following a 3-day medication regime of antibiotics due to relapse or reinfection, then the drug therapy should be a progressive stepwise approach with a 2-week course of therapy following the short-course 3-day therapy. The next steps would be to begin a 4- to 6-week course of therapy, followed by a 6-month course of therapy if that is unsuccessful. Recommended antibiotics include TMP-SMX, nitrofurantoin, cephalexin, trimethoprim, or a quinolone. If urinary tract infections are thought to be caused by other complicating factors, an evaluation for structural abnormalities may be warranted by ordering a voiding cystourethrogram. Third-generation cephalosporins (e.g., ceftriaxone) should not be given routinely, but rather should be given only when conditions demand and the UTI is severe and not responding. Unless the infections are severe or are complicated, intravenous antibiotics are not indicated.

43. (2) The symptoms of suprapubic discomfort, pyuria, dysuria, and bacteriuria greater than 100,000/mL of urine indicate an uncomplicated cystitis, which is a lower UTI that can be treated with a short course of antibiotics, especially if the symptoms began less than 7 days before starting the treatment. In this case the symptoms occurred during the past 24 hours and short-course therapy is indicated and is more effective than single-dose therapy and is preferred. A complicated lower UTI would be associated with some predisposing factor, such as renal calculi, an obstruction to the flow of urine, or an indwelling catheter. Upper UTIs often include severe flank pain, fever, and chills and are associated with acute pyelonephritis.

44. (2) Phenazopyridine (Pyridium) is a urinary analgesic and the medication does not treat the urinary infection but reduces the discomfort of dysuria. Nitrofurantoin and methenamine are urinary antiseptics. Trimethoprim (Primsol) is an antibiotic often used in conjunction with sulfamethoxazole (TMP-SMZ).

20

Mental Health

Disorders

1. Cocaine use during pregnancy is associated with:
   1. Abruptio placentae.
   2. Postdate pregnancy.
   3. Macrosomia infant.
   4. Maternal hypotension.

2. A patient delivers a healthy newborn with a cleft lip and cleft palate. Which action by the WHNP/midwife would promote maternal-infant bonding?
   1. Point out the newborn's normal characteristics.
   2. Explain to the mother how the problem is not significant.
   3. Have the mother begin taking care of the newborn immediately after delivery.
   4. Explain to the mother that orofacial surgery will completely correct the defect.

3. An older adult patient is experiencing a recent onset of confusion. The WHNP/midwife is trying to determine whether the confusion is related to depression or dementia. In evaluating the patient, what specific assessment finding would be helpful in making this distinction?
   1. Determining whether confusion worsens in the evening.
   2. Assessing early morning agitation, hyperactivity, and insomnia.
   3. Noting signs of anger, hostility, and loss of control.
   4. Assessing reality distortions and preoccupation with family matters.

4. QSEN A patient calls the clinic and asks to speak to the WHNP/midwife. When the WHNP/midwife answers the telephone, the patient states that she is going to commit suicide. The first action is to:
   1. Refer the patient to an appropriate treatment facility.
   2. Encourage ventilation of angry and depressed feelings.
   3. Assess the lethality of the suicide plan.
   4. Establish rapport with the patient.

5. An older adult woman answers the WHNP/midwife's questions by mumbling in low tones with answers that seem inappropriate. What would be initial findings associated with a diagnosis of dementia?
   1. Sees people floating across the ceiling of her room.
   2. Has problems with cognition and confusion.
   3. Hears voices at night telling her to change her clothes.
   4. Shows fear when the nurse makes any movements toward her.

6. An older adult patient is brought to the WHNP/midwife by her family for evaluation of increasing confusion over the past few days. The patient has a history of dementia; however, the family states that there is a definite change. What course of action would the WHNP/midwife consider?
   1. Help the family look for a nursing home.
   2. Order an MRI scan.
   3. Order a noncontrast head CT.
   4. Order a UA.

7. Which of the following statements regarding sexual assault is correct?
   1. Most women report the assault immediately to ensure the perpetrator is prosecuted.
   2. If women are coping well after an assault, they will not have any psychological symptoms later.
   3. All women who are sexually assaulted sustain significant injuries.
   4. Women often have difficulty remembering details as a result of the trauma.

8. When screening for intimate partner violence, the WHNP/midwife knows that:
   1. The WHNP/midwife should ask about violence only if the woman has obvious injuries.
   2. The WHNP/midwife only needs to screen pregnant women for violence.
   3. Screening all women should be a routine practice when taking a social history.
   4. Universal screening is not effective in identifying women who are experiencing violence.

9. **QSEN** Which of the following groups of patients fall under mandatory reporting laws for abuse and neglect in most states in the United States?
   1. Children, adult women, dependent older adults.
   2. Children, disabled individuals, adult women.
   3. Disabled individuals, adult women, dependent older adults.
   4. Children, disabled individuals, dependent older adults.

10. Physical findings of cocaine abuse include:
    1. Bradycardia, miosis, hypertension.
    2. Hypertension, tachycardia, tremor.
    3. Hypotension, bradycardia, abdominal cramps.
    4. Decreased level of consciousness, tachycardia, excessive salivation.

11. **QSEN** A 42-year-old woman presents to the office with her friend. The friend states that she found the patient confused with some shaking and was seeing things that were not there. The patient typically drinks two bottles of wine every day. The patient decided to stop drinking 2 days ago. Vital signs show elevated blood pressure, fever, and tachycardia. The WHNP/midwife transfers the patient to the hospital as she:
    1. Is overdosing on heroin.
    2. Has thyroid storm.
    3. Is septic from pneumonia.
    4. Has delirium tremens.

12. A patient has a controlling partner with a violent temper. She has just discovered that she is pregnant, and she is thrilled because she believes he will treat her better because of the pregnancy. The WHNP/midwife understands that:
    1. Intimate partner violence (IPV) often escalates during pregnancy.
    2. He is less likely to harm her because she is pregnant.
    3. Social services needs to be called immediately because the child will be in danger after birth.
    4. Have the patient encourage her partner to come to all prenatal appointments.

Pharmacology

13. **QSEN** A patient has been receiving fluphenazine (Prolixin) for the past 3 weeks and comes to the well-women clinic for an annual checkup. The WHNP/midwife's assessment notes the following: temperature elevated 105.8°F (41°C), marked muscle rigidity, agitation, and confusion. The WHNP/midwife understands these findings are often associated with the diagnosis of:
    1. Acute dystonia.
    2. Tardive dyskinesia.
    3. Neuroleptic malignant syndrome.
    4. Extrapyramidal disorder.

14. The preferred antidepressant for an older adult patient is:
    1. Amitriptyline (Elavil).
    2. Citalopram (Celexa).
    3. Trazodone (Desyrel).
    4. Haloperidol (Haldol).

15. The WHNP/midwife is prescribing an antidepressant medication for an older adult who recently lost her spouse. What is an important consideration regarding starting doses?
    1. Reduce starting doses by 50%.
    2. Reduce starting doses by 10%.
    3. Increase starting doses by 25%.
    4. Order the normal therapeutic dose.

16. What is the best initial treatment plan for a sleep disorder in the older adult patient?
    1. Medicate with amitriptyline (Elavil).
    2. Medicate with trazodone (Desyrel).
    3. Discuss the importance of naps daily.
    4. Decrease noise and light in the environment.

17. An older adult patient presents with a new symptom of acute confusion over the last 24 hours. Which assessment would be a priority for the WHNP/midwife to evaluate during the exam?
    1. Medication review.
    2. Electrocardiogram.
    3. Mini-Mental Status Exam.
    4. Thyroid profile.

18. Of the following antidepressants, which one has the most sedating side effects, making it a good sleeping agent?
    1. Fluoxetine (Prozac).
    2. Doxepin (Sinequan).
    3. Trazodone (Desyrel).
    4. Paroxetine (Paxil).

19. A patient is a 20-year, two-pack-a-day smoker with a history of chronic bronchitis. In addition to counseling, what is the prescription to give the patient who wishes to stop smoking?
    1. Nicotine polacrilex (Nicorette) gum 2-mg piece, chew for 30 minutes, q1–2h × 6 weeks, then q2–4h × 3 weeks, then q4–8h × 3 weeks, and then discontinue.
    2. Nicotine patch (Nicoderm) 21 mg/24 hr qd × 6 weeks, then 14 mg/24 hr qd × 2 weeks, then 7 mg/24 hr qd × 2 weeks, and then discontinue.
    3. Bupropion HCl (Zyban) 150 mg qd × 3 days, then 150 mg bid for 7–12 weeks, and then to stop smoking when medication is started.
    4. Nicotine patch (Nicoderm) 14 mg/24 hr qd × 6 weeks, then 7 mg/24 hr qd × 6 weeks, and then discontinue.

20. A young woman tells the WHNP/midwife that she no longer wants to be on sertraline (Zoloft). She had a traumatic event a few years ago but has been doing much better and has a strong support structure from family and friends. The WHNP/midwife advises her to:
    1. Stop taking the medication.
    2. Taper the dose slowly.
    3. Keep taking the medication.
    4. Switch to citalopram (Celexa).

21. An 82-year-old woman, who is on a stable dose of furosemide (Lasix) for heart failure, comes in with complaints of feeling down for the last year after losing her husband. After assessing the patient, the WHNP/midwife diagnoses the patient with depression and starts the patient on citalopram (Celexa). The WHNP/midwife knows the patient is at risk for:
    1. Hypernatremia.
    2. Hyponatremia.
    3. Hyperkalemia.
    4. Hypokalemia.

22. The WHNP/midwife understands the following regarding the use of benzodiazepines in the older adult:
    1. Withdrawal symptoms may occur within 24 hours of abruptly stopping the medication.
    2. Adverse effects are minimal and rarely lead to falls or other injury.
    3. Long-acting medications (e.g., chlordiazepoxide [Librium]) are preferred over the shorter-acting medications (e.g., lorazepam [Ativan]).
    4. Larger doses are needed to maintain therapeutic levels for the patient who is anxious or agitated.

20 Answers and Rationales

Disorders

1. (1) Use of cocaine during pregnancy is associated with placental abruption, spontaneous abortion, and preterm labor. Maternal blood pressure and heart rate are increased. The fetus is at risk for intrauterine growth restriction, fetal distress, seizures, and death.

2. (1) Initially after delivery, the mother needs an opportunity to accept that her newborn has a congenital defect. Pointing out normal characteristics of the newborn will allow her to put the problem in perspective. Often the mother will focus on the defect. Orofacial surgery will provide closure of the defect but will not completely correct it because scarring will undoubtedly occur.

3. (1) Confusion can occur in both dementia and depression. However, with dementia, symptoms worsen at night and are commonly referred to as sundowning. Additionally, the WHNP/midwife must also ensure that the increased confusion is not a result of an acute illness. Often the only sign or symptom the older adult with dementia may present with is confusion. Usually the culprit is a urinary tract infection (UTI). The WHNP/midwife should order a urinalysis (UA) to ensure that the confusion is not the result of an acute illness and is reversible.

4. (4) The WHNP/midwife must first establish trust and rapport with the caller before an assessment can be made. If rapport is not established, the patient will hang up the phone. The WHNP/midwife understands that, by keeping the patient talking, he or she is prevented from acting out the suicidal threat. On the side, while talking with the patient, the WHNP/midwife can signal for assistance to send additional emergency assistance to the home of the caller.

5. (2) Confusion and cognitive function problems (e.g., short-term memory loss) are initial signs of dementia. Other signs of early-stage Alzheimer dementia include time and spatial disorientation, poor judgment, personality changes, depression or withdrawal, and perceptual disturbances. The severity of the symptoms depends on what stage of cognitive degeneration the patient is manifesting. The other options are characteristic of hallucinatory experiences and may occur later. This patient may also be exhibiting signs and symptoms of an acute illness. The culprit is commonly a urinary tract infection (UTI) and the WHNP/midwife should order a urinalysis (UA) to ensure that the cause of the confusion is not related to a reversible cause.

6. (4) One of the most common reasons for an acute change in mental status in the older adult patient with dementia is an acute infection. This is usually a urinary tract infection (UTI). Usually the older adult patient with dementia is incontinent, and because of the changes of aging, does not recognize the normal signs or symptoms of a UTI (burning, urgency, frequency, and suprapubic tenderness). Older adults also do not typically run elevated temperatures. The WHNP/midwife should order a UA to ensure that an acute infectious process is not the cause of the acute confusion. The WHNP/midwife should also conduct a medication review to ensure that no new medications have been added or that no new over-the-counter or herbal medications have been added because this is the second major reason for acute confusion in the older adult patient.

7. (4) Women can experience a range of emotions after sexual assault and often have difficulty remembering details and recalling parts of the events before, during, and after the assault. Emotional and psychologic symptoms can manifest at any time, even if the woman appears to be coping well initially. The vast majority of assaults are not reported, and most women do not have significant injuries.

8. (3) Routine violence screening should be done with all women, regardless of age, relationship status, or any other sociodemographic factors. Many women who are in abusive and controlling relationships do not exhibit overt injuries. Screening is effective in identifying women who are victims of violence, and women are more likely to disclose if asked directly.

9. (4) The laws in most states require the reporting of suspected or actual abuse and neglect of any person considered to be dependent or with a reduced ability to make life choices. Children, disabled individuals, and dependent older adults fall into these categories. Very few states require reporting for adult women unless a weapon is involved; this is a different situation, requiring a report.

10. (2) Bradycardia and excessive salivation are not found with cocaine abuse. There are no drug antagonists that can be used for cocaine overdose, although benzodiazepines are used to treat effects of cocaine toxicity, such as seizures, tachycardia, and hypertension. Naloxone is given to reduce the concurrent toxic effects of other narcotic drugs that may be in the patient's body system but is not effective against cocaine toxicity.

11. (4) The history supports a diagnosis of delirium tremens. Delirium tremens is severe alcohol withdrawal that typically develops 24 to 72 hours after the last drink. The patient may be confused, disoriented, and have hallucinations, tremors, elevated blood pressure, tachycardia, a rise in body temperature, and tonic-clonic seizures. A patient with heroin overdose may also be confused, but he/she would have hypotension, slowed respirations, and a decreased pulse. A patient septic from pneumonia may present with cough, chills, low oxygen saturation, fever, hypotension, and tachycardia. Thyroid storm is severe hyperthyroidism that presents with elevated temperature, weakness, sweating, confusion, tachycardia, and gastrointestinal symptoms.

12. (1) IPV often escalates during pregnancy, placing women at risk for morbidity, mortality, and adverse pregnancy outcomes. The WHNP/midwife should discuss the patient's options for safety, including whether she is able to leave the relationship, along with community resources, such as shelters, law enforcement, and legal aid. Her partner is welcome to come to all prenatal appointments, but this may have no effect on his behavior.

Pharmacology

13. (3) The patient is experiencing a rare problem called neuroleptic malignant syndrome. The patient would require immediate referral and hospitalization. This can also occur with the medication prochlorperazine. Acute dystonia, parkinsonism, and akathisia are associated with extrapyramidal disorder or acute movement disorder. Tardive dyskinesia occurs late in therapy and is often irreversible. Slow, worm-like movements of the tongue are the earliest symptom, followed by grimacing, lip smacking, and involuntary limb movements.

14. (2) The favorable side effect profile of citalopram (Celexa), which is a selective serotonin reuptake inhibitor (SSRI), makes it a useful antidepressant in the older adult because it has a short half-life. Amitriptyline (Elavil) has the most anticholinergic and sedating side effects of the antidepressants. There may be pronounced effects on the cardiovascular system (hypotension). Geropsychiatrists agree it is best to avoid amitriptyline (Elavil) in the older adult; however, low dose (10 mg, PO every evening) is low cost and can be effective at controlling neuropathic pain. Trazodone (Desyrel) is very sedating for the older adult patient, which increases the risk for falls, but can be used for insomnia and for behavioral issues in patients with dementia. Haloperidol (Haldol) is an antipsychotic medication and is not to be used at all in long-term care facilities.

15. (1) It is important to reduce starting doses of antidepressants by 50% in older adults, people with impaired renal function, or those especially sensitive to side effects. Recommend re-evaluation in 2 weeks to assess tolerability, then begin to increase dose to target symptoms.

16. (4) Correction of environmental factors and treatment of underlying iatrogenic and medical problems should be addressed initially. Amitriptyline (Elavil) can cause excessive somnolence. Trazodone (Desyrel) may be of particular use when sleep disturbance is prominent; however, it does not address the best initial plan. The goal is to begin with good sleep hygiene before pharmacologic therapy. Eliminating naps during the day may be useful in facilitating sleep.

17. (1) Drug-drug interactions are a common cause of acute confusion in the older adult patient. This medication review assessment can minimize the need to do further costly interventions if the patient only needs medication adjustment. The other options should be included in the plan after the medication review history is completed and has been ruled out as a potential problem. The WHNP/midwife must always consider that an acute illness, such as a urinary tract infection (UTI), may be the cause of acute confusion. A urinalysis (UA) should also be obtained because the patient can quickly progress to sepsis.

18. (3) Trazodone (Desyrel) has sedation as a side effect, which has made it less popular as an antidepressant; however, it is commonly prescribed for insomnia.

19. (2) A highly nicotine-dependent patient benefits from intense counseling and prescription of alternative nicotine delivery during the smoking cessation process. The nicotine patch is usually the preferred form of replacement because the gum is noncontinuous and withdrawal symptoms may occur during nonchewing times. The nicotine patch delivers a fixed dose of nicotine on a continual basis, is applied once daily, and eliminates the gastrointestinal upset that often occurs with the gum. If this patient insisted on using the gum, the dose should be 4 mg, not 2 mg. A nicotine patch with 14 mg is too low a dose to start on this patient and is not the correct dosing schedule. Underdosing can cause patients to start smoking again. Zyban (bupropion HCl) would be used in conjunction with the nicotine patch, and patients are to quit smoking 1 to 2 weeks after starting the Zyban, not immediately, as noted in the option.

20. (2) When stopping a selective serotonin reuptake inhibitor (SSRI), such as sertraline (Zoloft), it is important to taper the dose over at least 2 weeks. Stopping the medication abruptly can lead to flu-like symptoms. There is no need to continue the medication or switch to a different

antidepressant because the patient was assessed for safety and it is reasonable to stop the medication. The WHNP/ midwife should make a follow-up appointment to assess how the patient is doing off the medication.

21. (2) Selective serotonin reuptake inhibitors (SSRIs), such as citalopram (Celexa), can lead to hyponatremia from syndrome of inappropriate antidiuretic hormone (SIADH). The patient is at particular risk because she is an older adult and is on furosemide (Lasix). The patient may be at risk for hypokalemia secondary to furosemide (Lasix), but it is not aggravated with the addition of citalopram (Celexa).

22. (1) Benzodiazepines should be tapered in all patients but especially in the older adult. If given longer than 2 weeks, withdrawal symptoms occur and may include sweating, vomiting, muscle cramps, tremors, and/or seizures. Rebound or withdrawal symptoms occur within 24 hours in patients taking the short-acting medications and may not occur for several days in patients taking long-acting medications. The adverse effects of oversedation—dizziness, confusion, and orthostatic hypotension—contribute to falls and other injuries in the older adult. Short-acting medications are preferred. Typically, larger doses are not needed but rather small initial doses with gradual increases.

Professional Issues (WHNP Only)

Research and Evidence-Based Practice

1. A WHNP has read a nursing research article in which there were no statistically significant findings. In interpreting these findings, what would be the WHNP's most appropriate response?
   1. "Because there were no statistically significant findings, there are no relationships between the study groups."
   2. "Because there were no statistically significant findings, there is no reason to conduct similar studies."
   3. "Because there were no statistically significant findings, further study is warranted to compare results."

2. The best explanation of the peer review process in research is to:
   1. Ensure that the manuscript is well written.
   2. Determine whether the manuscript provides additional information on the content subject area.
   3. To begin to learn how to analyze research and data findings.

3. What is the primary purpose of utilizing evidence-based practice (EBP) in clinical research and practice management?
   1. Increasing the amount of credible resources that can be used in clinical decision-making.
   2. To further advance the peer review process.
   3. To provide quality care to patients by closing the gap between theory, experience, and best practice guidelines.

4. When might a qualitative research design be employed over a quantitative or mixed methods research design?
   1. Qualitative research is the preferred methodology for exploring and understanding a particular phenomenon of interest.
   2. Qualitative research does not require rights of research subjects to be protected.
   3. Qualitative research will provide precise measures for statistical analysis.
   4. Qualitative research ensures tight control during data collection and data analyses.

5. Variance is a key statistical concept. How would current research methods change if there were no variance?
   1. Nurse researchers would need to increase the sample size in all research studies to 100 research subjects or greater.
   2. Because current research methods are based on the presence of variance, researchers would not be able to use current methods.
   3. Nurse researchers would need to decrease the sample size of all research studies to 15 research subjects.

6. What are the five major sequential steps in evidence-based practice (EBP)?
   1. Establish a patient relationship, perform a health assessment, make a diagnosis, devise a plan of care, perform prescribed treatments, and evaluate efficacy of the treatments.
   2. Identify the problem and generate a clinical question, conduct a literature review of scholarly research articles, critically appraise published research, implement useful findings in practice and clinical decision-making, and disseminate findings.
   3. Review the patient's lab reports, complete a thorough health assessment, diagnose, collaborate with the health care provider in developing a treatment plan, implement the treatment, and evaluate the efficacy of the treatment.

7. A WHNP is planning to conduct a study to examine the efficacy of a high-protein, high-fiber diet in weight reduction of obese patients. The WHNP develops the following research question to guide the study: *What is the effect on the weight of obese patients who follow a high-protein, high-fiber diet compared with the weight of obese patients who do not follow a high-protein, high-fiber diet over a 12-week period?* What is the independent variable and dependent variable in the research question?
   1. The independent variable is the 12-week time frame and the dependent variable is the high-protein, high-fiber diet.
   2. The independent variable is the high-protein, high-fiber diet and the dependent variable is the patients' weight.
   3. The independent variable is the high-protein, high-fiber diet and the dependent variable is the 12-week time frame.

8. The WHNP is evaluating research reports on the efficacy of cognitive-behavioral therapy (CBT) on anxiety in patients with fertility problems. When reviewing the literature, which type of research study does the WHNP recognize as the highest level of evidence?
   1. A qualitative research study using a grounded theory approach.
   2. A quantitative research study using a correlational research design.
   3. A quantitative research study using a randomized-controlled trial design.

9. The WHNP is working with a team of colleagues on a research study that will involve patients. The research team understands that which of the following must be included in the written consent to participate?
   1. Role of the primary research investigator.
   2. Anticipated date for publication of the completed research report.
   3. Assurance of patient privacy and confidentiality.

10. The WHNP is preparing to participate in a research study and is considering the key differences between qualitative and quantitative research designs. The WHNP discovers, on review, that the key differences between these two research designs include:
    1. Quantitative researchers employ controls during the research process to minimize impact to the results of the study.
    2. Qualitative research is a process in which the researcher attempts to stay far removed from the process to control for potential bias.
    3. Qualitative research methods utilize research questions and/or hypotheses to test for relationships or cause and effect.

11. The scientific method for conducting research uses the null hypothesis, which is statistically based. What is the correct format for stating the null hypothesis?
    1. There is no relationship between the independent and dependent variables.
    2. There is a significant relationship between the independent and dependent variables.
    3. There is an opposite relationship between the independent and dependent variables.

12. When evaluating claims made on advertisements, such as "Drug X has been used for 5 years with over 1 million doses administered in the United States, Canada, and Great Britain. Drug X stops premenstrual syndrome (PMS), aids in improving mood, and prevents anxiety and physical symptoms of bloating, breast tenderness, and is the 'treatment of choice' to relieve PMS," the WHNP realizes that the claim is:
    1. Invalid; there is no control or comparison group, and no statistics are stated.
    2. Valid; there are sufficient numbers of users who have had success.
    3. Valid; as the Hawthorne effect clearly demonstrates the relationship between the drug and the outcome.

13. Quantitative research articles provide a section containing descriptive findings because descriptive data analyses:
    1. Provides the basis for making inferences regarding the findings.
    2. May yield statistically significant findings that were unexpected.
    3. Provides a clearer understanding of study participants and variables.

14. A WHNP is evaluating research articles for a research utilization project. The majority of the articles report that randomization was used. The WHNP understands that the purpose of randomization in many quantitative research studies is to:
    1. Be sure that subjects can choose whether they receive the intervention or not.
    2. Attempt to control for threats to internal validity by randomly assigning research subjects to either a control or treatment group.
    3. Attempt to control for threats to internal validity by allowing research subjects to choose either the control or treatment group.

Legal and Ethical

15. Which authority regulates the scope of practice of WHNPs?
    1. Federal law.
    2. Academic institutions.
    3. Individual state law.

16. A WHNP is obtaining informed consent from a 78-year-old female patient with a clinical diagnosis of dementia for a minor vulvar incision and drainage procedure. Which option would provide best practice for obtaining informed consent?
    1. Have the patient sign the form.
    2. Inquire as to whether there is an individual who is a power of attorney (POA) for the patient.
    3. Have the patient sign the form in the presence of a witness who can substantiate informed consent and that information has been provided.

17. Early reporting of a potential professional liability claim is advantageous because:
    1. Insurance carriers have a 10-day reporting window, after which the coverage is cancelled.
    2. Documents and witnesses needed to defend the claim are more likely to be available at the time of the event.
    3. Insurance premiums will be reduced with a good-faith showing of cooperation with the carrier.

18. A 46-year-old woman who is mentally challenged has been diagnosed with ovarian cancer. Consent for the surgery should be obtained from:
    1. The patient herself.
    2. The patient's 84-year-old mother, who is her closest relative.
    3. The patient's court-appointed guardian.

19. A WHNP has a 75-year-old female patient with metastatic cancer. Her personal affairs are in order; she has arranged all her finances and her own funeral rites. She has systematically secured enough barbiturates to successfully end her life. The patient asks the WHNP to mix the drugs for her in some pudding to make them palatable for ingestion. What would be the WHNP's best course of action?
    1. Mix the medications as requested and stay with her while she consumes the preparation.
    2. Consult with the attending physician to warn them about the patient's proposed course of action.
    3. Sit down with the patient and conduct a physical and psychological assessment.

20. The Patient Self-Determination Act (PSDA) passed by the US Congress in 1990 resulted in which of the following policy changes?
    1. Hospitals are mandated to assist every patient to create a "living will."
    2. Federally funded managed care organizations (MCOs) are required to inform subscribers about their rights under state law to create "advance directives."
    3. Home health agencies are required to have "do not resuscitate" (DNR) orders on file for all terminally ill patients.

21. If served with a summons and complaint (lawsuit documents), the WHNP should take which of the following actions as the first step?
    1. Call the patient to determine the basis for the action and nature of the alleged wrongdoing.
    2. Confer with colleagues and review the chart to determine if notes need to be clarified.
    3. Call the insurance company for instructions on how to proceed.

22. A WHNP in an impoverished rural area frequently encounters a female patient in a situation of domestic violence with few community options for referral. To address the situation, the WHNP participates in community education forums and fundraising for a safe house. The WHNP's participation is an example of applying what ethical principle?
    1. Autonomy.
    2. Nonmaleficence.
    3. Justice.

23. Which population is not included in the definition of disability under the Americans with Disabilities Act (ADA)?
    1. Profoundly deaf employees.
    2. Persons who are wheelchair bound.
    3. Current users of illegal drugs.

24. Nurse expert witnesses are essential in the adjudication of most professional negligence claims against nurses. Which of the following criteria do attorneys use in selecting WHNP experts?
    1. Appropriate professional education, preferably at the technical level.
    2. Relevant and recent professional work experience.
    3. Ability to understand and articulate the legal issues involved in the claim.

25. What type of insurance coverage is purchased (or self-insured) by an organization to address employee job-related injuries?
    1. Professional liability insurance.
    2. Business interruption insurance.
    3. Workers' compensation insurance.

26. WHNPs with hospital privileges may be impacted by the part of the Health Care Quality Improvement Act known as the National Practitioner Data Bank (NPDB). Which of the following statements regarding the Data Bank is *not* true?
    1. Professional liability insurance claim payments made on behalf of WHNPs are reported to the NPDB.
    2. The facility granting medical staff privileges must query the NPDB before approving a practitioner's privileges.
    3. Insurance companies report all malpractice payments made on behalf of affected WHNPs within 30 days of the date the payment was made if the amount of the claim is in excess of $11,000, and no matter how it was settled.

27. In 1985, the US Congress acted against a phenomenon known as "patient dumping" by enacting what was known at the time as the Consolidated Omnibus Budget Reconciliation Act (known as COBRA) law, now referred to as the Emergency Medical Treatment and Labor Act. All of the following statements regarding the Emergency Medical Treatment and Labor Act are true *except*?
    1. The original purpose of the statute was to prohibit the transfer of uninsured and untreated patients from the emergency department of one hospital to another (usually the county hospital).
    2. Subsequent rules and case law have expanded the statute so that almost any unauthorized transfer of a patient from one facility to another is potentially problematic.
    3. To effect a proper transfer, the forwarding facility need not notify or secure the acquiescence of the receiving facility.

28. A WHNP who wants to effect change in the state's laws regarding the dispensing of prescription medications by WHNPs would take this case to the:
    1. State legislature.
    2. State board of nursing.
    3. Nursing specialty organization.

29. What is the common meaning of "gag clauses" or "gag orders" in managed care?
    1. The managed care organization (MCO) declines to publish in its subscriber contracts the treatments that are excluded from coverage under the plan.
    2. The MCO refuses to allow its member services personnel to answer certain subscriber questions about covered benefits.
    3. The MCO contracts with providers to disallow providers from offering treatment alternatives that the providers know are not covered by patient plans.

30. What is the primary reason that patients sue WHNPs for medical negligence?
    1. The care they received was substandard.
    2. The provider made an honest mistake.
    3. The patient was not "heard" when attempting to communicate with the provider.

31. Informed consent is based on the ethical principle of:
    1. Beneficence.
    2. Autonomy.
    3. Nonmaleficence.

32. The four elements of a professional negligence claim are:
    1. Duty, fulfillment of duty, professional relationship, and wrongful act.
    2. Professional responsibility, fault, harm to patient, and wrongful act.
    3. Duty, breach of duty, causal connection between act and harm, and harm to patient.

33. Why is an expert witness usually required in a nursing negligence case?
    1. Knowledge of medical or nursing facts is not considered intuitive to a lay jury.
    2. Jurors are allowed to use their "sixth sense" regarding the facts presented to them.
    3. Appropriately credentialed experts have more credibility in the eyes of lay jurors.

34. The standard of care for a WHNP will be established by an expert witness(es) in a trial. The expert opinion will be based on all the following *except*:
    1. National norms for the specialty.
    2. Facility policies and procedures.
    3. Opinions of other NPs.

35. The statute of limitations is:
    1. The state law that prescribes the time frames within which a nursing negligence action may be filed.
    2. The law that states that minors have no legal authority to sue nurses for malpractice.
    3. The law that limits the right of patients to sue WHNPs for negligent acts.

36. If a patient is under the "age of majority" for the state, all of the following are factors that would be considered to determine whether the patient is "emancipated" and able to consent to medical treatment *except*:
    1. The patient is married.
    2. The patient is in the military.
    3. A personal friend of the patient tells you that the patient has been emancipated by an order of the court.

37. A WHNP is helping out at a clinic for homeless women. A diabetic patient in her third trimester of pregnancy has been reasonably compliant with respect to insulin therapy. Now, however, she has announced her intent to abandon her insulin regimen because she has heard "on the streets" that some drugs are harmful to fetuses. Which option is **not** legally appropriate for the WHNP, as this patient's health care provider, to consider?
    1. Detain the patient in the homeless shelter and administer the insulin, with or without her consent.
    2. Attempt to engage the patient in dialogue to provide her with accurate medical information.
    3. Confer with social services to find an appropriate interim placement for the patient until her medical and legal issues can be addressed.

38. What is the purpose of the Americans with Disabilities Act (ADA)?
    1. "Level the playing field" with respect to employment and other opportunities for disabled persons.
    2. Create a federal entitlement program for AIDS patients.
    3. Guarantee wheelchair access to every residential and commercial building.

39. As a result of the US Supreme Court's ruling on assisted suicide, which of the following is the current state of the law on this topic?
    1. Assisted suicide is still a criminal offense in most jurisdictions.
    2. A physician may prescribe a fatal dose of medication with the concurrence of the ethics committee.
    3. A WHNP may prescribe a fatal dose of medication with the concurrence of the supervising physician.

40. A professional negligence or medical malpractice case is a civil action. What is the difference between a civil lawsuit and a criminal lawsuit?
    1. The damages sought in a civil suit are monetary; one private party sues another for money.
    2. If convicted in a criminal case, you are still covered by your professional liability insurer.
    3. In a criminal case, your state sues you for money; other penalties do not apply.

41. The WHNP understands which of the following about the Health Insurance Portability and Accountability Act (HIPAA) of 1996?
    1. The HIPAA provides easier access to all providers to obtain secure and private health information.
    2. A National Provider Identifier and Employer Identifier facilitates enrollment, eligibility, and claims processing and provides a mechanism to identify a specific provider, insurer, or patient.
    3. Health care organizations, insurers, and payers using electronic storage of patient data and performing claims submission must comply with the Final Rule for National Standards for Electronic Transactions.

42. Bioethical practice dilemmas are best described as situations in which proposed treatment alternatives are:
    1. Ranked from most acceptable to least acceptable.
    2. Less-than-perfect approaches to the situation.
    3. Lacking acceptance by anyone.

43. What is the difference between the electronic medical record (EMR) and the electronic health record (EHR)?
    1. There is no difference.
    2. The EHR is more efficient and effective.
    3. The EMR is more comprehensive.
    4. The EMR communicates information within a facility.

44. What should the WHNP do to reduce liability while using either an EHR or EMR system?
    1. Clone or copy and paste notes and details from a previous exam or patient history into a current visit record.
    2. Avoid making late entries and changes in the EHR or EMR.
    3. Share your log-in ID with colleagues who are also entering information into the EHR or EMR.

45. All of the following are true regarding obtaining prescriptive authority *except*:
    1. Requires an additional pharmacology course for continuing education after graduation.
    2. Requires a Drug Enforcement Administration (DEA) number for prescribing controlled substances.
    3. Requires an application for a National Provider Identifier (NPI) number.

46. The WHNP understands the following regarding Drug Enforcement Administration (DEA) number:
    1. DEA numbers are site-specific and issued by the federal government.
    2. DEA number is automatically provided on receiving prescriptive authority.
    3. DEA numbers are required for all prescriptions.

47. The WHNP understands that the following illustrates a breach in patient confidentiality:
    1. Using the electronic health record to document clinical findings.
    2. Having health care records subpoenaed by a local court.
    3. Discussing a patient's laboratory findings with the patient's family.

Patient Safety

48. What priority action should the WHNP take when assessment findings on an older adult patient indicate potential physical abuse during a scheduled office visit?
    1. Admit patient to the hospital for observation.
    2. Review patient's chart to see if there were any other documented findings that would indicate abuse.
    3. Report case to appropriate agency based on state law.

49. A family member calls the office to speak to the WHNP who is taking care of her mother. The family member asks for specific information related to the patient's medical history and clinical diagnosis. What action should be taken at this time by the WHNP?
    1. Answer all of the questions that the family member has with regard to the patient.
    2. Acknowledge the family member's concerns but do not answer any questions as there is nothing listed on the chart to indicate that the patient has given consent to release information.
    3. Call the patient at home and ask if the patient gives consent to answer the family member's questions.

50. Under the Safe Medical Devices Act of 1990, which of the following health care providers or organizations are required to report the death of a patient to the US Food and Drug Administration (FDA) if the death is related to the use of a medical device?
    1. Physician office staff.
    2. Hospitals, home health agencies, and ambulance companies.
    3. Nurse family members treating patients without compensation.

51. Which activity could be considered grounds for a sexual harassment claim?
    1. A female employee tells an off-color joke to another female employee. The joke is overheard by another female coworker who seems to appreciate the humor in it. The joke telling is an isolated incident.
    2. A nurse supervisor conducts an employee performance review. The supervisor does not mention a prior social relationship with the employee. The ratings are appropriate for the level of performance, and the employee receives a salary increase.
    3. A co-ed locker room is decorated with multiple centerfold photos from a popular men's magazine. The female employees find this offensive and have filed several complaints.
    4. A nurse is complimented on her appearance and asked on a date by her coworker.

52. What is the primary purpose of a preemployment physical exam?
    1. Identify existing health problems that might adversely affect the company's insurance rates.
    2. Determine the mental status of the applicant.
    3. Determine if the applicant is physically capable of doing the job.
    4. Document any existing disabilities and recommend accommodations.

53. In the clinic, the WHNP must resolve a conflict between two medical assistants. The nurse has observed that one assistant is usually pleasant and helpful, and the other is often abrasive and angry. What is the most important guideline that the WHNP must observe in resolving such a conflict?
    1. Require the medical assistants to reach a compromise.
    2. Encourage ventilation of anger and use humor to minimize the conflict.
    3. Deal with issues, not personalities.

54. A WHNP approaches her friend, another WHNP, and tells her that a male physician at the clinic often follows her into the supplies room and tells her how "good looking" she is. Yesterday he patted her hand and said, "I wish we would get to know each other better. I would make it worth your while; better benefits at the clinic, more money." The WHNP asks her friend, "What do I do? I don't want to date him, but I don't want to lose my job. I just want him to leave me alone." What would be the friend's best reply?
    1. "Tell him that his behavior makes you feel uncomfortable and that you want him to stop."
    2. "Go for it; date him and see if you get what he promises."
    3. "Go to the human relations office at the agency right away and relate to them the entire situation."

Issues and Trends

55. An older adult patient with metastatic ovarian cancer has decided to start hospice care. What is the eligibility criteria for hospice care as required by Medicare?
    1. Continue with curative care and chemotherapy.
    2. Have a terminal illness and a prognosis of 6 months or less to live.
    3. Choose to continue to use Medicare benefits.

56. Considering the four advanced practice roles of the clinical nurse specialist, nurse practitioner, certified nurse midwife, and nurse anesthetist, which role became accepted by and included into the practice arena without significant controversy?
    1. Clinical nurse specialist.
    2. Nurse practitioner.
    3. Certified nurse midwife.

57. Who started the Frontier Nursing Service program?
    1. Hildegard Peplau.
    2. Mary Breckenridge.
    3. Loretta Ford.

58. Who is credited with the development of the nurse practitioner role?
    1. Mary Breckenridge.
    2. Loretta Ford.
    3. Agnes McGee.

59. In the early formation of the women's health nurse practitioner role, what was the title given to nurses specializing in women's health, obstetric, and neonatal care?
    1. WHNP.
    2. FPNP.
    3. OGNP.

60. Which is the most important action in developing health policy skills in the WHNP?
    1. Develop political allies in the US Congress.
    2. Work on a campaign.
    3. Write letters and editorials.

61. According to the APRN Consensus Model, the WHNP is categorized as:
    1. An APRN role.
    2. Representing a specialty.
    3. Specifies a practice population focus.

62. To obtain reimbursement, the WHNP must understand which of the following?
    1. ICD-10, CPT, and HCPC codes.
    2. HCPC codes and NANDA diagnoses.
    3. MNDS codes.

63. What was the major impetus for WHNP development?
    1. Need for an expert nurse clinician.
    2. Feminist movement in the 1960s.
    3. Trend for specialized nurses to diagnose and manage unstable acute and chronic patients.

64. The WHNP understands that Medicare B provides:
    1. Hospitalization costs for insured patients.
    2. Outpatient laboratory services, radiography services, and skilled nursing care in appropriate facilities.
    3. Benefits that cover physicians, WHNPs, medical equipment, and outpatient services.

65. What was the impact of the Balanced Budget Act of 1997 on WHNP practice?
    1. Authorized all states to provide WHNPs prescriptive authority.
    2. Prevented a physician from billing 100% for an WHNP's services.
    3. Allowed direct Medicare payments to WHNPs in both rural and urban settings.

66. What is the purpose of the Agency for Healthcare Research and Quality (AHRQ)?
    1. Produce evidence to make a safer health care that is equitable and affordable.
    2. Provide assessment and treatment protocols and algorithms.
    3. Promote health care policy by lobbying efforts.

67. In 1999, the Institute of Medicine (IOM) reported that at least 44,000 people die in hospitals each year as a result of which of the following?
    1. Hospital-acquired infections (HAI).
    2. Medical errors.
    3. Falls.

68. Which course is required in an advanced practice education program to comply with the APRN Consensus Model?
    1. Informatics.
    2. Advanced health assessment.
    3. Social policy and political action.

69. What is the purpose of the Technology Informatics Guiding Education Reform (TIGER) competencies as applicable for a WHNP?
    1. Identify tools and procedures to address specific quality outcomes and metrics in health care agencies.
    2. Improve nursing practice, education, and delivery of patient care through the use of health information technology (HIT).
    3. Set the stage to increase awareness of WHNPs needing a national provider identifier number.

70. Which of the following is a common competency for all doctorally prepared advanced practice nurses?
    1. Provide care to children through young adult.
    2. Perform a comprehensive evidence-based assessment.
    3. Advocate only for the patient.

71. For quite some time, there has been an increased number of studies comparing nurse practitioner care to physician care. What have been the findings of these studies?
    1. Nurse practitioner care is equivalent to physician care.
    2. Nurse practitioner care is inferior to physician care.
    3. Nurse practitioner and physician care are mostly equivalent with the indicator of patient satisfaction higher for nurse practitioners.

72. What type of advanced practice nursing care did the Frontier Nursing Service (FNS) provide?
    1. Pediatric well-care.
    2. Older adult home services.
    3. Midwifery services.

73. Which of the following is covered under Medicare Plan A?
    1. Ambulance services.
    2. Diagnostic testing.
    3. Skilled nursing facility care.

74. According to the American Association of Colleges of Nursing (AACN), the clinical hour requirements for completion of the DNP program are:
    1. 500 supervised clinical hours.
    2. 900 supervised clinical hours.
    3. 1000 supervised clinical hours.

75. All of the following are purposes for reporting patient outcomes *except*:
    1. Increase revenue stream and expenditures.
    2. Improve patient care outcomes.
    3. Required by state and federal regulatory agencies.

76. All of the following are accurate statements regarding quality improvement (QI) *except*:
    1. QI needs to be realistic and achievable.
    2. QI involves large-scale projects for best outcomes.
    3. QI generates new ideas and knowledge.

77. Which of the following legislation changed Medicare payments beginning January 1, 2019, away from the existing fee-for-service system to one that is based on the quality and effectiveness of the care the health care provider delivers?
    1. Medicare Access and CHIP Reauthorization Act (MACRA).
    2. Consumer Assessment of Health Care Providers.
    3. Sustainable Growth Rate Formula Values-Based Modifier.

78. What is the purpose of clinical practice guidelines?
    1. Generally accepted set of practice recommendations.
    2. Recommend evidence-based practice based on research.
    3. Fixed protocols that must be followed.

79. The WHNP participates in a clinic-based quality improvement project on management of obesity. When the WHNP records a body mass index (BMI) score using the BMI Protocol Template from the Agency for Healthcare Research and Quality (AHRQ), this process is:
    1. Peer review.
    2. Risk analysis.
    3. Benchmarking.

21 Answers and Rationales

Research and Evidence-Based Practice

1. (3) The lack of significant findings is an important piece of information in the study findings. Particularly when findings are not statistically significant, additional studies need to be conducted regarding this topic to determine if the data are inconclusive. Threats to validity may cause a relationship to exist between study groups with no statistically significant findings. Ideally, changes in practice are based on the findings of more than one study, and a small sample size makes it more difficult to find statistically significant findings, not a large sample size.

2. (2) The peer review process exists across all disciplines in that the expectation is that it will help to determine if the provided research adds to the body of knowledge, is logically presented, well designed, and scientifically based. Although a manuscript should be well written, an excellent writing style alone in contrast to a research design with flaws is not acceptable. Individuals who participate in the peer review process do not have to provide editorial edits for grammar and formatting. Additionally, requirements in terms of clinical, research, and/or academic experience are required to be able to participate in the peer review process, thus it is not a beginning learning activity to understand how to analyze research and data findings.

3. (3) The primary purpose of utilizing EBP in clinical research and practice management is focused on the ability to provide quality care to patients by closing the gap between theory, experience, and best practice guidelines. Although credible resources are important, this relates more to the systematic process and ranking of research. The peer review process is also used in conjunction with EBP, but again this relates to the evaluation process rather than the primary purpose. Finally, arriving at a consensus of opinion relates to the overall evaluation of the presented research. It is not an expectation of purpose.

4. (1) The purpose of qualitative research designs is to learn more about a particular phenomenon of interest by exploring the beliefs, values, and experiences of individuals. Qualitative designs do not yield precise measures, are usually not analyzed statistically, and carry the same concerns regarding the rights of subjects as all other research designs. Quantitative research designs ensure tight control over data collection and analyses.

5. (2) All current research and statistical analysis methods rely on the presence of variance or variation. Variance is a statistical measure used to identify how spread out scores are from the mean. If variance is no longer present, current methods could no longer be used. If there is no variance, a sample of one would be adequate.

6. (2) Identify the problem and generate a clinical question, conduct a literature review of scholarly research articles, critically appraise published research, implement useful findings in practice and clinical decision-making, and disseminate findings contain the published steps of evidence-based practice (EBP). All other options are nursing actions taken on behalf of the patient (in no particular order).

7. (2) The independent variable is the measure that can be manipulated in a study: the high-protein, high-fiber diet. The dependent variable is the response from the independent variable and is measurable, for example, the obese patients' weight. The population of interest is the obese patient and the length of the study is 12 weeks.

8. (3) A randomized-controlled trial is one of the highest levels of evidence in determining if a cause and effect relationship exists between an experimental intervention (treatment) and dependent variable (outcome). By randomizing participants into either a control or treatment group, rigor is increased. A quantitative correlational research design examines the relationship between one or more variables; correlational research does not predict causality. Qualitative research designs are lower on the hierarchal level of evidence pyramid as they do not attempt to predict causality or determine the effectiveness of an intervention.

9. (3) By federal law, the rights of human research subjects must be protected. Patients must be assured of their privacy and confidentiality through informed consent. The researchers may include the other information; however, it is not required by federal law.

10. (1) Quantitative researchers remain as removed from the research process as possible and employ controls to mitigate influencing test results or introducing potential bias. Quantitative research tests for relationships and cause and effect through a statistical analysis and reporting to test hypotheses or research questions. Qualitative researchers are integrated into the research process and through analysis of dialogue and observations search for themes.

11. (1) The correct format for the null hypothesis is "There is no relationship between the independent and dependent

variables." If a relationship does exist, the null hypothesis would be rejected. The alternate or research hypothesis may take the other forms.

12. (1) Even though the claims detail extensive use of "Drug X," there must be statistical evidence reported. Additionally, randomization, as demonstrated through the use of control or comparison groups, should be implemented that will render a level of significance. The Hawthorne effect is a limitation and threat to a study's validity, as the study participants' behaviors and responses are changed because of being in the study, not necessarily from the intervention or treatment performed.

13. (3) Descriptive data analyses organizes the data and facilitates understanding of those who participated in the study and variables of the study. Descriptive statistics cannot be used for significance testing or for making inferences; inferential statistics are used. Predictions or causality are made from studies that use inferential statistics.

14. (2) Randomization is a research technique used to increase the amount of control and reduce potential threats of internal validity in any research design. The other three options do not decrease potential threats to internal validity.

Legal and Ethical

15. (3) WHNPs' scope of practice is regulated by individual state law. Federal law does not address scope of practice. Academic institutions provide the necessary training for individuals to obtain an academic degree and assist in preparation for required certification in the specialty area. Scope of practice is not regulated by individual practice settings.

16. (2) A clinical diagnosis of dementia for a patient indicates that to provide and obtain informed consent an individual who has been designated as a health care surrogate and/or is acting as a power of attorney (POA) should be contacted to provide informed consent. The WHNP should not allow the individual patient to sign the form, as informed consent process cannot be verified. Having a witness present when signing the form does not convey informed consent has taken place. Delaying medical treatment would not represent prudent practice.

17. (2) Fact witnesses and necessary paperwork are always easier to discover the sooner they are sought after a medical misadventure. Memories are fresh, and documents are less likely to be misplaced or destroyed. No rigid reporting window is required by insurance carriers, although they do want to be notified in a timely manner. Insurance premiums may be reduced if the insured's track record is clean (i.e., no claims), but not by mere compliance with policy requirements. Risk management employees prefer early notification so that damage-control efforts may be implemented promptly, not for regulatory reasons.

18. (3) The patient's capacity to consent is questionable, so alternatives must be sought. If the patient has a court-appointed guardian, that person is the decision-maker. The court has already determined the patient's legal incapacity and appointed the person to whom the WHNP will look for consent. If there was no guardian, the WHNP would analyze whether the patient herself may be able to consent or whether to look to her mother as the most appropriate surrogate decision-maker. The group home employee has no automatic legal authority to consent to treatment for any resident.

19. (3) Assisted suicide is still a criminal activity in most states (and in legal limbo in others). Circumventing the patient may seem to be an appealing option, but it substitutes paternalism for the autonomy we all claim as our due. A diagnosis of depression cannot be made with inadequate data; the necessary information can be determined only by conferring with the patient herself.

20. (2) Managed care organizations (MCOs) are one group of health care organizations impacted by this law. All subscribers must be provided with the stated information at the time of enrollment. Advance directive documents, although extremely helpful in the health care setting, are never mandatory.

21. (3) Insurance carriers are thoroughly familiar with the processes of handling a claim. They will assist with every step, first by meeting their obligation to put the WHNP in contact with a lawyer. Conferring with the patient or the patient's lawyer is never a wise move. Colleagues can only offer moral support at this stage; the lawyer is the professional of choice at this time. The WHNP must never consider altering a record; it can turn a defensible case into a nondefensible one.

22. (3) Lobbying for underserved patients is an example of justice, which is the duty to treat all patients fairly, without regard to age, socioeconomic status, or other variables. Autonomy is the patient's right to self-determination without outside control. Nonmaleficence is the duty to prevent or avoid doing harm, whether intentional or unintentional.

23. (3) The Americans with Disabilities Act (ADA) does not protect this population. In fact, employers may test for illegal drug use; this is not considered a medical exam, which ordinarily is subject to specific requirements under the law.

24. (2) The level of education preferred is that of a master's or Doctoral of Nursing Practice (DNP) degree with WHNP specialization, not an associate's degree conferred on the technical nurse. The legal issues are the province of the attorneys and the judge; the nurse is expected to be the expert in the clinical issues.

25. (3) Workers' compensation is the line of coverage that protects employees after on-the-job injuries. It is a no-fault system (negligence is not a factor) that covers employee medical bills and pays a percentage of wages while an employee is unable to work. Liability insurance is acquired to protect the organization from suits by patients arising from negligent acts of employees. Business interruption coverage is usually purchased in tandem with fire insurance. It reimburses an organization for losses sustained while the business is partially or completely shut down after a catastrophic event.

26. (3) The intent of the NPDB is to improve the quality of health care by encouraging state licensing boards, hospitals, and other health care entities and professional societies to identify and discipline those who engage in unprofessional behavior and to restrict the ability of incompetent physicians, dentists, and other health care practitioners to move from state to state without disclosure or discovery of previous medical malpractice payment and adverse action history. Adverse actions can involve licensure, clinical privileges, professional society membership, and exclusions from Medicare and Medicaid.

27. (3) The forwarding facility needs to know whether the receiving facility has space for the new arrival and, more importantly, the ability to treat the particular illness for which the patient needs therapy. The receiving agency needs to be contacted and agree on the transfer. The transferring agency must send the patient's medical records. The transfer must be with qualified personnel and transportation equipment. A familiar example of a patient transfer is that of the burn victim, for whom specialty care is mandatory, and the locations of that specialty care are usually limited.

28. (1) Health care policy within the states is codified or enacted into law by the respective state legislature. The state boards of nursing and pharmacy should have significant input in the process, providing the research data and expert "testimony" that the legislature needs to make informed decisions. Nursing organizations should also be willing to provide background information and nurse experts to educate the lawmakers.

29. (3) The managed care organization (MCO) cost-containment strategy is enhanced if providers practice within the treatment guidelines suggested by the plans. Providers who inform patients that a certain treatment regimen is the preferred alternative create difficulties if that alternative is excluded from coverage. MCOs usually clearly set out the exclusions in the plan documents, and member services personnel are expected to be able to explain the coverage to subscribers. Experimental treatment, if excluded, would be listed as such in the plan documents.

30. (3) Patients are often unable to evaluate the quality of the care they receive, but they do react to the way in which the care is delivered. Patient perceptions of rudeness or "uncaring" actions by the provider often spur patients to pursue legal action. Patients tend to be more forgiving of less-than-optimal outcomes if they have been involved in the process and are treated with respect.

31. (2) Making one's own decisions is the basis for informed consent and the ethical underpinning of the Patient Self-Determination Act. "Doing good" (beneficence) and its corollary, "avoiding harm" (nonmaleficence), are ethical principles that are usually cited as the basis for other health care activities, such as maintaining professional competency.

32. (3) Usually phrased as duty, breach, proximate cause, and damages, these are the four elements of proof required to prevail in a medical negligence action. Intentional acts are not synonymous with negligent acts. Duty presumes a professional relationship and obligation to provide services. The breach is the error or mistake ascribed to the provider that results in the harm to the patient.

33. (1) Lay jurors are not expected to know the clinical facts and circumstances involved in a professional negligence claim. The expert witness is necessary to educate the jurors regarding the medical facts and to testify to the standard of care to be applied. Witnesses with direct involvement in the case are no less credible because of their involvement; their testimony and personal bias, if any, will be evaluated by the jurors in the context of their roles.

34. (3) With respect to nursing specialties, the standard of care is usually a national one. Facility policies, books, and journals are important to review, and physician input may be sought. In some cases, physicians may even be allowed to testify regarding the standard of care. Opinions of other NPs and current events are not considered a component of expert opinion.

35. (1) Statutes of limitations set out each state's rules for the timing of the filing of lawsuits, including malpractice actions. These statutes are procedural laws in that they describe the "how-to" parameters within which legal rights may be exercised. Minority is considered a legal disability; other state laws usually define it and describe

its effects. Rights to sue are not governed by statutes of limitations.

36. (3) Two of these factors enter into an analysis of whether it is appropriate to accept a minor's consent to treatment. Another factor to consider is the type of treatment sought. Some states have statutes allowing minors to consent to specific therapies, such as treatment for a sexually transmitted infection. A statement from a third party without supporting documentation to show that the patient is emancipated is not a factor.

37. (1) The option of detaining the patient would create liability potential for the WHNP under at least two legal theories: battery and false imprisonment. Talking with the patient would be the first prong of a planned approach to convince this patient that she needs the prescribed medical therapy. Conferring with social services would be the next choice. Court-ordered treatment is a consideration with a viable fetus.

38. (1) This is the overall goal of the Americans with Disabilities Act (ADA). It is not an entitlement program, and it cannot impose wheelchair ramp requirements on every building owner in America. Access ramps and interpreters may be required as a "reasonable accommodation" to qualified people in certain defined circumstances. No across-the-board mandate exists for these types of aid to the handicapped population.

39. (1) The US Supreme Court essentially deferred to the states to legislate on this topic. In most states, the activity is not permitted. In one of the states involved in the high court's case, a statute permitting assisted suicide is being challenged. WHNPs need to look at their state laws on this topic for guidance. The providers referenced in the other options would act at their peril if their state laws followed the current majority view.

40. (1) The purpose of a medical malpractice action is to make the claimant whole by the awarding of money damages. The award compensates the claimant or plaintiff for the wrong (or tort) he/she has suffered at the hands of the defendant. On the criminal side, the state sues on behalf of society for violations of society's criminal laws. The punishments are fines, imprisonment, or both. Professional liability insurance usually excludes criminal and intentional acts, so coverage for these types of activities is unlikely.

41. (3) The four major goals of the Health Insurance Portability and Accountability Act (HIPAA) of 1996 are to ensure health insurance portability by eliminating "job-lock" because of preexisting medical conditions, reduce health care fraud and abuse, enforce standards for health information, and guarantee security and privacy of health information. Because of protests from civil libertarians and others concerned about privacy issues, the National Individual Identifier has been put on hold until some compromise can ensure that no abuses of such an identifier system will occur. The first compliance HIPAA rule relates to national standards for electronic transactions.

42. (2) The crux of a bioethical dilemma is that the proposed solutions are not perfect, and therefore create some aspect of moral conflict.

43. (4) The electronic medical record (EMR) communicates information within a facility and the electronic health record (EHR) communicates information among multiple facilities. They are both efficient and effective.

44. (2) It is important to maintain the integrity of the electronic medical record (EMR) or electronic health record (EHR) because it is a legal and medical record and must meet federal and state regulations. By avoiding late entries or changes to the record, such as postvisit addendums, corrections, retractions, deletions, or other late entries to the electronic record, can reduce the WHNP's legal liability exposure. Cloning records or copying and pasting information from previous visits can lead to inaccurate documentation and should be avoided. The log-in ID should never be shared with other colleagues. The EHR or EMR is a legal document and must reflect the accurate entry of information related to the patient and their care whether or not the WHNP agrees with it.

45. (1) Most states and all certification programs require a core advanced pharmacotherapeutics course during the advanced practice program, which is a requirement of the APRN Consensus Model. An additional pharmacology course after graduation is not required. Requirements for obtaining prescriptive authority vary among states, along with specific requirements to maintain licensure. The Drug Enforcement Administration (DEA) number, as required by federal and state policies, is issued to nurse practitioners to prescribe or dispense controlled substances. In addition to prescriber and DEA registration, APRNs will need to apply for an National Provider Identifier (NPI) number, which is issued by the National Plan and Provider Enumeration System that collects identifying information on health care providers.

46. (1) A Drug Enforcement Administration (DEA) number authorizes prescription of controlled substances and are applied for by the WHNP. DEA numbers are site-specific. WHNPs practicing at more than one site will need to obtain an additional DEA number for each site. The DEA's authority is federal; states have specific regulations pertaining to controlled substance authority. A WHNP who does not prescribe controlled substances

is not required to obtain a DEA number, but will need a national provider identifier (NPI) number for general identification purposes for other prescriptions.

47. (3) The Health Insurance Portability and Accountability Act (HIPAA) of 1996 mandates confidentiality regarding and protection of patients' personal health information. The legislation defines the rights and privileges of patients for protection of privacy. The release of a patient's medical information to an unauthorized person, such as a member of the press, the patient's employer, the patient's family, or online, is a breach in patient confidentiality. The information that is in a patient's medical record is confidential and may be shared with health care providers for the purpose of medical treatment only. A patient must authorize the release of information and designate to whom the health care information may be released.

Patient Safety

48. (3) If the WHNP suspects that physical abuse has occurred, then she is legally obligated to report the case to the appropriate agency based on state law. Admitting the patient to the hospital is not indicated unless confirmation of injury or trauma is justified. Reviewing the patient's chart for past history of abuse may be warranted but it is not the priority action.

49. (2) Release of medical information by a patient to others requires documentation of intent and approval within the patient's chart. As the patient has left the office and there is no documentation related to medical release of information, the WHNP is bound by patient confidentiality and privacy laws (Health care Insurance Portability and Accountability Act [HIPAA]) to not answer any questions.

50. (2) These are three of the agencies required to report. Events occurring in the other settings are exempt from reporting requirements under this federal law.

51. (3) The co-ed locker room with centerfold photos seems to fit the criteria for a hostile environment, a form of sexual harassment. The harassment seems to be pervasive and longstanding; the women have complained, and apparently no action has been taken. The individuals did not find the actions of an off-color joke or being complimented and asked on a date objectionable, and job performance was not affected. Although the potential was there for the supervisor nurse to use the prior relationship either to downgrade the employee or to deny a benefit during the employee performance review, this result did not occur.

52. (3) The purpose is to determine the appropriateness of the applicant for the job. Identifying health problems to prevent hiring an individual is discriminatory. The mental status and disabilities may also be a part of the preemployment physical but are not the primary purpose.

53. (3) Conflict must be addressed directly by the WHNP. The personal characteristics of the medical assistants must not enter into the conflict resolution process. The WHNP should determine the issue of conflict, and then work on possible solutions to resolve the issue. Compromise, in which both parties must be willing to give up something, is only one method of conflict resolution.

54. (1) There are two ways to deal with sexual harassment at work: informally and formally through a grievance procedure. The harassed person should always start with the direct approach and ask the person to stop. The female WHNP should tell the male physician in clear terms that his behavior makes her uncomfortable and that she wants it to stop immediately.

Issues and Trends

55. (2) If a patient has Medicare Part A and meets all of the following conditions, the patient can receive hospice care: (1) health care provider must certify the patient is terminally ill (with a life expectancy of 6 months or less); (2) patient accepts palliative care instead of curative care; and (3) patient must sign a statement choosing hospice care instead of other Medicare-covered benefits to treat the terminal illness and related conditions. Patients do not pay for hospice care. There may be a small copayment (less than $5) for prescription medications.

56. (1) According to the National Commission on Nursing (1983) and the Task Force on Nursing Practice in Hospitals (1983), the clinical nurse specialist (CNS) role was accepted quite rapidly. The psychiatric CNS role is considered the oldest and most highly developed of the CNS specialties and helped initiate the growth of other CNS specialties.

57. (2) Mary Breckenridge established the Frontier Nursing Service in the depressed, rural mountain area of Kentucky, which led to training nurse midwives. Loretta Ford, RN, PhD, and Henry Silver, MD, established the first pediatric nurse practitioner program at the University of Colorado. Hildegard Peplau started the first psychiatric clinical nurse specialist (CNS) program at Rutgers University.

58. (2) In 1965, Loretta Ford, RN, PhD, and Henry Silver, MD, established the first pediatric nurse practitioner program at the University of Colorado and are credited with the development of the modern nurse practitioner role. Mary Breckenridge established the Frontier Nursing Service in the depressed, rural mountain area of

Kentucky, which led to training nurse midwives. Agnes McGee is credited with offering the first postgraduate program for the nurse anesthetist role at St. Vincent's Hospital in Portland, Oregon.

59. (3) Obstetric gynecology nurse practitioner (OGNP) was the early credential used by nurses who specialized in women's health, obstetric, and neonatal care. The Association of Women's Health, Obstetric, and Neonatal Nurses (AWHONN), as a leader in championing women's health issues, has worked to expand the role of the OGNP into the more holistic care role of the WHNP. The Planned Parenthood (PP) Federation of America created in-house nurse practitioner programs. Nurses in these programs were trained in 8 weeks to become family planning nurse practitioners (FPNP), which had a limited scope of practice, that is, family planning. Advanced practice registered nurse (APRN) is the term used to identify a nurse who has a master's, postmaster's certificate, or practice-focused doctor of nursing practice (DNP) degree in one of four specific roles: nurse practitioner, clinical nurse specialist, nurse anesthetist, or nurse midwife.

60. (1) Although all these answers are important for the WHNP in developing policy skills, the most important is developing political allies. Having political allies in decision-making places (legislature) will enable the WHNP to be active and informed regarding issues of regulation, limitations on admitting privileges and prescriptive authority, and managed care.

61. (3) According to the APRN Consensus Model, there are four APRN roles: nurse anesthetist, nurse-midwife, clinical nurse specialist, and a nurse practitioner. Specialty areas include but are not limited to clinical areas of practice/health care needs (family practice, pediatrics, adult-gerontology, women's health, psychiatric/mental health, neonatal, etc.) rather than patient populations. The WHNP represents a practice population foci that addresses specific populations across the lifespan.

62. (1) The International Classification of Diseases (ICD-10) diagnostic codes identify the condition, illness, or injury to be treated and are used for billing insurance carriers. Physicians' Current Procedural Terminology (CPT) codes specify the procedure or medical service given. The Health Care Financing Administration Common Procedure Coding (HCPC) system is used for reporting supplies and medical equipment. Minimum Nursing Data Set (MNDS) is a classification system of a set of items of essential nursing data with specific definitions and categories related to nursing and nursing care. NANDA diagnoses are not involved with reimbursement.

63. (2) The feminist movement in the 1960s had a profound effect on the advancement of women's health from both a political and health care perspective. In addition, women-specific alternatives, including abortion clinics, women-controlled health centers, self-care information and publications, and freestanding birth centers, began to flourish in the 1960s and 1970s.

64. (3) Medicare is regulated by the federal government, and Plan B includes the services described (services or supplies that are needed to diagnose and treat a medical condition and preventive services), plus outpatient laboratory, radiography, durable medical equipment (DME), ambulance services, mental health care (both inpatient and outpatient services, along with partial hospitalization), and obtaining a second opinion before surgery. Hospitalization costs, skilled nursing facility care, hospice care, and home health care are covered under Medicare Plan A.

65. (3) The Balanced Budget Act is a crucial piece of legislation that allows direct payments to WHNPs at "80% of the lesser of either the actual charge or 85% of the fee schedule amount of the same service if provided by a physician." This does not change the "incident to" rule, which allows a physician to bill for 100% of a WHNP's services, provided the physician is in the suite at the time of the service and readily available to assist.

66. (1) The Agency for Healthcare Research and Quality's (AHRQ) purpose or mission statement is to produce evidence-based practice and research to make health care safer for all individuals that is of higher quality, more accessible, equitable, and affordable. The AHRQ works within the US Department of Health and Human Services (USDHHS) and with other agencies to make sure that the evidence-based research is understood and used.

67. (2) The 1999 IOM report *To Err Is Human: Building a Safer Health System* revealed that at least 44,000 and as many as 98,000 people die in hospitals each year due to preventable medical errors. Medical errors were defined as failure of a planned action to be completed as intended or the use of a wrong plan to achieve an aim.

68. (2) The APRN Consensus Model stipulates that an APRN education program must include at a minimum of three separate comprehensive graduate-level courses known as the APRN core, which are advanced physiology/pathophysiology, advanced health assessment, and advanced pharmacology. Social policy and political action and ethical/legal issues would be included in other courses and are not part of the APRN core.

69. (2) The Technology Informatics Guiding Education Reform (TIGER) initiative was formed in 2004 to bring together nursing groups to collaborate to improve nursing practice, education, and delivery of patient care use

of health information technology (HIT). This included recommendations for basic computer competencies, information literacy, and information management (including use of an electronic health record). In 2011, the group published a landmark report titled *Informatics Competencies for Every Practicing Nurse: Recommendations from the TIGER Collaborative.*

70. (2) The doctorally prepared advanced practice nurse performs a comprehensive evidence-based assessment and demonstrates competent and efficient assessment of patients with multiple comorbidities. Advanced practice nurses advocate not only for the patient, but for other populations, as well as advancing nursing practice in general. They also advocate for improved access, quality and cost-effective health care, and ethical policies that promote access, equity, quality, and cost. Providing care to children through young adult focuses only on the pediatric nurse practitioner. The WHNP provides obstetric, gynecologic, and primary care to women within inpatient and outpatient settings.

71. (3) Multiple studies over the past 10 years have shown that nurse practitioner care as compared with physician care is equivalent and in some outcome indicators, such as patient satisfaction, nurse practitioner care is higher.

72. (3) The FNS founded in Kentucky in 1925 by Mary Breckenridge initially provided Appalachia with nursing services and obstetric services in this economically depressed rural setting. British nurse-midwives and American public health nurses provided midwifery and nursing care through a decentralized network of nurse-run clinics.

73. (3) Hospitalization costs, skilled nursing facility care, hospice care, and home health care are covered under Medicare Plan A. Medicare Plan B includes the services described (services or supplies that are needed to diagnose and treat a medical condition and preventive services), plus outpatient laboratory, radiography, durable medical equipment (DME), ambulance services, mental health care (both inpatient and outpatient services, along with partial hospitalization), and obtaining a second opinion before surgery.

74. (3) To achieve the DNP competencies, advanced practice programs should provide a minimum of 1000 hours of supervised clinical practice as part of the academic program. The credentialing body, the American Academy of Nurse Practitioners (AANP), requires a minimum of 500 faculty-supervised direct patient care clinical hours for eligibility to take the certification exam. The credentialing body, the American Nurses Credentialing Center (ANCC), requires completion of school required faculty-supervised clinical practice hours for degree completion. In addition, the ANCC states, "All practice requirements must have been met while holding an active professional license (RN licensure for nursing certifications or applicable license, certification, registration, or organizational documentation for interprofessional specialties) in a US state or territory or the professional, legally recognized equivalent in another country."

75. (1) Measuring outcomes is a required component of health care by federal and state regulatory agencies, practice guidelines, employers, and consumer groups. Health care organizations monitoring outcomes of patient care as a means of evaluation, as well as meeting requirements, for accreditation and certification. Measuring outcomes does not correlate with additional revenue, but instead with the maximum revenue available and should reduce expenditures.

76. (2) Quality improvement (QI) needs to be realistic and achievable. Large QI studies are not necessary and can be intimidating or overwhelming to those engaging in a QI project; small projects with available resources and tools are best. QI can generate new ideas and knowledge to change and improve nursing practice and patient care.

77. (1) The Medicare Access and CHIP Reauthorization Act (MACRA) took effect on January 1, 2017, with final implementation on January 1, 2019. MACRA repeals the Sustainable Growth Rate Formula that has determined Medicare Part B reimbursement rates for physicians and replaces it with new ways of paying for care. MACRA combines three existing programs: Physician Quality Reporting System, Value-Based Payment Modifier, and meaningful use into one system that provides both financial incentives and penalties based on quality of care, outcomes, and efficiencies. The initial 2 years are focused on collecting and analyzing data, and for hospital systems and providers to see the future impact of their reimbursement.

78. (2) According to the Institute of Medicine (2011), clinical practice guidelines are "statements that include recommendations, intended to optimize patient care, that are informed by a systematic review of evidence and an assessment of the benefits and harms of alternative care options." Clinical practice guidelines define the role of specific diagnostic and treatment modalities that health providers use in the diagnosis and management of patient conditions. The statements contain recommendations that are based on evidence from a rigorous systematic review and synthesis of the published medical literature. They are not fixed protocols and do not apply to every patient situation. According to the IOM, a set of practice recommendations not explicitly informed by a systematic review of research should no longer be considered a clinical practice guideline.

79. (3) Benchmarking is an important component of a quality improvement project because it helps identify when performance (measuring BMI at each clinic visit) is below an agreed-on standard, and it signals the need for improvement. If the score falls below a set standard, interventions can be initiated. In addition, after an intervention is implemented, changes as can be tracked using the BMI score to determine whether the interventions were effective in weight management. Using standardized measurement tools can inform the WHNP when changes in care are needed, and whether implemented interventions have resulted in actual improvement of patient outcomes. Peer review is an evaluation of work by another person with similar competencies. Risk analysis is the process of identifying and analyzing potential issues that could negatively impact key initiatives or critical projects to help organizations avoid or mitigate those risks.